"A powerful compendium of Hakomi philosophy and body techniques that wonderfully highlights how fundamentally mindful body work is and has always been, well before mindfulness rose to popularity. I highly recommend this to all readers interested in what life is all about and how to make its possibilities realized."
    —**Albert Pesso**, author of *Experience in Action* and *Psychomotor Psychology*

"This anthology is indeed destined to be a landmark volume, not only in the advancement of the healing arts of Hakomi, but also in the wider fields of somatic psychology and body-mind therapy. The articles presented here are clearly written, deeply thoughtful, and readily accessible to both student and seasoned practitioner. The book comprises a beautiful balance of theory and clinical practice, of philosophical grounding and therapeutic application. In short, this volume is invaluable, and one of the top ten 'must read' books for anyone committed to mindfulness and somatic psychotherapy."
    —**Barnaby B. Barratt, PhD, DHS**, former professor of Family Medicine, Psychiatry, and Behavioral Neurosciences at Wayne State University, and author of *The Emergence of Somatic Psychology and Bodymind Therapy* and *Psychoanalysis and the Postmodern Impulse*

"In reading this volume about Hakomi I find myself thinking that it aims to bring infants' multi-level meaning-making processes—how infants understand themselves in the world through a simultaneous integration of every level of their being (metabolic, immunologic, physiologic, stress regulatory, emotional, behavioral), which we all still possess—into the co-creative exchange of adults who now have expansive capacities for mindfulness, reflection, and symbolization. It is also working at one and the same time to overcome these adult capacities' tendency for imperialist dominance and constriction of somatic multilevel experience. Thus this book challenges each of us both personally and professionally to try to make meaning of our own changes and therapeutic change processes. Taking on this challenge is more than worth the effort."
    —**Ed Tronick, PhD**, University of Massachusetts Boston, Director of the Infant-Parent Mental Health Program, and author of *The Neurobehavioral and Social Emotional Development of Infant and Children*

"This book has finally arrived! The Hakomi Method is one of the earliest efforts to integrate mindfulness into therapy, beginning in the 1960's. It is a fascinating approach that includes body awareness, investigation of core beliefs, compassionate presence of the therapist, embracing the unconscious, and collaborative investigation. A unique contribution of Hakomi to mindfulness-oriented therapy is the emphasis on exploring the structure of the personal 'self' and the causes of its suffering. This book is comprehensive in every way—historical background, theory, method, interventions, case illustrations, clinical applications—and deserves to be read by anyone seriously interested in psychotherapy and its many wonderful expressions."
    —**Christopher Germer, PhD**, Clinical Instructor, Harvard Medical School; author of *The Mindful Path to Self-Compassion* and co-editor of *Mindfulness and Psychotherapy*

"I started *Hakomi Mindfulness-Centered Somatic Psychotherapy* wondering if I would just be learning about mindfulness as has often been expressed by therapists turning East. What I found instead was a profoundly complex understanding of the human self and the healing process, rooted in the wisdom of Lao Tzu. Nothing has been lost in how these authors translated Taoism into the world of psychotherapy. The image of therapists exploring the unconscious through the body and gestures with non-judgmental awareness of the self is refreshing. But more so, the book offers a critique of the current world operating on the capitalistic assumption. Hakomi is much more than a therapeutic corrective of what has gone wrong. It is a way of being in this complex reality. Philosophically and existentially therapeutic, *Hakomi Mindfulness-Centered Somatic Psychotherapy* is provocative, informative, and simply refreshing for shepherds of the souls."
—**Siroj Sorajjakool, PhD**, professor of Religion, Psychology, & Counseling, Loma Linda University; author of *Do Nothing: Inner Peace for Everyday Living* and *Wu Wei, Negativity and Depression: The Principle of Non-Trying*

"Read this book! In this era of cookie-cutter therapy, *Hakomi Mindfulness-Centered Somatic Psychotherapy* stands head and shoulders above the fray. Drs. Weiss, Johanson, and Monda have assembled a masterful collection of writing about the Hakomi method, distinguishing this approach to healing from many other works and depicting how it is being illumined by current psycho-neuro-biological research. The beauty of this volume is its attention to the integration of a strength-focused perspective, which emphasizes that people are not problems but rather stories and struggles that need to be heard and allowed to heal. The way mindfulness is utilized here maintains its integrity as a profound experience that reconnects the client and therapist to their true and common humanity. It is when an individual feels truly joined by another on their healing journey that the depth of healing is realized. Weiss, Johanson, Monda, and the contributing authors have elegantly captured this essence!"
—**Thomas Roberts, LCSW, LMFT**, Director/Psychotherapist, Innerchange Counseling, Onalaska, Wisconsin; Owner, Thomas Roberts, LLC: Retreats, Workshops, Training; author of *The Mindfulness Workbook*

"Weiss, Johanson, and Monda have brought forth a deeply rich volume reflecting the best of Ron Kurtz and the Hakomi Therapy that is his legacy. This book reflects a deep emotional-spiritual orientation reflected in interfaces with neuroscience, mindfulness practices, systems theory, object relations, and more, as each of the 28 chapters takes on an aspect of that interface. A rare combination of theoretical and case material makes it intellectually stimulating and at the same time delightfully enlivened. Described variously as a textbook and a reader in Hakomi, it is a path-breaking compendium. And, it even includes a glossary, an index, and lots of meaty references. I hope that other modalities of body psychotherapy will shortly follow this auspicious lead."
—**Jacqueline A. Carleton, PhD**, editor of *International Body Psychotherapy Journal: The Art and Science of Somatic Praxis*

Hakomi Mindfulness-Centered
Somatic Psychotherapy

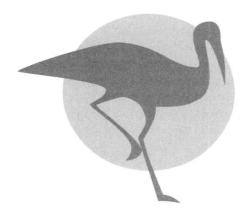

Hakomi
Mindfulness-Centered
Somatic Psychotherapy

A Comprehensive Guide to
Theory and Practice

Halko Weiss, Greg Johanson, and Lorena Monda

Editors

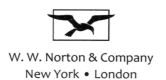

W. W. Norton & Company
New York • London

For information about permission to reproduce
selections from this book, write to Permissions,
W. W. Norton & Company, Inc., 500 Fifth Avenue
New York, NY 10110

For information about special discounts for bulk
purchases, please contact W. W. Norton Special Sales at
specialsales@wwnorton.com or 800-233-4830

Manufacturing by Edwards Brothers Malloy
Production manager: Christine Critelli

ISBN: 978-0-393-71072-4 (pbk.)

W. W. Norton & Company, Inc.
500 Fifth Avenue, New York, N.Y. 10110
www.wwnorton.com

W. W. Norton & Company Ltd., Castle House, 75/76 Wells
Street, London W1T 3QT

1 2 3 4 5 6 7 8 9 0

To Ronald S. Kurtz

(1934–2011)

Originator of Hakomi therapy

Hakomi (Hah-*co*-me)

A Hopi Indian word meaning, "How do you stand
in relation to these many realms?"

Contents

Foreword

Richard C. Schwartz

RON KURTZ LIVED 77 years and spent the second half of his life developing and teaching what he came to call Hakomi. He was a brilliant theorist, integrator, and clinician with whom I collaborated and exchanged ideas for many years. I am so glad that this book follows closely after his death. So many psychotherapies have faded away after the charismatic leader died. This book will help ensure that Hakomi will continue to thrive—continue to touch and heal so many lives—especially because the book is so well referenced with the mainline psychological literature.

Somewhere around 1992, Greg Johanson came up to me during a workshop I was doing on the model of psychotherapy I developed called internal family systems (IFS) and asked excitedly if I'd ever heard of Hakomi. I said, "Isn't that some kind of sushi dish?" Greg introduced me to Ron and, through Ron, I met much of the Hakomi community. I was blown away. At the time, I was an academic and as such, very intellectual and concerned about appearing professional. Sitting in on Hakomi conferences and training sessions, I found myself surrounded by lovely people of all stripes (psychotherapists, bodyworkers, dance-movement therapists, and psychodramatists, as well as many nontherapists) who looked to me like they were constantly dancing, emoting, hugging, and "probing" each other.

While my science-oriented skeptical parts were on guard, I couldn't deny the power of the work and the way it both paralleled and complemented the path I was on. Decades before mindfulness became the rage that it is now in psychotherapy, Hakomi therapists were helping clients into a mindful state to observe their inner reactions to various stimuli, and then following the trail of emotion or belief that came up in those experiments to find and release core, often unconscious, beliefs. In addition, they highly valued a quality of therapeutic relationship they called "loving presence" that they practiced so that clients would feel safe and held. Through this process, they were helping clients access what I call the exiled parts of themselves—vulnerable, young, hurt parts that I was trying to get to in a different way. Once getting to an exile, they helped a client remain in that emotional part even when it looked like he or she was experiencing a scary regression or abreaction. Then, through experiencing the loving presence of the therapist or other group members, the part's beliefs would be released.

This collaborative period greatly enriched both the theory and technique of IFS and, I'd like to think, Ron and other Hakomi therapists were helped to appreciate systemic aspects of the world of inner parts they were exploring and the power of what I call the client's Self as a primary healer.

As one swims in the currents of psychotherapy's mainstream, one still rarely hears Hakomi mentioned, despite the fact that it has flourished outside that mainstream, with training courses around the world and a plethora of Hakomi-inspired books and thematic variations. With psychotherapy's increased appreciation of mindfulness, emotion, the body, the loving presence of the therapist, and trauma, the field has been moving closer to where Hakomi (and IFS) has been for decades. I hope this book will help Ron and the Hakomi community get the credit they deserve. I know that it will provide Hakomi with a needed body of collected wisdom and technique that will ground this remarkable approach for years to come, at the same time that it introduces the work to the larger professional psychotherapeutic community.

Acknowledgments

SINCE IT IS axiomatic that editors and writers are never singular players, but always selves-in-relation, embodied in multiple contexts, a publication such as this reveals an underground of communal significance.

So many people have been involved on myriad unseen levels. Supposedly solitary participants should perhaps take a poll of all those who are part of their immediate communions before embarking on such prolonged endeavors: partners who organize years of their lives around endless publishing concerns; children who wonder why a parent is so preoccupied; relatives who worry about where one's life is headed; friends who feel they are on a never-ending cheering squad and get worried about writer-clinician-teaching-community members being stretched out in too many directions; colleagues who get antsy waiting for energy to be made available for other projects; and more. Decisions matter for individuals. They carry significant weight for the communities individuals comprise.

Certainly, a major acknowledgment we have as editors is to the faculty, organizers, administrators, and committed Hakomi therapists of the Hakomi Institute in Boulder, Colorado, who have striven since 1980 to preserve, build upon, and teach Hakomi therapy throughout the world to professional psychotherapists and others in cognate disciplines. We thank our current administrator, Laurie Adato, for her enthusiastic encouraging of this text.

Hakomi Institute faculty who contributed chapters to this volume are all scientist-artist, mind-body practitioners dealing with the demands of working with clients as well as offering the time, skill, and energy to teach Hakomi therapy, often far from their homes. A number of them are not professional writers, but agreed to take their part of a major project that meant engaging in the demanding processes of researching, composing, rewriting, and meeting ever-moving deadlines. Likewise, we want to thank the faculty of the Hakomi Educational Network, those who worked closely with Ron Kurtz as he sought to simplify the Hakomi method in his later years to make it available to a larger public, for their willingness to contribute to this common project.

Our gratitude extends to those who actually make teaching Hakomi therapy possible, namely our students of these many years who recognized something significant in what we were doing, and trusted us to teach them a unique, and, for many seasons, new kind of psychotherapy whose name they needed to learn to pronounce.

The references in this volume reflect the larger community of learning of which this contribution is part of a long, ongoing dialogue. As editors and contributors we have had opportunity to study with some in this great cloud of thinkers and writers that have gone before. Some we have only met in print, and have been enriched by the opportunity to compare our experiences with theirs.

For helping this volume itself to become a reference, we want to thank Deborah Malmud of W. W. Norton, who had the generosity to look at a manuscript by multiple authors not attached to a household name, and then support us with high-level professionalism, energy, and appreciation.

This work is dedicated, of course, to Ron (Ronald S. Kurtz), the brilliant, charismatic originator and core professional inspiration of the work before we ever found the name Hakomi, and the founder of the Hakomi Institute. He served as mentor, friend, and colleague to many of us, though his lasting contribution is that he encouraged others to take stewardship of the work and to train people around the world. There are now over three generations of Hakomi trainers in many countries all over the world who are able to pass on the work to people who never had the opportunity to study with Ron directly. We are grateful that Ron was able to contribute a chapter on his latest thoughts to this book before he died, and we want to mention his beloved wife, Terry, and daughter, Lily, who hold his memory dear. We trust that this book will be a suitable legacy to the healing Ron fostered in the world.

As he invited us to check out the wisdom of how he was learning to help people with our own wisdom, so we now invite the greater professional therapy community to do the same in relation to this volume.

Hakomi Mindfulness-Centered Somatic Psychotherapy

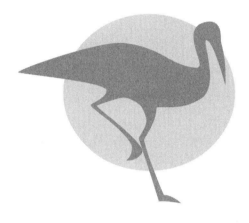

Overview

CHAPTER 1

Introduction

Maci Daye

MINDFULNESS HAS GONE viral. Open any psychotherapy journal or conference brochure and you will likely find something with "mindfulness" in the title. So pervasive is this trend that an issue of *Psychotherapy Networker* magazine was dedicated to the "mindfulness explosion." It's hard to remember when the term "mindfulness" entered the vernacular of psychotherapy, but in recent years it has spread to every therapeutic modality, many of which now allege to be "mindfulness-based," simply to establish land rights on this fruitful turf. But, in 1980, when the Hakomi Institute was formed, only Buddhists and forward-thinking physicians training in Jon Kabat-Zinn's mindfulness-based stress reduction knew the term.

Now, with enough publications on the subject to fill a virtual warehouse, one wonders, "What more can be said?" While many authors cite growing evidence that a regular mindfulness practice can regulate emotions, increase happiness, and inoculate against stress, few describe how mindfulness can promote deep characterological transformation. As pioneers in the use of mindfulness in psychodynamic therapy, Hakomi therapists do just that.

Hakomi is a form of guided self-study that uses mindfulness to access the memory system where our most fundamental, wide-reaching beliefs are implicitly encoded. These beliefs, which lie below the level of conscious choosing, condition our perceptions and responses to all aspects of life. New research suggests that we can reshape our neural hardware and shift these organizers of experience through the function of attention. This book will show you how.

Hakomi began with one man's vision, found its name in another man's dream (see Appendix 3) and was refined and expanded upon by a cadre of passionate pilgrims who set forth on a journey that has spanned five continents and three decades. Thousands of practitioners now make their living using Hakomi, as trainers and therapists, so why isn't our approach better known?

Like many indigenous teachings, Hakomi has been transmitted to clients and practitioners who are drawn to our purported willingness to welcome rather than reject the qualities that make us most human: vulnerability, uncertainty, contradiction, and pain. Our guiding mantra—pause and study, rather than fix—is a balm for road-weary seekers of healing and personal growth, who have attempted to eliminate rather than befriend their troublesome parts.

It sounds counterintuitive, but Carl Rogers once said, "The curious paradox is that when I accept myself just as I am, then I can change." He was echoing Lao-tzu, who some 2,600 years earlier wrote in more poetic terms: "If you want to shrink something, you must first allow it to expand. If you want to get rid of something, you must first allow it to flourish. If you want to take something, you must first allow it to be given. This is called the subtle perception of the way things are."

Hakomi integrates the perennial wisdom of Buddhism and Taoism with modern scientific findings on how the brain changes itself through experience rather than reflection. It also balances the aware and compassionate qualities of larger self-states with the realities of the historically conditioned ego. Simply put, our knowledge often outpaces our readiness to put this knowledge into practice, and our self-acceptance can be obscured by feelings of unworthiness.

Hakomi is at once idealistic in its belief that humans have the capacity to be aware of themselves and, therefore, less bound by their automatic reactions; and simultaneously realistic, in that we accept that it takes time and a particular attitude and state of consciousness to do so. This attitude requires going beyond judgment, toward understanding and integration, since the "war on self" is clearly not working. Instead of polarizing against the parts of the self that seem to sabotage our happiness, we may need to befriend all parts, especially the most difficult and intractable.

The first step is to slow down and turn inward in a calm and curious way. Admittedly, step one may be a hurdle for those of us who function at Mach speed or prefer to turn away from or, worse, eliminate the parts of ourselves that give us trouble. What's more, our species has never been great at relaxing into and embracing discomfort. Our preference for anesthetizing ourselves via distraction, or sidestepping rather than encountering difficult experience, is legendary.

Second, we must suspend attachment to what we think we already know, choosing instead to learn from the pregnant mystery of the not-yet-named aspects of our felt experience. This requires exploring the many realms of our existence instead of granting favor to cognition. For too long, under the sway of our Cartesian heritage, we have attempted to know ourselves by splitting wholes into parts, focusing more on our thoughts than our feelings and bodies. However, as Rob Fisher asserts in the section that follows, "People are adept at using words to dissemble, but the body is far more direct in communicating our inner states to those who are willing to listen."

Fortunately, the tides are beginning to turn: As we move into what might be termed the age of integration, many people are beginning to appreciate that the part can only be informed by the whole. This integrative ontology is the crux of Hakomi, whose principles of mind-body holism and unity acknowledge our multiply determined selves and the larger context within which they relate.

Consistent with our integrative approach, this book is a symphony of voices rather than a solo composition. Since differentiation promotes integration, several members of the Hakomi faculty have coauthored this book. Some writers have chosen to explore the tail, others the trunk of the Hakomi method, each trying to provide as good an understanding as words on a page can give of the felt sense of this experiential approach.

We began soliciting submissions in 2005, and then bit our knuckles as more books on mindfulness and psychotherapy hit the shelves. To quiet our anxiety, we reminded ourselves that to know oneself requires slowing down and trusting the intrinsic readiness to move forward. Now, after nearly 10 years of reflective writing about thirty-plus years of clinical and training experience, we are ready to move Hakomi into the forefront of the mindfulness explosion, by showcasing our considerable expertise on core-level change. Toward this end, we offer readers a guide to our unique mindfulness-centered, somatic approach with plentiful references to the mainline literature in psychology and counseling.

Specifically, this volume provides:

1. An understanding of how the perennial wisdom traditions and the sciences of complexity can help clinicians establish the requisite conditions for deep transformation and characterological change.
2. A view of human change processes that embraces the coexistence of contradictory impulses both to maintain a stable and coherent core and to grow to higher levels of complexity.
3. A way to join with our clients' organic impulses to heal, by working nonviolently with their barriers to change, and by gently integrating new potentialities into their everyday lives.
4. A rationale and specific guidelines for integrating the body in psychotherapy, including instances of trauma.
5. An understanding of how the early learning system stores memories subcortically, and a detailed process to transform a person's relationship to these preconscious memories.
6. Guiding principles that increase trust in each person's internal blueprint for growing and becoming that also shape the personhood of the therapist to be a compassionate and healing instrument of change.

For those who want to jump in and learn the technique, we direct you to Section IV, which outlines our basic skills and therapeutic process (Chapters 14–24). For those who prefer to read about the overarching principles and theoretical underpinnings of the method, go to Sections II and III (Chapters 4–13). For the social scientists, who like to know what historical developments shaped the method, go to Appendix 3. To get a glimpse of the Hakomi method in clinical practice, view the section that follows: "Psychotherapy Beyond Conversation: The Psychodynamic Use of Mindfulness and the Body," as well as Appendix 2.

As there is no substitute for direct experience, we invite you to participate in a workshop if what you read here interests you. To access a worldwide calendar of Hakomi events, go to the Hakomi Institute website (www.hakomiinstitute.com or www.hakomi.org).

A Hakomi Case Illustration: Psychotherapy Beyond Conversation— the Psychodynamic Use of Mindfulness and the Body

Rob Fisher

As I opened the door to my office for our first appointment, Jane said a curt hello before I could greet her, and walked in ahead of me.[1] There was a soldierly rigidity to her walk that immediately left me feeling a bit shut out. She greeted my smile with a slight scowl as she told me, without preamble, what had brought her to therapy. She was tired, she said, of being so alone in her life.

"Even when I'm with my husband, I'm alone," she said. She had tried talk therapies and appreciated the insight she'd gained, but said, "I just keep doing the same things I've always done to push people away from me."

Successful in her career as a physician in a small town, 57-year-old Jane found herself returning to her house in the evenings to watch TV alone while her husband tinkered in the garage. She routinely rebuffed kindly overtures of support from others without really knowing why—which enabled her to say, truthfully, that she got "very little help from anyone." For instance, before dinner was finished, she would jump up from the table and wash the dishes, feeling resentful while preempting her husband from helping her. Of the implicit, but ironclad, rules that dominated her somatic and emotional life, however, she was almost entirely unconscious.

She spoke with an air of independence, and I had the distinct impression that she suspected that I would only be marginally useful to her, if at all. Her straight posture, stiff carriage, and severe mouth communicated—more than her words could—that she was struggling to rely only on herself.

As typically happens with clients in a first session, taking in Jane's verbal pace, posture, and facial expression, I found myself formulating some initial questions about the formative experiences and inner templates that shaped her approach to life and her habit of

---

1. Originally printed in *Psychotherapy Networker*, July/August 2011. Article entitled "Psychotherapy Beyond Conversation: The Psychodynamic Use of Mindfulness."

removing herself from contact. What must her world be like that she walked with such purpose and didn't respond to my smile? What had happened to her that made it a good idea for her to be so tough?

Accessing Implicit Knowledge

Hakomi gently and safely encourages clients to use the power of present emotional and somatic experience to explore the unconscious models of reality that dictate how they live their lives and engage in relationships. It relies on a form of body-based mindfulness as a primary tool to explore the implicit beliefs that organize life experiences and address attachment injuries that shape our emotional realities. While people are adept at using words to dissemble, the body is far more direct in communicating our inner states to those who are willing to listen. Through the way we move and hold ourselves, we reveal the internalized working models of the world and self that are unconsciously encoded in our brains, which govern our behavior, perceptions, and feelings.

One such cardinal, implicit rule Jane had learned early in life was never to rely on others. In her unconsciously established worldview, nobody could be trusted to give her what she needed or wanted. Jane's dismissive style and rigid posture were part of a character strategy designed to protect her from the wounds of massive disappointment—not needing or depending on others was an attempt to save herself from further injury. As I watched Jane caught in the tyranny of her toughness, it was clear to me that while she knew how to be strong, she didn't know how to be connected to people. In some ways, her strategy of insulation was functional, but overused. It had become a life sentence of separation. Part of the job of therapy would be to make Jane's implicit and somatically held knowledge consciously available to her, then to provide experiences in the present that would challenge some of her self-limiting beliefs, and finally, to offer new options for both perception and behavior.

Attachment in the Present Moment

Clients' attachment styles originate in early interactions with primary caregivers and often endure into adulthood. Deficiencies in attachment can be transformed later in life as a consequence of nourishing and attuned relationships with partners, friends, and therapists, but this requires experiential events, not just word-bound conversations. One of the most powerful ways for a therapist to establish an experiential, relational state of attunement is through mindfulness—both the clinician's and the client's.

While mindfulness starts with the ability to attend to the many details that make up the present moment, most of us can easily be transported away from the experience of the moment, especially by the content of conversation. Studies have shown that 70–80% of communication occurs through mostly unconscious somatic signals—pace, posture, gestures, voice quality, breathing patterns, changes in energy, and skin coloration. These signals arise directly from the core beliefs and models of the world that the client holds. By not allowing ourselves to be carried away with the content of a client's story, we can begin to notice the many other ways in which a client communicates. The process of noticing and joining with a client at this level generates the kind of nonverbal attunement—normally supplied by good early parenting—that can build secure attachment and begin to address the early injuries that occur often in preverbal life.

During our first session, Jane told me in a flat voice that her husband had decided, without consulting her, to accept a more "responsible position" (meaning many more hours away from home) at his law firm. She roughly pulled a tissue from the box. Noticing the vehement gesture, I said, "You're mad at him, huh?" "Yes," she replied, "he's always like this." There was a flash of grief on her face, followed by a dismissive movement with her hands as she turned away her face.

Rather than following the content by asking, "He's done this before?" I responded by reflecting back her current experience again, saying, "You're pushing away with your hands, huh?" I left it to her to tell me what she was pushing away—her husband or her feelings. What she offered was a gesture, a demonstration of the impulse to push away and turn away. It seemed important, as it was performed with some energy, and it was consistent with her predisposition toward self-reliance.

Focusing on the gesture caught her attention. I suggested she could do it again, but slowly, really taking time to notice the details of her experience, the subtleties that get lost in ordinary consciousness and conversation. As she did so, she said, "You just can't count on anyone." She grimaced as if the words tasted bitter.

I responded, "You feel betrayed and bitter, huh?" I wanted to contact what was stirring inside, beneath the impulse to push away. Contacting her emotional experience here opened a door—her eyes welled up with tears and her lower lip began to quiver. I responded, "These are some strong feelings. It looks like you're fighting with them a bit." As she tried to answer, something softened inside her, and she began to weep.

Part of the process of healing for someone who's been entranced by a belief structure like Jane's is risking the emotional vulnerability that can lead to a response from another person that supplies a missing experience different from the neglect of childhood. Without pushing in any way for increased abreaction, this recognition of the internal battle between expression and containment shifted the balance toward the former, and allowed Jane to show me more of her vulnerability.

Much of trauma's impact stems from isolation. Telling one's story to an attentive, warm listener will begin, in and of itself, to reconsolidate how the memory is held. While we can't change the past, we can offer a place in which it's no longer held alone, but in relationship. This also builds attachment.

Studying in Mindfulness

Studying an experience while it's happening presents many opportunities that are missing in ordinary conversation. One important element in Jane's internal model of relationship was how she held herself apart from others. In a later session, I wanted to construct a therapeutic experience of mindfulness that would enable her to experientially explore her need to be invulnerable.

"Jane, I have an idea," I said. "I'll say something to you, and you can notice where it lands inside. Notice the response. It could be a thought, a feeling, a sensation, an impulse, a memory, a fantasy, music, or nothing at all. Would that be okay?"

Asking permission is always important in establishing a genuinely collaborative relationship based on safety and equality. Once she agreed, I let myself shift into a slower, more mindful state in which I could begin to notice the details of my own internal world and start to even more precisely track her moment-to-moment experiences. With the help of limbic resonance and the activation of mirror neurons, she began to let her attention focus inwardly.

"Okay," I said, "let your attention go inside so you can notice whatever happens when I say these words . . . [pause]: 'Jane, your needs are important.'" I said this not to elicit agreement, but quite the opposite: I was looking for the parts that disagreed. Again, this was guided by the knowledge that people who have a set of implicit rules of relationship like Jane's have a tendency to protectively deny their needs. I wanted to bring this into Jane's conscious awareness.

She opened her eyes for a moment. "Yeah, sure!" she mumbled sarcastically, more to herself than to me. Now, emerging in consciousness, we had the part of her that dictated toughness.

"Great!" I said. "Let's invite that part to be here. It sounds like a street fighter."

"Yeah," she replied. "Needs are the same as disappointment."

I asked Jane to turn her attention inside and let her own words echo—"Needs are the same as disappointment"—and notice what experience emerged. In this kind of mindful exploration, the therapist can track external signs of internal experience in the fine changes in the client's face, emotional temperature, breathing, and voice quality. As both participants carefully attend to present experience, something deeper than left-brain conjecture can occur.

In this case, Jane said, "I feel really hot!" She looked down, and her shoulders and the top of her chest were turning red. As with many clients beginning to explore unfamiliar territory, it was easier for her to recognize the sensation than the underlying emotion. I encouraged her to stay with the heat and the redness, and asked her to notice the mood that went with it. She said, with surprised consternation, but also curiosity, "Oh, I'm ashamed . . . of my needs!"

There are, of course, contraindications to this procedure. Immersing a client in a trauma memory, for instance, risks his or her hyper- or hypoarousal—becoming flooded or immobilized—and retraumatized. It's important for the therapist to carefully track the client, be alert to signs of dissociation and disconnection from the therapist, and titrate the immersion in immediate experience to avoid overwhelming the client. Exploring experiences slowly in homeopathic doses, and noticing the fine grain of sensations and motor activity in particular, can yield more information and change in the long term than dramatic, multiple-tissues-in-the-garbage-can sessions that raise explosive emotions. Before, and alternating with, immersion in traumatic or negative memories, clients should be focused on the felt experience of their own resources—the places, people, things, and experiences that bring comfort, a sense of self-confidence, and expansiveness.

Every experience we have, conscious or unconscious, is a mix of other, underlying experiences—many of which are unconscious—stored in the neural networks of implicit memory. Jane's sense of invulnerability was composed of many associated cognitive, emotional, and somatic experiences, including tension in her muscles, a rigid posture, a belief that to show softness exposed her to danger, and a memory of being shamed for her vulnerability. Consciousness of one part of the neural network tends to evoke related parts.

"Let's make lots of room for shame," I said. "We can hold it gently. Just let a little bit of it be here. Go ahead and stay with it, and let's see where it takes you."

I was intending to follow her lead, but the suggestion took us to what appeared to be a dead end. The feelings stopped and she sat up straight, wiping her eyes. As Jane started to explore the feeling of shame, something inside her obviously shut down. On a somatic level, her posture shifted—she sat up straight, no longer resting against the back of the couch.

Drawing on Jane's immediate present experience for clues about where to go next, I said, "You're sitting really straight, and it seems like your feelings just went away. Let yourself be with that uprightness, feel all the muscles involved, and notice what they remember." Eliciting a memory, in effect, from the feeling in her muscles, she saw the memory of when her father taught her about the limits of trust: he told the seven-year-old Jane to jump from a kitchen counter into his arms, and then purposefully let her fall, without trying to catch her. "Never trust anyone," he instructed her. She learned this lesson well.

To ensure that no one ever had the same kind of power over her again, she'd adopted a strategy, a relational model, requiring her to rely only on herself and no one else. While superficially functional—she could protect herself from being hurt—this strategy also sentenced her to the feeling of lonely disconnection that had finally brought her to therapy. In fact, this kind of strategy tends to recruit others to act in predictable ways that reinforce the underlying beliefs—Jane preempted anybody from doing anything generous toward her, which reinforced her distrust of others.

As her feelings began to ebb, I commented, "You learned not to rely on anything or anyone, huh? Not even the back of the couch. How about we start by supporting your back, so it doesn't have to hold you up all on your own?"

I was speaking somatically and metaphorically here. Could she risk taking in support after many betrayals of her trust? This experience was designed to challenge the habitual neural pathways that led her to self-reliance, and to help her develop a new set of neuronal firings that would permit greater nourishment and support in her life. Jane began to experiment with just leaning back and trusting the couch. While she explored the simple, metaphorical act of leaning, I encouraged her to slowly and mindfully notice her subtle internal reactions. As she did so, I could see her gradually relax her body, as she realized she could lean a little on the couch without losing herself.

Transformation and Integration

Several weeks later, I noticed that as Jane talked to me, she looked at me slightly out of the corners of her eyes. I was still looking for signs of the old patterns—compulsive self-reliance and the dismissal of human warmth—so I said, "Sometimes you look right at me, and sometimes you look from the side of your eyes. How about we explore the difference between the two looks?"

She agreed, and I asked her to turn her attention inward, noticing the thoughts, feelings, sensations, memories, and images that arose as she tried each way of looking. She reported that when she looked directly at me, she felt vulnerable, and when she looked at me somewhat sideways, she felt more protected, though lonely. I told her that she was entitled to look at me any way she wanted, and that she could decide which she wanted to do now, to exercise her choice. She decided to look directly at me, and as she did, she smiled and then started to chuckle.

She said, "I feel a bit scared, but this is really what I want." Next, the goal was to help her stabilize this resourceful experience. I asked her to really take her time, to make room for this mirth bubbling up and the sense of connection, to notice how it lived in her body, and the words and impulses that came with it—this was more important to follow than fear. By having the client immerse herself in the new experience, new neural pathways can be built. Immersion in expansive experiences is as, if not more, important than immersion in the experience of wounds and limitations.

During ensuing sessions, we returned many times to this constellation of issues. Each new pass helped Jane to clarify the implicit beliefs structuring her reality and the risks she could take to create new experiences and generate new models of the world. She practiced allowing herself to depend more on me without losing her self-reliance. She looked at me directly without losing her choice to withdraw when she wanted. Then Jane became increasingly able to transfer the vulnerability she showed in sessions to her relationship with her husband. She gained the ability to ask him for more time and closeness in a way that engaged him because of its genuineness and lack of hostility, which previously accompanied her demands. He started to find her more interesting than the car engines he'd previously found so absorbing.

At this point, she suggested it might be helpful to invite him to one session to help consolidate her gains in therapy. This is the integration stage, in which it is important to assist clients to weave their newfound options and ways of behaving into the fabric of their social and professional lives. Frequently, relationship partners have a homeostatic reaction to changes in their relationship and can undercut therapy. When Charles arrived, his eyes looked big and hypervigilant, unsure of what to expect. I welcomed him warmly. He seemed more scared than oppositional to his wife's new way of being. After checking in with him conversationally about how he experienced the changes in Jane, she brought up the feeling that she "could not lean on him." Unsure whether she was referring to her inability to lean or his inability to support her, I suggested we try this out in mindfulness to see what the effect might be on each of them—to have her actually practice leaning physically on him. It turned out that it was hard for her to do this as it involved facing the demons of disappointment in all the people who had failed her in the past. When she finally succeeded and let her head come to rest on his shoulder, he breathed a big sigh of relief. I said, "Feels good, huh?" He said, "Yeah, I finally feel useful to her and less like she is looking for trouble." I asked him to tell this to her directly, which was challenging to his tendency to withdraw, but he was inspired by her smile and able to tell her about his discomfort. As it was beyond the work of an adjunctive session, I gently suggested that it might be helpful for him to continue with this theme in individual therapy with someone else. As she became more able to hold a new model of support in her life and integrate it into her relationships, it was time to start thinking about bringing therapy to a close.

Conclusion

Jane arrived in therapy determined to feel less isolated. We could see how her implicit belief in the unreliability of support, and her tendency to look tough and pretend that she had no needs, pushed others away. This guided the interventions over the next few months. Rather than being remote and barely accessible, her unconscious spoke of its implicit models of the world in many ways: in gestures, posture, in the style of her relating to the therapist in the present moment. Each session exposed new experiential doorways to this material. Over time, we continued to assess the progressive changes that eventually translated into her personal life. I was also able to create an experience of attunement that slowly allowed her to feel safe and held in the therapeutic relationship, something that hadn't happened for her as a child. By asking her to mindfully explore her organizing beliefs as they revealed themselves in the present moment, she accessed memories and resources that touched her deeply and allowed her to experiment with new ways of being inside and outside of therapy.

CHAPTER 2

Characteristics of Hakomi

Halko Weiss

HAKOMI IS A psychodynamic and experiential approach that systematically uses the ancient tool of mindfulness and integrates the body into the psychotherapeutic process. Four hallmarks of Hakomi therapy—psychodynamic, experiential, mindfulness-centered, and body-inclusive—are outlined below, and then discussed in the context of the therapist's attitude and the therapeutic relationship created.

The Psychodynamic Perspective

The psychodynamic tradition assumes that there are dynamic unconscious processes, rooted in individual development, that shape our experience and behavior. These processes are thought to be partly accessible to consciousness, where they can be explored and influenced. Though not the only benefit, just making them conscious is already a highly relevant step toward healing and freedom from the ties of powerful forces shaped by the individual developmental process.

Hakomi stands in this tradition. We believe that the early environment provides formative experiences that determine one's understanding of the world and of oneself. A child starts to create implicit models of the world (beliefs) from the start—an inherent trait of all self-organizing living systems (Holland, 1998; Kauffman, 1995). These implicit beliefs and meanings help the growing individual anticipate external events and orient in the world, and make up the base of how experience and behavior are organized. Most of these beliefs are held outside consciousness in implicit memory, and—as body psychotherapists generally assume—as "affect-motoric schema" or "micropractices" (Downing, 1996, 2015), patterns of somatic and emotional processes that are used habitually.

Psychodynamic theories assume that a person is somehow structured intelligently by "forces," "parts," "voices," "internal objects," and so forth that have the capability to self-organize. For a Hakomi therapist, the central questions of psychotherapy are: How does the particular self-organization of my client work? Can we explore essential aspects of the client's habitual information processing, even though these are mostly unconscious? Can we understand the meaning that the client has made of his experience? Therefore, as a core constituent trait of Hakomi therapy, the therapist consistently tracks for nonverbal signs of how self-organization seems to be engaged in a specific moment, rather than mainly listening to the content of what a client is saying. The unconscious self-organization of a client is the focus of attention and the object of research within the therapeutic session.

Many of the chapters in this book relate to these questions, and those of Section II (Theory) in particular, for instance, Chapters 4, 5, 7, and 8. In later sections, specific psychodynamic issues, like defenses (Chapter 17), regression (Chapter 18), working through (Chapter 19), transformation (Chapter 20), or transference (Chapters 22 and 23) are addressed.

The Experiential Perspective

Ron Kurtz, the founder of the Hakomi method, understands beliefs to be the key to therapeutic transformation. Transformation occurs when formative core beliefs, activated along with their deeply ingrained and complex, original experiential patterns, are expanded by new experiences. With reexamined and expanded beliefs and experiences, the world literally looks different and offers new options. This perspective on transformation is a foundational piece of the method.

Thus, the Hakomi method is designed to bring alive formative experiences and the beliefs held within them. Those experiences are coaxed forward, examined, and understood in a cooperative process between client and therapist. New, "corrective" (Alexander et al., 1946), or "missing" (Kurtz, 1990a) experiences are then conceived and introduced to the client. When taken in by the client as felt experience, they are thought to affect the related, highly habitual, activation patterns of self-organization and their representations in the neuronal architecture.

As an experiential therapy (a term defined by Greenberg, Watson, & Lietaer, 1998), Hakomi builds the psychotherapeutic process around the art of preparing for, evoking, and examining experiences that shed light on a person's self-organization and its sources. Experiences always happen in the "here and now" (Perls, 1973). Clients are guided to become aware of a specific element of a meaningful experience, focus on it, and stay with it for extended periods of time. As a result, these sessions have the potential of becoming highly emotional, with an option toward carefully guided, regressive states. This is one of the reasons why the tool of mindfulness is essential for this kind of work.

The experiential aspect of the work is, therefore, one of the threads that the reader can follow throughout the book. Chapters 4, 7, 10, 11, and 16 through 20 shed light on different perspectives of this trait of the method.

The Perspective of Mindfulness

Ron Kurtz had long considered including the term "mindfulness" in the name of the method he created, because of the extraordinary meaning mindfulness has for the essence, feel, and process of Hakomi work. As early as the 1960s, Kurtz began to pioneer a way of working with this ancient Buddhist technology of consciousness in therapy (Johanson, 2006; Nyanaponika, 1972; Weiss, 2008). By the time the Hakomi Institute was formed in 1980, the use of mindfulness was already deeply integrated into a psychodynamic process and had shaped the character of the work. Certainly, this approach had its predecessors. Gestalt and other methods used special forms of awareness, rooted in Eastern practices, in their work. Kurtz, however, became quite specific about several characteristics of the traditional methodology. He created processes around

1. the conscious regulation of attention processes inward,
2. the conscious regulation of attention processes in relation to time,
3. the establishment of an internal observer with a number of critical characteristics,
4. a therapeutic approach that consequently would have to let go of goals and become experimental instead, and
5. a therapeutic relationship that would have to become nonviolent in order to not interfere with mindfulness and a naturally unfolding therapeutic process.

All of these characteristics are discussed in detail later in this book. Combined, they create the typical Hakomi flavor that distinguishes the work so clearly from other forms of psychotherapy.

Mindfulness serves several essential objectives of Hakomi work. Its use is primarily based on pragmatic considerations, rather than ideological or spiritual ones. The key advantages are the following:

1. For work with the body, a powerful tool for observing internal, somatic processes is needed, especially if that tool can deepen with practice. From within the traditions of spiritual practice, mindfulness constitutes a deeply tested and powerful method of self-study.
2. Mindfulness allows for comparatively easy, conscious regulation of attention processes that do not follow the automatic and habitual patterns of already established pathways of self-organization. Instead, it allows for the directed exploration of hitherto unconscious processes.
3. Mindfulness supports a nonjudgmental exploration of self. It creates a gentle and accepting relationship toward parts of a person that were previously seen negatively or have become dissociated.

4. Mindfulness strengthens reflexive ego functions or, in the terminology of Schwartz (1995), "Self"-states that serve progressive objectives and give protection from the dangers of regressive therapy processes.
5. Establishing a stronger and stronger internal observer over time is already a transformative element of therapy. The observer allows for a process of "disidentification" from the trancelike pull of limiting states of being, such as depressive states (Beck, Rush, Shaw, & Emery, 1979; Linehan, 1993; Segal, Williams, & Teasdale, 2002).

Of course, this list cannot yet reflect all the benefits that mindfulness practice offers for the therapist (Breslin, Zack, & Mcmain, 2002; Hick & Bien, 2008; Grepmair & Nickel, 2007; Grepmair et al., 2007). In Hakomi therapy, mindfulness becomes the very basis of what Kurtz calls "loving presence," a being state that carries the fundamental qualities a Hakomi therapist can bring to the therapeutic relationship.

Cognitive-behavioral therapists in particular have recently begun to include mindfulness training in their therapeutic programs (Orsillo, Roemer, Block Learner, & Tull, 2004). In their methodology, mindfulness mainly serves the objective of disidentification, or helping clients to distance themselves from overwhelming and ingrained automatic patterns of experiencing. Clients learn to do mindfulness meditation, often in a parallel and separate process. In the Hakomi method, instead, mindfulness is deeply integrated into a moment-to-moment explorative and experiential psychodynamic process.

Consequently, a number of chapters in this book devote themselves to different perspectives on mindfulness: a more general and philosophical one (Chapter 6), one on the use of mindfulness in a psychodynamic context (Chapter 10), two on specific Hakomi interventions embedded in mindfulness (Chapters 16 and 23), along with chapters on some special benefits of working with mindfulness—regressive processes (Chapter 18) and transformation (Chapter 20).

The Perspective of the Body

Being aware of and using the body in psychotherapy is closely connected to the experiential aspect of Hakomi. The body is the place where emotions and feelings are experienced (Damasio, 1999), and where the unconscious often first shows us signs of emerging content on a sensing level (Gendlin, 1996). It is the place in the here and now, where self-organization manifests in ways that can be observed and directly experienced, rather than merely being talked about. Bodily experience is also deeply rooted in the precognitive, nonverbal, and implicit realms of memory, and sheds light on how we learned to respond to the world as we got to know it early in life (Downing, 1996; Roth, 2003).

There is no doubt that Freud was right in his assumption that those early years are most formative for the way a person experiences the world and relationships, even today. Moreover, it is implicit memory and the emotional-somatic levels of the self that hold the impressions and lessons from those times. Infant research has shown how strongly first relationships are encoded somatically and how their abstractions (called "representations of interactions generalized" or RIGs [Stern, 2002]) are reinforced through repetitive experiences that shape the neural architecture.

When in the business of reconnecting, uncovering, and understanding the deeply held models of reality that form in those years, it is the body that can most clearly and most quickly bring them into awareness, both emotionally and mentally. One just needs appropriate therapeutic relationship, technique, and process to bring them alive.

Staying in contact with how emotions are experienced in the body also allows those formative experiences to emerge in a live fashion. They become present, palpable, and evident. They can be studied for their exact makeup, for their consequences, and for what models of reality were established early on. Even if the connected memories have not been stored (infant amnesia, for example), have faded, or were repressed, their traces can be studied through the way the emotional body responds habitually. Understanding and meaning can be created by examining those traces.

Some authors (for instance, Becker, 2006) have called the body the "royal road" to the unconscious. For them, the future of psychotherapy is unimaginable without the inclusion of the body in the psychotherapeutic process. Hakomi, therefore, stands in the tradition of Reich, Lowen, Pierrakos, and others who, more than half a century ago, began to compose theories about how emotional, behavioral, mental, and somatic realities are interconnected and shape complex systems of self-organization in a human being (Marlock & Weiss, with Young & Soth, 2015). Today, even cognitive-behavioral therapists are thinking about the body in a new way, accepting the notion that there may be emotional and somatic schema in addition to cognitive ones (Sulz, 2015).

In this book, the body is addressed again and again: in the theory section (Chapter 4); in Chapter 23, on character-based interventions; and, of course, in many of the chapters in the technique section (Chapters 14, 16 through 19, and 24).

Therapeutic Attitude and Therapeutic Relationship

Before Kurtz simplified his concept of the therapeutic relationship to what he called loving presence, there was a thorough learning process about what works when using mindfulness and bodily experience as core ingredients in psychotherapy.

One aspect was clear early on: the use of mindfulness does not go along with a goal-directed approach. Mindfulness requires an accepting attitude on the part of the client and consequently on the part of the therapist. An emphasis on what needs to change destroys the quiet and curious observation of what is happening inside (Weiss, 2008).

Additionally, deep insights about the nature of change that Kurtz garnered from the Taoist traditions reinforced the understanding of the therapist as being in a midwifing role where existing forces are followed and used rather than confronted or challenged (Johanson & Kurtz, 1991).

Together with the conviction that a therapeutic path that is supposed to lead to the very foundations of self-organization needs to offer an absolutely safe environment (Porges,

2003), the pragmatic teachings of Buddhism (mindfulness) and Taoism (nondirectivity) have established a strong understanding of the therapist's presence in the relationship: mindful and "contactful," slow, accepting, compassionately curious, precise, nonviolent, observant, warm, and genuine (Hick & Bien, 2008). This list could be extended, but gives a first sense of what a therapist would have to find in herself when doing a Hakomi session. In many ways, Hakomi training can be looked upon as teaching the trainee a special state of being, designed to be supportive of a self-healing process. This state of being is understood to be more important than all the artful technique and specific therapeutic knowledge learned in the process as well. Chapters 5, 6, 9, 11 through 14, 17, 22, and 23 include a special eye on this aspect of the Hakomi method.

CHAPTER 3

The Essential Method

Ron Kurtz

I DO NOT, and cannot, speak for all Hakomi therapists. I am writing here about how I work now and how I now understand the method. I'm fairly sure that what I do is similar to what other Hakomi therapists do. Still, I began to develop and teach the work over 40 years ago. Some of my original students have themselves been teaching it for 35 years or more. Each of them has modified it in some ways. And I certainly have. However, the most essential elements of the Hakomi method have changed little. Those elements are what this chapter is about.

Though based on the best science available, the Hakomi method is not only science. The intimate and delicate exchanges the work gives rise to can be as beautiful as poetry or song. The skills needed are as much those of the heart as of the head. As theory, the method is reason, form, and tools; the use of them, however, is an art. As in any art, there is both freedom and constraint. And I am grateful for them both, for they have led me to whatever understanding I now enjoy. They have kept me interested and productive. They are a great blessing.

For me, the method is a living thing. For over 40 years, my vision of the work has continuously evolved, shifting, slowly, like a tectonic plate, under the whole endeavor. Occasionally, an earthquake of an idea has radically altered my understanding of the process. Three of these ideas are (1) the realization of the importance of the therapist's state of mind; (2) an understanding of the method, not as working to cure disease, but as assisting another in his or her search for self-knowledge (the method can be described succinctly as assisted self-study); and (3) an understanding of the unconscious as adaptive (Wilson,

2002), that is, intelligent, aware, working to benefit the whole and, without our conscious knowledge, automatically handling most of our daily actions.

The adaptive unconscious operates on the basis of assumptions, expectations, habits, and implicit beliefs about ourselves, others, and the world of which we are part.

> Whatever particular theory is subscribed to, all agree that expectations of other people and how they will behave are inscribed in the brain outside conscious awareness, in the period of infancy, and that they underpin our behavior in relationships through life. We are not aware of our own assumptions, but they are there, based on these earliest experiences. (Gerhardt, 2004, p. 24)

These assumptions were created by our earliest and strongest formative experiences. They are not available to consciousness through the usual processes that retrieve memories. They must be accessed using special techniques. The Hakomi method employs unique techniques, developed over many years, to accomplish just that.

In a very real sense, we start out ignorant of who we are. To gain understanding and control requires deliberate effort. Self-study is a powerful path to change and it is most powerful when we can discover our unconscious assumptions, when we can examine them with a more mature, experienced, and reasoning mind. The whole world is not the same as the limited one we spent our childhood learning to live in. To act as though it is usually results in suffering. The kinds of assumptions that cause such suffering are inaccurate, usually overgeneralized, and emotionally charged. Because of this, the suffering they cause is, in principle, unnecessary. It can be lessened or even completely eliminated by changing the assumptions.

Not all formative experiences cause suffering. Positive experiences of love, protection, caring, and enjoyment can also be formative. And, of the negative ones, not all are inaccessible because they occurred too early in life. Some simply happened when the person was vulnerable. They overwhelmed the nervous system. The person simply lacked the inner resources and the external support needed to integrate them. The experiences were "encapsulated" and repressed:

> During these periods of *abaissement* [a lowering of psychic energy], Janet found, our psyche seems to lose some of its capacity to synthesize reality into a meaningful whole. If we encounter a traumatic or strong emotional event during these periods, the mind lacks its usual ability to make sense of it and fit it properly into a meaningful, secure whole. . . . During abaissement, we tend to be emotionally vulnerable and easily overwhelmed; we can register the life experiences, but we cannot properly "digest" them. The emotional experience floats in our unconscious, unassimilated, in effect, jamming the gears of the mind. (Rossi, 1986, p. 125)

The Hakomi method is designed to access these "undigested" experiences and the habits that keep them outside of consciousness. We bring these experiences into consciousness and we find ways to integrate them. And, though the process is at times emotionally painful, it consistently accesses the adaptive unconscious. Doing so makes completion and transformation possible. And this reduces unnecessary suffering.

These ideas have reshaped my vision and the way I work. And while there have been radical shifts, some things have not changed at all or at least not very much. Though new techniques have been added, the old techniques remain central. The original underlying principles—of unity, organicity, mindfulness, mind-body wholeness, and nonviolence—also remain, though my understanding and appreciation of them have deepened. The core of the method has not changed.

The essence and uniqueness of this method remains a simple combination of two things: the client's state of mind (mindfulness) and the therapist's ability to create experiments that trigger reactions while the client is in that state of mind. These reactions are indications of unconscious assumptions. (These assumptions are not verbal, but are implicit in the habits that express them.) The therapist looks and listens for signs of these assumptions and tries to discern the nature of the emotionally nourishing experiences the assumptions are preventing. The therapist makes a guess about this and uses it to create an experiment that will trigger a reaction. The experiment is simply an offering of some potentially nourishing statement or action, something the therapist guesses will be automatically rejected. The experiment is done while the client is in a mindful state. The client notices the reaction. The reaction, when it is allowed to unfold into an integrative process, provides an opportunity to access and examine the operations and assumptions of the adaptive unconscious that produced it. It provides an opportunity to complete, in a positive way, the old, painful experiences that led to those assumptions in the first place.

Mindfulness entails a change in the quality of attention. Attention is directed inward, toward the flow of present experience; it is receptive, open, and allowing. This quality has been described as "a change in the quality of attention, which passes from the looking-for to the letting-come" (Depraz, Varela, & Vermersch, 2000, p. 126). This combination of an open, vulnerable client and a therapist who is attempting to trigger reactions is exactly what makes the method work. Of course, clients know that this is the process. They understand what can happen. The procedure is voluntary and a completely cooperative effort. If the therapist is adroit enough, a client's reaction will be a source of insight—long-buried feelings and memories will emerge. If the therapist is compassionate, then new experiences—of comfort, safety, hope, and happiness—may become possible.

An example of an experiment might be a simple statement such as, "You're completely safe here." Or it could be the client looking away and then looking directly at the therapist. The variety of such experiments is effectively infinite. The experimental statements or actions are always positive and are meant to offer something emotionally nourishing. "You're a good person" is another example. If the therapist has guessed well, the statement will run counter to the client's implicit beliefs and foundational experiences. It will be the kind of emotional nourishment that the client has never been able to receive. It can evoke a longing that the client suppressed (another word is "encapsulated") long ago. Offering such a statement can trigger strong emotions, painful memories, and the realization of what's been missing. At this point, new beliefs about what is possible can be entertained and new experiences—the missing ones or something close to them—become possible. This simple process is the core of the method.

Several other important elements of the method support this core process, including:

1. the client's commitment and ability to enter into the process consciously and willingly, and
2. the therapist's ability to be present and compassionate, and to
3. understand nonverbal expressions as signs of present experience, and to
4. notice and understand the client's nonconscious, habitual behaviors as indicators of implicit beliefs and formative experiences, and to
5. create experiments that will trigger reactions, which can lead to emotional release and self-understanding, and to
6. enable positive emotional experiences that were previously extremely rare or entirely missing.

The Client's Commitment: Mindfulness and Honesty

I give prospective clients a document that makes clear what will be expected of them. It says in part:

> This method is not about talking out your problems. There won't be long, speculative conversations about your troubles or your history. This method is designed to assist you in studying the processes that automatically create and maintain the person you have become. It is a method of assisted self-study. It requires that you enter into short periods of time where you become calm and centered enough to observe your own reactions, as if you were observing the behavior of another person, a state called mindfulness. The therapist assists your self-study by creating "little experiments" while you are in mindfulness. These experiments are always nonviolent and basically are designed to evoke reactions that will be reflections of the habits and beliefs that make you who you are. The implicit beliefs and relationship habits with which you meet the world automatically shape your present behavior. Aspects of your behavior, the aspects that reflect your deepest beliefs, are what the therapist uses to create the experiments.

The document goes on to say:

> The process works best: (1) if you can follow and report on your present experience; (2) if you're able to get into a calm, inward-focused state and are relaxed enough to allow reactions; (3) if you're willing to experience some painful feelings and speak about them; and (4) if you have the courage to be open and honest about your experience. That courage will be your greatest ally.

I have come to recognize that the method requires these four things of a client. Of course, some clients won't be able to do all this at first. There will have to be a "pre-study" phase in which other methods will have to be used. Such methods might be simply listening sympathetically without talking much, just indicating that you understand what the client is going through. It may take some time doing things like this to build the client's trust and to gain the cooperation of the client's adaptive unconscious, enough time to bring the client to the stage where he can enter mindfulness and allow reactions. I also tell clients about the rewards that are there for those who practice self-study. Zen master Dogen said, "To study the Buddha Way is to study the self, to study the self is to forget the self, and to forget the self is to be enlightened by the ten thousand things" (in Keown, 2006, p. 109). Of course, the work we do is only a small step on that journey. And though the method is different, the attitude and direction are the same. Release from unnecessary suffering is release from an identity that includes habits and ideas that are not only old and outworn but fundamentally flawed as descriptions of reality.

The Therapist's State of Mind: Loving Presence

The phrase "state of mind" has much more precise meaning nowadays than it had just a few decades ago. Neurological research has revealed much about exactly what states the brain can be in when people interact (Lewis, Amini, & Lannon, 2000). Much has been written on the interaction of caregivers and the infants in their care (Schore, 2001; Gerhardt, 2004; Cassidy & Shaver, 2010). Adults in relationship also affect each other's states of mind. For the very intimate relationship between a therapist and client, the therapist's conscious awareness and deliberate control of his or her state of mind is essential. The effect of the therapist's state of mind on the process of this method is without a doubt the single most important factor in its success.

To best serve others in their self-study, the therapist must be able to sustain both presence and compassion. The therapist has to maintain a constant focus on present activity and present experience, both her own and that of the client. That's what presence means. A feeling of compassion is also essential. When presence and compassion are combined and constant, the therapist's state of mind can be called loving presence. (In training people in this method, the development and practice of this state of mind have become primary goals.) This aligns the Hakomi method with the most universal spiritual teachings: agape in Christianity, compassion and mindfulness in Buddhism, nonviolence and non-separation in both.

In a very short time, loving presence can establish in the client a sense of being safe, cared for, heard, and understood. Self-exploration, especially when using mindfulness, places clients in extremely vulnerable positions. A therapist in loving presence helps clients to allow this vulnerability and provides the best context for assisted self-study to happen. Here's a quote:

> Loving presence is easy to recognize. Imagine a happy and contented mother looking at the sweet face of her peaceful newborn baby. She is calm, loving, and attentive. Unhurried and undistracted, the two of them seem to be outside of time . . . simply being. Gently held within a field of love and life's wisdom, they are as present with each other as any two could be. (Martin, n.d., p. 1)

For the therapist to develop this state of mind, she must first look at others as living beings and sources of inspiration. As one therapist put it, "If you cannot see anything lovable in this person that you can respond to in a genuine way, then you are not the right person to help this person." It is this intention and habit of seeing something lovable in the other that creates the feeling state necessary for loving presence. The first thing I instruct students to do is to create this habit as the primary thing in any interaction. Create it and sustain it throughout your sessions.

Any number of things will support this intention. First, one must avoid being drawn into a conversation about abstractions—ideas, explanations, the meaning of the past, and such. The first goal is to establish a relationship that will support assisted self-study; the habit of gathering information by asking questions and considering answers is not the way to do it. The therapist's words and actions must demonstrate that he is paying attention to what the client is experiencing right now, cares about what the client is feeling, and understands what that means for the client. This connection through present experience is the key to limbic resonance. So the therapist searches for what there is about the client that is emotionally nourishing or inspiring of appreciation and connection. Another thing that helps build the right relationship is realizing the process as a cooperative enterprise where feelings of partnership, teamwork, and mutual respect are basic. The idea that we are not separate, that we are inescapably parts of a whole infinitely greater than each of us alone, is the root of loving presence.

Present Experience, Implicit Beliefs, and Procedural Memory

A picture has emerged of a set of pervasive, adaptive, sophisticated mental processes that occur largely out of view. Indeed, some researchers have gone so far as to suggest that the unconscious mind does virtually all the work and that conscious will may be an illusion.

TIMOTHY WILSON, *Strangers to Ourselves*, 2002

All living organisms from the humble amoeba to the human are born with devices designed to solve automatically, no proper reasoning required, the basic problems of life.

ANTONIO DAMASIO, *Looking for Spinoza*, 2003

The one thing we most want to help clients discover and change is the habitual ways they create unnecessary suffering for themselves and others. The logic is this:

1. Experience is organized by habits that function outside of consciousness.
2. The most significant of these organizing habits are those that were learned early in life and developed in reaction to compelling, formative experiences.
3. Such habits are stored in implicit memory and are not normally accessible to consciousness.

> Implicit memory [sometimes called procedural memory, sometimes emotional memory] involves parts of the brain that do not require conscious processing during encoding or retrieval. When implicit memory is retrieved, the neural net profiles that are reactivated involve circuits in the brain that are a fundamental part of our everyday experience of life: behaviors, emotions, and images. These implicit elements form part of the foundation for our subjective sense of ourselves: We act, feel, and imagine without recognition of the influence of past experience on our present reality. (Siegel, 2003, p. 29)

4. They are automated procedures, triggered by perceptions of internal and external realities, perceptions which themselves are influenced by organizing habits.
5. They are the functional equivalents of implicit beliefs.

These implicit predictions and beliefs exert a profound influence over everyday life without any simple, direct way to modify them. They influence all ongoing experience, whether it originates internally or externally, by producing the habitual reactions that result. They shape all manner of experience—perception, mood, thought, feeling, and behavior. Thus, present experience is a reliable, immediate expression of unconscious habits and beliefs. For that reason, we focus on present experiences and use them to bring what is normally unconscious into consciousness.

Nonverbal Indicators and Formative Experiences

Accessing the kinds of beliefs that pervasively and unconsciously influence experience requires that the therapist get ideas about what the client's formative early experiences were or what implicit beliefs the client's behaviors are expressing. To gather this information, the therapist focuses attention on the qualities of the client's habitual posture, tone of voice, facial expressions, gestures, eye contact, speech patterns, and such. (Some examples include ending verbal statements with the inflection of a question or a habitually sad-looking face or tilt of the head.) Many of these qualities are habitual nonverbal expressions of implicit beliefs. We call them indicators.

As you may imagine, there are many such indicators. Some can be completely obvious in what they say about the client. Others require that the therapist learn them over time. In bioenergetics, for example, the indicators are often postural. A sunken chest and locked knees for a bioenergetic therapist would be indicators of "an oral pattern" (Lowen, 1975). Given that pattern, the therapist has both a diagnosis and a way to proceed with treatment. Almost all methods of psychotherapy use particular sets of indicators this way and usually refer to them as "symptoms." In this method, we use indicators differently. We use them to get ideas for experiments.

As we interact and relate to others, we don't normally focus on their little, seemingly insignificant habits. In an ordinary interaction, conversation is most important; we might not consciously think about a person's subtle nonverbal behaviors. We might ignore a slight feeling of discomfort (about not being believed, for example) that results from the way the other person is looking at us with her head always turned to one side. Odds are she won't be consciously aware of either the angle of her head or the skepticism it indicates. This level of interaction is usually handled by the adaptive unconscious. In Hakomi, we consciously search for indicators, and the turning of the head is a common one. Through experimenting with it many times, I have come to expect that it can indicate formative experiences of not being told the truth or not being understood. The emotion associated with it is usually hurt. Though the hurt is not being felt at the moment, it is an expression of an implicit belief: "I must be careful about what people are telling me! I could get hurt again." Though not conscious, this belief is controlling present behavior and experience. Indicators are the external expressions of this process.

In Hakomi, we use indicators to create experiments, experiments designed to trigger reactions. This is a vital piece of the method. It is our clear intention to study a client's behavior not for symptoms of disease but for sources of experiments. We anticipate that the experiments we carry out will bring the unconscious, adaptive processes driving that behavior into the client's awareness. A therapist using this approach is thought of as having an experimental attitude. We are evidence seekers—evidence that is gathered on the spot, evidence that clients can use to understand themselves. The basic idea is this: (1) indicators suggest experiments; (2) experiments create reactions; and (3) reactions are evidence of implicit beliefs. Gathering evidence is what experiments are all about, and that's exactly why we do them.

For instance, if the client's habit is to hold her head a little bit off center and turned slightly away, we might do an experiment where the client, while in a mindful state, slowly turns her head back toward center. Most such clients, when doing this movement deliberately and carefully, will react with fear. This fear is about being emotionally hurt, and it is associated with memories of that happening and beliefs about how to avoid it. The habitual turning of the head is only one indicator and the experiment only one that could be done. There are endless possible indicators and experiments that can be done. Finding indicators and devising suitable experiments are some of the things that make this work so interesting. It is a combination of searching for clues like a detective and testing them like a scientist. It is a long way from the "talking cure."

Using Mindfulness and Little Experiments

The procedure that is used is as follows:

1. Find an indicator.
2. Imagine and decide what experiment to use.
3. In a gentle way and at a suitable time, shift the client's attention to the indicator and ask if it would be okay to do an experiment.
4. If the client agrees, set up the experiment by asking for mindfulness and a signal from the client when she is ready.
5. When the signal is given, do the experiment.

6. Watch for and, if necessary, ask the client about the outcome. (I often have to remind new students, "It's an experiment. So, get the data!")

Several general types of outcomes are possible:

1. The experiment could have no effect whatsoever. In that case, either the indicator wasn't significant, there was something wrong with the way the experiment was conducted, or, in some sense, the client wasn't ready.
2. The experiment evokes an image, memory, or idea, but without an accompanying emotional reaction.
3. It evokes an emotional reaction. For each case, the process unfolds differently.

This procedure is how we assist clients to study themselves. The experiments we do are meant to evoke reactions that will lead to discoveries. The most important discoveries are those that tell a client about herself: who she has become; that much of her suffering is unnecessary; how her old habits and hidden beliefs are preventing positive emotions and nourishing relationships; that these habits and beliefs that shape her everyday experiences began in childhood; and that there is a path that leads out of that past into an easier, more fulfilling present. With good experiments and the right follow-through, all that becomes possible.

A frequently used experiment is one in which the therapist offers a simple statement. The statement is designed to offer a nourishing idea that will be automatically rejected by the client. For example, with the indicator mentioned above, the head turned slightly away, the therapist might offer a statement like, "You can trust me" or "I won't betray you." In experiments like that, the first reaction might be a thought like, "I don't believe it!" Often it will be followed by an emotion, such as anger or sadness.

Experiments like this reveal the connections between beliefs, memories, and habitual behaviors. When clients experience such connections, accessing the unconscious material becomes possible. Mindful observation of triggers and reactions accesses memories of formative events, the experiences they created, and the habits that still manage those experiences.

Supporting Spontaneous Emotional Management

The Hakomi method is inspired by Buddhist principles. It is the principle of the primacy of consciousness that leads to the use of mindfulness. And it is the principle of nonviolence that leads to the particular way the method deals with emotions. When emotions are triggered by an experiment, clients very often react by containing them in a habitual way. They change posture, tense muscles, restrain breathing, and hold back expression. Some therapeutic methods think of such reactions as defensive—resisting the process as the therapist would like it to happen. Ideas like this are based on an adversarial attitude: the therapist versus the disease.

We, on the other hand, see such reactions as habits intended to manage the intensity and expression of an emotional experience. Where some methods attempt to break down the "defenses" and overcome the "resistance," we do the opposite: instead of pushing for a breakthrough, we offer and provide support for the reactions. For example, if a client has reacted by drawing her shoulders up and in—to contain her fear—we might help the client to maintain the tension by holding her shoulders up and in for her. In doing this, we are demonstrating understanding and compassion. In what may seem a paradox, this kind of support helps the client allow the emotional process to unfold. As we support the client and wait, the client very often relaxes voluntarily and allows the painful feeling and its expression. This supportive approach has been part of Hakomi since its inception. The techniques involved are referred to as "taking over" and they are the second major thing that is unique to Hakomi. (The first is the use of mindfulness in the evocation of experience.)

Almost all management behavior involves muscle tension of some kind. It is often possible for the therapist to offer and, with permission, provide actual physical support for that tension. For example, when the emotion is intense, clients will spontaneously tighten their diaphragms, abdominals, and chest wall muscles. They may wrap their arms tightly around themselves. Holding the client tightly will provide support for this way of managing. What can happen then, and what often does happen, is that the emotion being contained is released. In the case of fear, it might be a scream. In the case of sadness, it would be sobbing. Taking-over techniques consistently lead to the voluntary release of emotion and they contribute a great deal to the effectiveness of the method.

Providing Positive Missing Experiences

The release of contained emotions is extremely satisfying and healing. But even more, it is the prelude to insight. Support for management leads to release and, when handled properly, release leads to insight and integration. The habits of containment, when relaxed, allow an alternative path to unfold—the path of expression and relief. Support for this path is the simplest of all. The first simple thing to do is to maintain contact by continuing to hold or touch the client, the touch that was already present in the taking over. Only at this point, when expression has subsided, should the pressure involved in taking over be relaxed. Contact is continued, perhaps by keeping a hand on the client's back or by holding the client in one's arms. This provides the kind of comforting that didn't happen during the painful formative experience. This lack of comfort prompted containment rather than expression. This is a basic missing experience. Imagine a child playing and in his playing, he stumbles and falls, hurting himself. He cries and runs to his mother, who drops whatever she is doing and holds the child and dries his tears and whispers soft words of sympathy and reassurance. That's the universal treatment for distress. In some way, all mammals do something similar (other species, too).

After release and while comforting is available, clients will very often quiet down and look away. From their very slight head movements and facial expressions, one can tell that they are thinking, remembering, and making sense of what just happened. This is the integration phase. This is the reconciling of oneself to what was. This is the time of letting the past be past. This is how one moves on. It is how habits are changed and freedom of choice is gained. This is how painful experiences are resolved, how completion is accomplished. During this time of integration, the therapist continues to provide contact and, most important, the therapist remains silent—present and attentive, but without interfering with the client's inner work of making sense of her experience and coming to completion. It may take five or even ten minutes.

When the client is complete, she will open her eyes and look at the therapist. It is best to stay silent, even then. Best to just wait. She will slowly begin to talk about what she has discovered. That is also part of integration—telling your story to a concerned friend. Her understanding is shared and confirmed. She is now known to another as she has come to know herself. She feels relief and the warmth of being with a caring, helpful person. She feels a new sense of freedom and hope—the possibility of satisfactions previously missed. Such are the rewards for those with the courage to take the journey.

The Shifting Vision

My way of working was a fly-by-the-seat-of-your-pants affair back when I began. Over the years, it has evolved. It has clarified and changed through sessions, workshops, training, reading, and interacting with students and colleagues. The long process of learning my craft brought refinements. The biggest ones are these:

1. When I started out, I was influenced mostly by the psychotherapy approaches that were academically based, like behavior modification and Rogerian therapy. But slowly, after several years and with the help of friends, I realized that the information I needed to move the process could not be obtained by conversational means. Discussion, stories, and questions actually interfered with the process I was developing. I learned to search for indicators and to do experiments. Friends versed in character theory and the body therapies provided the original inspiration for this shift.

2. I learned to think of the work as assisted self-study. In this, I changed from being the doer, responsible for everything that happened, to the helper who only supported what the client did for himself. Elements of my support were necessary, but all of them together were not in any way sufficient. The client did the work.

3. I learned to maintain a strong focus on present experience and to shy away from "taking a history." Reich pointed out that a person's history, at least what's still significant about it, is present in everything about him. You only have to look.

4. I learned, in one dramatic moment, to shift from breaking down defenses to offering support for management behavior. It was my personal experience with the kind of force used in some therapies and my devotion to the Buddhist principle of non-violence that inspired this change. Since that moment, I have developed ways to move the process forward gently.

5. I learned to place a strong emphasis on providing positive experiences and moved away from emphasizing the expression of painful emotions. When painful emo-

tions arise spontaneously, I make an effort to help them complete in a natural way. The process became more and more a matter of following and supporting what wanted to happen and less and less of making it happen. As a result, the work became faster and easier.

6. I learned to emphasize nourishment and comforting as ways to support the ongoing process. And I learned to be silent and to recognize when silence was called for. I realized that the most important work is what the client does.

7. I shifted away from the Freudian image of repression and libidinal impulses. I learned to accept the unconscious as a potentially strong, positive player in the healing process. I learned to recognize the activity of the adaptive unconscious and, by honoring it, create a satisfying working relationship with it (Wilson, 2002; Gladwell, 2005).

8. Again, in one dramatic moment, I learned about loving presence and the power it has to support healing. I learned to deliberately establish a felt state of compassion and to present myself as, first of all, just another human being (Gerhardt, 2004; Lewis et al., 2000).

9. I learned that following is another way of leading, that supporting natural processes is more fruitful than trying to control them. The inspiration here is Taoism. This way of working grew more and more satisfying as my understanding and respect for the adaptive unconscious grew.

10. I also gained, as we all have these last 10 years, a greater understanding of the neurological bases of all behavior, and especially of emotions and beliefs (Calvin, 1997; Goleman, 2004; Damasio, 2003; Hobson, 1996; Llinás, 2001; Panksepp, 1998; Pinker, 2002; Rossi, 1996; Schore, 1994; Schwartz & Begley, 2002; Shlain, 2003; Siegel, 1999, 2009; van der Kolk, McFarlane, & Weisaeth, 1996).

Appreciation

So many people, so many open, loving hearts have shared themselves with me. I have witnessed tears shed and joy given and felt. I cannot imagine a more rewarding journey. For every inspiring book and every conversation, for all my students and colleagues, more than I can list, I offer thanks. I have built a life around this work. My sincere hope is that what I have contributed will help all those who wish to begin or to continue on this journey.

Theory

CHAPTER 4

The Central Role of the Body in Hakomi Psychotherapy

Marilyn Morgan

Andrew sits back in the chair, his legs crossed, his arms behind his head. He oozes confidence. "I know I deserve the promotion," he says, "and I just can't understand why I haven't asked for it." His brow crinkles as he tries to work it out. I suggest that Andrew imagine asking for his promotion, and turn his attention mindfully to his inner responses as he does so. He takes a few moments, and then reports a tight, heavy sensation in his solar plexus. I say to him, "You deserve the promotion." Andrew notices the sensation intensifying. He stays with the experience in his body, and fierce words come to him: "No you don't! You are not worthy!" Tears sting at his eyes and he feels small and shamed. Focusing his attention on his body sensation has rapidly taken Andrew to a deeper awareness of parts of himself that hours of thinking and talking did not.

WE HAVE BECOME accustomed to dissociation from the body (Leder, 1990). Damasio calls it "the abyssal separation between body and mind" (1994, p. 249). This split was articulated clearly by the French philosopher René Descartes in 1637, and has since profoundly influenced Western thought, including Christian doctrine, psychoanalysis, science, and medicine. Cognitive functioning has been accorded a status separate from other dimensions of our being—those very dimensions that give our lives significance, pleasure, and passion. The pulse, movement, and wildness tend to be stiffly constrained, and our bodies become foreign, even an embarrassment, a nuisance—alien objects to be tolerated at best, or abused and controlled at worst. This is like the Freudian concept of the rational ego trying to dominate the unruly id. So much in modern life supports this separation from embodiment—frantic busyness, the television and computer, emphasis on appearance, efficiency, and the intellect. Discomfort and dis-ease bring people to consult a therapist.

Hakomi is a body-inclusive therapy, giving a central place to somatic experience (Kurtz, 1990a, 2004; Kurtz & Minton, 1997). This position has been supported by clinical observations during therapy sessions, and is grounded in a lineage dating back to Reich, and influenced by Feldenkrais, Lowen (1958), Pierrakos (1990), and others (Boadella, 1987; Crisp, 1987; Greenberg & Rhonda, 1988). The role of the body in self-awareness, relationship, life satisfaction, and therapeutic change is now supported by a growing body of writing and research in neuroscience and attachment (Caldwell, 2011; Cozolino, 2006; Lewis et al., 2000; Porges, 2006; Rossi, 1986; Schore, 2003; Siegel, 1999, 2003). Trauma therapists affirm the importance of body experience in trauma recovery (Ogden, 1997; Rothschild, 2000; Scaer, 2001; Siegel, 1999, 2003; van der Kolk, 1994), and this perspective continues to scientifically inform and enrich Hakomi practice.

Staying in Contact With the Body Is Staying in Contact With a Deeper Knowing

It is not uncommon for people to believe that rationality and deciding what we want in any given moment are functions emanating from the head. However, our experience is located in the body, of which the head is only a part. As Kurtz says, "your mind is hooked up to your physiology" (2004, p. 78). Damasio describes how we use body sensations to assist us in decision making. In fact, he argues, reasoning and efficient decision making would otherwise be well-nigh impossible. Sensations generated by the emotional brain, based on prior experiences, give us immediate messages about the significance of options we are considering for the future. Damasio calls these sensations "somatic markers" (1994, p. 174). For example, when thinking of going to a social event, you might perceive a sinking in the stomach. It doesn't feel right to accept the invitation, so you decline. It saves hours of weighing the pros and cons. The negative somatic marker has acted like an alarm bell, giving a warning. On another occasion, you think of going out with a friend and you feel a warm expansive feeling in the chest. After some thinking about practicalities, you decide to go. You have experienced a positive somatic marker, which acts as an incentive. Frequently, somatic markers influence our decisions, even when we are unconscious of their operation (Damasio, 1994).

The Body as a Royal Road to the Core Unconscious

To understand the role of somatic markers and the body in therapy, we need to know about memory. "The body is alive with meaning and memory" (Kurtz, 2004, p. 78).

Important remembered experiences are embedded in emotion, and emotion arises in the body. Damasio differentiates between emotion as bodily response, and feeling as conscious perception of the emotion: "Emotions play out in the theatre of the body. Feelings play out in the theatre of the mind" (2003, p. 28). A person can have a disconnection between the conscious experience of feeling and emotion. This can occur after head injury and in avoidant attachment experiences such as occur in sensitive/withdrawn, tough/generous, and charming/seductive character styles (see Chapter 8). Due to this disconnection, conscious memory of important events may be sparse, and it is possible these events have not been encoded into autobiographical memory (for a good discussion on this topic, see Siegel, 1999, p. 94; Caldwell, 2011). Clinical experience and some research suggest that unrecognized emotions are still occurring on a bodily level and can be accessed somatically (Lambert & Kinsley, 2005).

In Hakomi, the focus is on assisting the person to self-study and explore his own truth at all levels of organization. A person like Andrew, described earlier, can gain an understanding of himself that is not just conscious, intellectual knowledge, but is an awareness of the deeper, unconscious aspects of self. This includes core material, which is composed of beliefs, nervous system patterning, sensations, memories, images, emotions, and attitudes about the self and the world. Core material shapes our patterns of behavior, our bodily structure, and our experiences—and is mainly unconscious. In fact, it may be in complete contradiction to our conscious beliefs and aspirations, but tends to "run the show" (Blakeslee & Blakeslee, 2007).

Core material not only is about memory, behavior patterns, and beliefs, but also influences the ongoing experience and expression of self. Damasio says, "At each moment the state of self is constructed from the ground up" (1994, p. 240). Daniel Stern (1985) describes the core self, the foundation of which is formed in the first two years, as essentially somatic in nature. Kurtz comments, "[The] job of observing bodily expressions and inferring core beliefs from them is one of the more important tasks of the body psychotherapist" (2004, p. 62). He also says, "understanding the expressions of self through the body is one basic component of body psychotherapy" (Kurtz & Minton, 1997, p. 54).

The Body May Remember What the Mind Cannot

During infancy, and under conditions of threat, we may not make conscious memory, but experiences at these times can continue to influence us long after. The body and associated emotional circuits are imprinted. Implicit, intuitive knowledge is memory that is encoded functionally in the nerve circuits, and structurally in the brain and body. Implicit memory does not require attention for encoding and is not experienced as a remembering. Our unconscious can process information very rapidly, below the threshold of awareness, and this information is held in implicit memory. (For a discussion on rapid unconscious acquiring and utilizing of intuitive knowledge, read Malcolm Gladwell's [2005] book, *Blink*.) The infant can make implicit procedural and emotional memories from birth. She can also start forming memories for features of things and snapshot images. The right hemisphere and amygdala, the brain areas most connected to implicit memory and the body, are "online" at birth. However, the hippocampus, which is necessary for encoding the sequence and context of explicit memory, is not developed until about three years of age, hence the commonly observed infantile amnesia. The left hemisphere, necessary for verbal encoding and developing conscious narratives, is not functioning until around the same time (Badenoch, 2008).

In traumatic and very stressful situations, the amygdala increases its function and the hippocampus shuts down. The hippocampus is particularly sensitive to cortisol, secreted during stress, which causes damage to the neurons there. For a child enduring ongoing high stress, even one old enough to form narrative memories, this function could be suppressed. If explicit memory is not encoded in the first place, then it can never be retrieved. Many clients may never remember, in a conscious, narrative way, some of the traumatic events of childhood. As discussed above, some people also have difficulty being mindful or sensing the body. Effects on brain development for a neglected and traumatized child, such as fewer fibers connecting the corpus callosum and smaller frontal lobes, can make body awareness problematic later in life (Teicher, 2002). The therapist may need to work for some time with a client to allow for sufficient repair to occur before accessing core material is feasible (Schore, 2003).

The Body Places Us in the Here and Now Where Change Happens

When the client focuses on the body in the present moment, unconscious material can surface into awareness. Implicit memory doesn't feel like memory—it is perceived in the present. Unconscious memory related to core material seems to come in packages, similar to the complexes described by Carl Jung and the COEX systems detailed by Stanislav Grof (1975). There will be images, memories, phrases, affect, behavior, impulses, and states of consciousness, all related to a theme. Each is tied in with particular somatic markers. As Kurtz says, "Finding the meanings [bodily sensations] embody is an important part of changing them" (2004, p. 63). Touch one aspect of the package—use mindful attention and stay with the experience—and the rest will emerge into awareness. Often it is experiencing the somatic marker that is the doorway opening to awareness and change. This is a difficult process for some who want to have meaning before experience. Tony Crisp says, "[People] want to know in advance what is going to emerge, so they can edit it, change it, or make it socially acceptable" (1987, p. 26).

The good news for psychotherapy is that memory and brain structure are much more plastic than previously thought (Fuchs, 2004). We are constantly storing, activating, and restoring memories. Lynn Nadel (1994), a researcher on the function of the hippocampus, found that when a memory trace is activated, it is vulnerable for a short time and can be changed before it is recoded. Further research is confirming this finding (McCrone, 2003). This would affirm the importance of working in the here and now. The hippocampus can make a new memory, based on a different experience, this time putting it in context and time sequence. Sleep and dreams, along with neural communication between the left and right cerebral hemispheres, are thought to help turn the new memory into a permanent one (Siegel, 2003).

Mindfulness and Body Awareness

Mindfulness is an essential foundation of Hakomi and necessary to utilize bodily wisdom (see Chapters 6 and 10 for a full discussion). The attention is taken inward, and time is spent in quieting internal noise. Scanning body sensations lowers arousal and allows more subtle signals to come to awareness. Body signals are usually missed when the attention is in outer, task-focused mode or sufficient time is not given. Signals may be changes in the felt sense of the body, impulses, small movements, and tension in the muscles. These can evoke words, images, memories, and so on. Candace Pert (1999) suggests that paying mindful attention to an aspect of body experience releases molecules in that area that are carriers of information upward to the brain.

Finishing Unfinished Business Held in the Body

Fritz Perls described unfinished business as unprocessed memory that pushes for attention through symptoms or unwanted impulses, thoughts, and behavior. Bringing unconscious material to consciousness begins a differentiating and integrating process (Wilber, 1977, 2000), where things settle and complexity grows. In narrative terms, this could be described as moving from a thin story to a rich story. Peter Levine and Pat Ogden have developed somatic sequencing, in which "frozen" experience is released and can be sequenced through the body (Ogden, Minton, & Pain, 2006). This method is useful for working with trauma, and can be helpful and safe for distressing, "undigested" emotional issues that clients bring to therapy.

> *As a child, Martha inhibited her impulses to ask for help or to reach out. She feels the block in her throat and tension in her arms. During her sessions, she reconnects with these bodily "stuck places" and moves with what her body wants her to do. She says what she wants to say, voicing requests to the mother of her childhood, then to her husband, represented by a chair. She feels the impulses within the tension in her shoulders and slowly reaches her arms out for touch and support. Later she feels anger impulses coursing down her arms. Her fists tighten, and she realizes how angry she is at being the one who had to do most of the work.*

In the present moment, when the old circuits are active and the client is experiencing the memory and decisions that were made at an earlier time, a missing experience can transform the memory. This missing experience is frequently relational, involving limbic connection and revision (Lewis et al., 2000). As the new experience is deeply felt and embodied, it becomes nourishing and transformative. By keeping mindful attention on the somatic dimension, the experience feels real to the client, and is anchored in the body. The new experience can then become a positive somatic marker for the future. Change can occur very quickly, as Gay and Kathlyn Hendricks describe: "The great advantage of body-centered therapy is that it goes immediately to where people live: the reality of their somatic experience. People feel actual shifts in their inner experience as the work proceeds from moment to moment. And it works with a speed that is often astonishing" (Henricks & Hendricks, 1993, pp. 4–5).

Supporting Bodily Defenses Allows for Deepening Awareness

Among many somatic interventions a Hakomi therapist might employ is physical taking over. When body sensations, impulses, or tensions become manifest, the therapist, with permission, can physically support them, allowing the client to pay attention to deeper layers of experience. This is a nonviolent approach, in contrast to the idea of "breaking down defenses," which may lead to further resistance or to the client feeling overwhelmed. Taking over, in a variety of forms, can be very powerful, providing the support and safety to allow hidden parts to emerge (Kurtz, 1990a; Weiss & Benz, 1989). The following illustrates one style of taking over.

> *Martha was the eldest child of six, and now is a mother caring for her children and elderly parents. In her therapy session, she is holding her head with her hand. As she talks of stresses in her family, her head becomes lower, and her body droops to the left. I offer to support her head, and she accepts. Immediately after Martha allows me to take the weight of her head with my hands, she starts to sob. "I'm tired of being the strong one," she says. "I want someone to care for me for a change!"*

Bodily Expression as Information for Client and Therapist

Hakomi therapists give primacy to the body in every aspect of the therapeutic process. Contact between therapist and client, where the therapist is compassionate and attuned, leads to a limbic resonance (Lewis et al., 2000) that creates the "bubble" of connection within which the therapy proceeds. This allows for what we call the cooperation of the unconscious, where core material can start to emerge in an organic way. The therapist may feel in his own body particular sensations that mirror those of the client. Mindful, curious attention to these sensations, without identification, can provide valuable information, which assists the empathic contact. By carefully tracking body signals and bringing them to the client's attention, the therapist can deepen the process. The body structure, posture, and movement of the client can indicate the characterological defenses that have been developed, opening a window to the vulnerabilities beneath (Caldwell, 1997, 2011). Kurtz says, "the body reveals psychological information" (2004, p. 78). This can serve as a guide for formulating sensitive ways of working with a particular client (Kurtz, 1990a; Morgan, 2004b; Weiss & Benz, 1989). Ken Dychtwald vividly described his experience of being deeply seen and understood by John Pierrakos:

> I realized who and what my informer was. It was my body—the body I had taken with me to the workshop, the body that had been with me since birth, the body that I had trained and nurtured throughout my life. Somehow, this body, my body, was presenting information about me to John Pierrakos that he was noticing and reading back to me. (1987, p. 5)

Shaping the Bodymind: Child as Mapmaker

Ron Kurtz described the child as "the mapmaker" (1990a, p. 133). Neuroscience emphasizes that the connections formed within the brain depend on experience. The child is born with approximately 100 billion neurons. If these nerve cells were placed end to end, they would stretch 2 million miles. Many nerve connections are already in place at birth, the brain being hardwired to seek connection with caregivers, and to allow basic bodily functions. However, the major growth of neurons and the wiring of neuronal circuits are yet to take place, depending on the experiences to come. Eventually each nerve cell is likely to have up to 10,000 connections. Even if a child will never consciously remember his early childhood experiences, his brain and body are being shaped by them. Daniel Siegel (2003) describes the brain as an anticipatory machine. The child's interactions with his world are imprinted in his brain circuitry, which is reflected in the body. He is "wired up," and his body shaped to suit his particular situation. This bodily held "memory" will profoundly affect later emotions, behavior patterns, beliefs, and abilities to process information. In Hakomi, we recognize that this core material shapes character styles (see Chapter 8).

The Felt Shift: How Change Is Felt in the Body

Eugene Gendlin, who developed the focusing method, argues for the importance of the border zone between conscious and unconscious: "A direct sense of the border zone occurs *bodily*, as a physical, somatic sensation" (1996, p. 18). His process of focusing on what he terms the "felt sense" leads to awareness and therapeutic change. The client comes with an issue. She turns her attention to something she directly senses in the body, which initially may be murky and puzzling. She turns away from the known information and feelings toward the unclear, and waits. This may be uncomfortable, but the felt sense starts to constellate. It is physical, in the moment, and has a feeling of complexity and wholeness. Often an organic shift is felt from within the sensation, a kind of opening, which brings some relief. The client keeps a witness state present and does not identify with the felt sense. After the felt shift, it is likely that the client will have a new perspective on the original situation. She then can retrospectively think about what has emerged. Leslie Greenberg works with the felt sense in his process experiential psychotherapy, describing how in a safe, attuned setting, markers—experienced as an unclear felt sense—emerge. Emotions are seen as organizing bridges to core issues, as well as for reorganization (Greenberg & Goldman, 1988).

Being Embodied Is Being Alive, Able to Grow, and Be Intimate

The Hakomi principle of organicity is related to the natural growth processes innate within us as complex systems. Bruce Lipton (2005), a molecular biologist, has asserted that we cannot be in defense mode and growth mode at the same time. The impact of stress on the body is detailed in an excellent book by Gabor Mate (2003), *When the Body*

Says No: The Costs of Hidden Stress, which asserts that core beliefs, which can keep us defended, are imprinted at a cellular level.

A number of writers have commented on the importance of attuned relationship and safety in bodymind therapy involving accessing and transformation (Gendlin, 1996). Kurtz emphasized the therapeutic importance of loving presence. The social engagement system, as described by Stephen Porges, gives us useful information on the somatics involved in safety and relationship, and the ability to feel the sensations of the body. Porges emphasizes that the ability to relate is heavily dependent on physiological factors and is not a conscious process, although we can learn to apply consciousness to activating the relevant nervous system. The social engagement system allows us to sense our bodies, feel grounded, and be in contact with our self and others. This system can be "offline" but is able to be awakened with the right stimulation. It helps for the therapist to activate in herself the part of the nervous system that regulates social connection: a calm behavioral state. Body awareness is integral to this state. The therapist can then, through limbic mirroring processes, help the client who feels stressed or fearful move to a more grounded, contactful place, where therapy can constructively proceed (Lewis et al., 2000; Porges, 2006).

Increased body awareness enables access to our more essential self, and we can thus make life decisions in keeping with our deepest wants. We feel more, which gives life texture and meaning. We can bring core beliefs into awareness and change patterns that are now limiting us. Feeling our bodily sensations allows us to attune more intimately to others, and to give and receive satisfying nourishment. Deep down there is hunger for knowing our embodied selves, to reconnect with that wisdom—those quiet, wise rhythms of life that guide us and are the breath of our wholeness and growth. As Mary Sykes Wylie says, writing in *Psychotherapy Networker*, "it is through and in the language of the body that we most fully and completely express our human *being*" (2004, p. 33).

I will end with a quote from Paul Tillich:

> We are in constant motion and never stop to plunge to the depth. We talk and talk and never listen to the voices speaking to our depth or from our depth. . . . Like hit and run drivers, we injure our souls by the speed with which we move on the surface. . . . We miss, therefore, our depth and our true life. (1948, pp. 55–56)

CHAPTER 5

Hakomi Principles and a Systems Approach to Psychotherapy

Greg Johanson

HAKOMI IS AN integrative approach to psychotherapy, growth, and healing that can eclectically incorporate a range of methods and techniques, in addition to the ones it has pioneered. However, it is a highly principled eclecticism and integration. The answer to what might or might not be considered Hakomi is whether the process embraces the foundational Hakomi principles of unity, organicity, mind-body holism, mindfulness, and nonviolence.

These guiding philosophical principles with their clinical implications can be explored from a variety of vantage points. The approach taken here is to view the principles in relationship to systems theory, broadly conceived. Kurtz (1990a, 2008) not only studied widely in the experiential psychotherapies, Taoism, and Buddhism, he spent noteworthy time exploring the new sciences of complexity, the study of living, organic, self-organizing, dissipative systems, and more (Cowan, Pines, & Meltzer, 1994).

Contemporary systems theory provides a framework for understanding the core principles of Hakomi and translating material from other realms, such as scientific research,

With special thanks to Sid Kemp.

the philosophy of science, and spiritual traditions into working concepts that guide thera-peutic tools and processes. This chapter refers to important and accessible literature in the philosophy of science and psychotherapy dialogue. The large volume of material available precludes anything more than a brief introduction to essential elements of this material. See Johanson (2009a, 2009b) for a more extended discussion and additional references.

Unity

In the early days of Hakomi (the 1970s), one particularly fruitful source from the philoso-phy of science literature that held up well was the book *Mind and Nature* by Gregory Bateson (1979). Here, Bateson outlined 10 propositions that characterize a living organic system, which can be said to have a mind of its own, including nature itself. These propo-sitions were tied directly to the fundamental principles that defined Hakomi, beyond its specific method and techniques (Kurtz, 1990a).

Bateson's first proposition is that living organic systems with a quality of mind are made of parts organized into wholes. Atoms join to make molecules; molecules join to make complex organisms; organisms join to form larger communities; and so forth. Lao-tzu said, "Tao produced the One. The One produced the two. The two produced the three. And the three produced the ten thousand things" (Johanson & Kurtz, 1991, p. 1).

There is good news here. Things are building up and coming together. In the old New-tonian paradigm, things were more depressing. The second law of thermodynamics spoke of entropy, the notion that the universe is breaking down, running out of energy. But Ilya Prigogine (Prigogine & Stengers, 1984) won the Nobel Prize for demonstrating that there is another force within organic life that builds up, that moves parts to organize into greater wholes, namely negentropy.

This was the basis for Hakomi's unity principle, the notion that we are joined with many other parts in increasing levels of complexity. We live in a participatory universe, as Morris Berman (1990) notes. Laszlo suggests our "informed universe is a world of subtle but constant interconnection, a world where everything informs—acts on and interacts with—everything else" (2004, pp. 5–6). The most fundamental unity of reality according to Arthur Koestler (1967) is a holon—a shorthand designation for a whole that is made up of parts, which in turn is part of a larger whole (Nowak & Vallacher, 1998).

Unity has many implications for psychotherapists. For one, it means we can be lazy, in the sense that we can have faith that whenever people are fragmented, there is a force that wants to move things in the direction of greater wholeness. We do not have to engineer or create a new person. Many therapists who come to Hakomi training are overly stressed, holding too much responsibility for their clients' growth, and too little trust in their innate impulse to move toward wholeness.

Laszlo points to a second connotation when he says our interdependent world should be apprehended "with our heart as well as our brain" (2004, p. 6). Compassion, as Thomas Merton noted, is the profound awareness of the interconnectedness of all things. Clients who stand across from us are not totally other. They are us as well. Thus, Hakomi therapists find it both scientifically and clinically necessary to develop that sense of compassion or loving presence that honors and embodies the communion between living systems (Germer, 2006; Kornfield, 1993). This is foundational for facilitating core transformation, as well as normal, healthy attachment (Cozolino, 2006; Davidson & Harrington, 2002; Shaver, Lavy, Saron, & Mikulincer, 2007; Siegel, 2006; Siegel & Hartzell, 2003).

A third implication, sad for psychotherapists and their pocketbooks, is that we cannot be imperialists. If we are holons composed of subsystems that participate in suprasystems (Skynner, 1976), then all those levels will be important and need proper attention. For example, to be holistic and responsible, if people present themselves as depressed, we might need to attend to metabolic issues through nutrition, biochemistry, movement, deep-tissue work, and so forth, as well as the developmental, psychological issues that psychotherapy traditionally addresses, as well as family, labor, spiritual, community, political, and/or economic issues in some cases (Graves, 2008). Since single practitioners do not have skills in all these areas, it means we need to work in interdisciplinary ways as much as possible. Hakomi therapists affirm full psychosocial assessments as outlined in such books as *Metaframeworks* (Breunlin, Schwartz, & Mac Kune-Karrer, 1992).

Ken Wilber was an early resource for Kurtz, and an ongoing one for Hakomi. The unity principle is where Wilber's all-quadrant-all-level model of integral psychology recommended itself. While feminist psychotherapists emphasized holons by saying the self is always and only a self-in-relation (Herlihy & McCollum, 2007; Jordan, Kaplan, Miller, Stiver, & Surrey, 1991), Wilber (1995) expressed it by saying that psychology is always also sociology. Wilber agrees that the meaning of something is intimately related to its context, one of the main points of postmodernism (Graves, 2008; Harvey, 1989).

Wilber (1995), as well as Habermas (1979), clarified that a human holon not only has an individual and a communal aspect, but also an internal-subjective and external-objective aspect. Laszlo concurs: "What we call 'matter' is the aspect we apprehend when we look at a person, a plant, or a molecule from the *outside*; 'mind' is the readout we get when we look at the same thing from the *inside*" (2004, pp. 147–149). Following Wilber in plotting the individual-communal versus the interior-exterior results in a four-part grid, or four quadrants (Figure 5.1).

These quadrants suggest that the intentional, cultural, social, and behavioral aspects of a holon are inseparably intertwined, with no one quadrant able to reduce the others to itself. Internal-individual consciousness (II quadrant) has a degree of autonomy, but is highly influenced by internal-communal dispositions (IC quadrant), namely the values of the multiple cultures in which we are immersed (Helms & Cook, 1999; Johanson, 1992; McGoldrick, Giordano, & Pearce, 1996; Wilber, 2006). These values might or might not have strong support through actual social structures that embody them in the external-communal (EC) world of laws, educational systems, housing arrangements, legal systems, economic policies, and so forth. These three quadrants work in terms of mutual, reciprocal influences with the external-individual (EI) quadrant of one's objective underlying physiology and observable behavior. Wilber's inclusion here of an interior dimension as well as a cultural-social dimension goes a long way toward addressing what has been the inadequate or shadow side of systems theory (Berman, 1996).

	INTERIOR .	EXTERIOR
	+Dialogical	+Monological
	+Hermeneutical	+Empirical, Positivistic
	+Consciousness	+Form
	Sigmund Freud	*B. F. Skinner*
	C. G. Jung	*John Watson*
INDIVIDUAL	*Jean Piaget*	*Empiricism*
	Aurobindo	*Behaviorism*
	Plotinus	*Biochemistry*
	Gautama Buddha .	*Neurology*
	(II) Intentional Aspect (I)	(EI) Behavioral Aspect (It)
	(IC) Cultural Values (We)	(EC) Social Structures (Its)
	Thomas Kuhn	*Systems Theory*
	Wilhelm Dilthey	*Talcott Parsons*
COLLECTIVE	*Jean Gebser*	*Auguste Comte*
	Max Weber	*Karl Marx*
	Hans-Georg Gadamer	*Gerhard Lenski*

Figure 5.1. Wilber's Four Quadrants With Representative Theorists

While unity was the term chosen in the Hakomi context, the principle also relates to the Buddhist philosophical terms nonduality and interbeing (Coffey, 2008). This teaching, which dates back to the Buddha (Macy, 1991) and is also integral to contemporary Buddhist thinking (Hanh, 1987; Wallace, 2007), is that it is erroneous to think that we are separate from one another, and detrimental to think that we are all one and the same. Rather, interconnected diversity is seen as a model for how holons interact (Stolorow, Brandchaft, & Atwood, 1987). This model suggests that people should interact with one another as different, yet not entirely separate, which can be a guide for the therapeutic relationship as well as healthy family and social relationships.

Organicity

Following the implications of the unity principle results in John Muir's observation that if we pick up a stick, we discover it is connected to everything in the universe, which makes being succinct problematic. To return to Bateson's propositions, his second one is that what makes a system organic is not simply that it has parts, but that the parts are connected and communicate within the whole (Nowak & Vallacher, 1998). Wilber (1979) notes that a broad-spectrum way of thinking about therapy is that it is a matter of healing splits—splits between one part of the mind and another, between the body and the mind, between the whole self and the environment, and a final transpersonal split that overcomes all division.

Trouble, therefore, for living organic systems may flow from a lack of communication. When the liver is not interacting with the pancreas, pituitary, and heart, there are problems. When the family doesn't talk within itself, the football team doesn't huddle, production is out of touch with sales, the designers who are doing the dashboard don't talk to those engineering the heater, and governments don't stay in touch, there is potential for great harm. Various therapies tend to address a particular split. Hakomi therapists, working out of this integral systems approach, treat their clients in ways appropriate to each split, and/or seek to refer them to specialists who can (Johanson, 2009b).

When the communication and information exchange is happening, the system is self-organizing, self-directing, and self-correcting, characterized by complex, nonlinear determinism, meaning it has a mind of its own based on its own internal wisdom—Bateson's third proposition. A living, organic system is not a machine where one input will mechanically translate into a predictable outcome. It has decider subsystems, which take any input and process it in unique ways that organize both its experience of the input and its expression in response to the input (Nowak & Vallacher, 1998).

The second Hakomi principle, organicity, is respectful and trusting of a living system's inner wisdom and integrity as it participates in and interacts with its environment. Organicity distinguishes the qualities of living systems from those of nonliving systems (Vallacher & Nowak, 1994a, 1994b). The organicity principle acknowledges that, as opposed to a machine that can be fixed from without, a living organism can only be healed from within, through enrolling its own creative intelligence when dealing with issues of worldview and meaning (Juarrero, 1999; Murphy & Brown, 2007).

The implication for psychotherapy is that it looks for and follows natural processes, inner movements, inner rhythms, and spontaneous, nonverbal signs of the collaboration of the unconscious (Kurtz, 1990a) orienting toward increased wholeness; this, as opposed to artificially prescribing structures or agendas from without. In everyday life, parents adapt to the differing needs of their children as teachers take into account the various learning styles of their students. This is organically necessary and natural.

Another way of saying this is that organic systems display emergent properties that cannot be predicted or controlled (Clayton, 2004; Deacon, 2006). The solutions needed often cannot be known before they happen. Therapists need to wait in patience and trust. The best leader follows, according to Lao-tzu.

Embracing the principle of organicity clearly moves us toward giving up white knight models of riding in and saving people, in favor of more organic midwife or gardener models that talk less extravagantly of coaxing nature.

Lao-tzu seconds this implication in many places:

> [The sage] only helps all creatures to find their own nature, but does not venture to lead them by the nose. . . . He simply reminds people of who they have always been. . . . Because he has given up helping, he is people's greatest help. . . . The highest form of goodness is like water. Water knows how to benefit all things without striving with them. (Johanson & Kurtz, 1991, pp. 33, 134)

Self-healing holons are complex and unpredictable. They cannot be effectively modeled by reductionistic models. It is possible to model the consequences of kicking a football by creating a simplified representation of the foot, the football, and the force applied. However, the consequences of kicking a living being cannot be represented in the same way. If a dog is kicked, for instance, its interpretation of the meaning of the kick comes into play. Is the kick perceived as hostile or playful? Is the person doing the kicking known to the dog, or a stranger? The dog has an internal perspective that must be considered in order to make sense of its actions. Bateson and Bateson (1987) and Wilber (1995) recognize that complex, self-healing holons have an internal perspective that interprets meaning. To support the healing of a therapy client, the therapist must honor and receive information that reflects the person's internal wisdom (Knight & Grabowecky, 1995).

Mind-Body Holism

It is common in Western thinking to separate the mind and body. This separation, proposed by René Descartes, has not stood up well in recent centuries in philosophy, and has been thoroughly disproved by research in neuropsychiatry and psychoneuroimmunology (Damasio, 1999; Lakoff & Johnson, 1999; Shusterman, 2008). Hakomi embraces a unified view through its principle of mind-body holism, which is actually a subset of organicity, and the principle that development occurs by envelopment of previous levels (Andersen, Emmeche, Finnemann, & Christiansen, 2000), resulting in a compound individual of subatomic, physical, biological, psychological, cultural, and transcendent levels (Emmeche, Koppe, & Stjernfelt, 1997; Graves, 2008; Wilber, 1995).

Common understanding assumes that a mind processes information and a body processes physical energy. However, no aspect of human experience can be described as purely mental or purely physical. Wilber's four quadrants derive from distinctions between interior and exterior combined with individual and communal, but he is careful to say all four are constitutive of a holon and cannot be separated. A thought is meaning, and also is an electrochemical impulse in the brain. A feeling contains meaning, and is also a combination of neuromuscular tension and hormonal balance. A sensation is the translation of a physical change, such as pressure, heat, or cold, into a neural impulse. That impulse is immediately interpreted, perhaps as comforting or hostile, by the person receiving it. A person is a bodymind system, with mind (information) and body (energy and matter) so intertwined that they can only be thought of as one (LeDoux, 1996; Schwartz & Begley, 2002).

It is therapeutically powerful to work with the mind-body interface. The body is a reflection of mental-emotional life (Kurtz & Prestera, 1976; Marlock & Weiss, 2001, 2006; Marlock & Weiss, with Young & Soth, 2015). It is immediate and present, and has not been overused in therapy, as has verbal exchange (Johanson, 1996). The body's revelations are more closely connected with the deepest levels of the tripartite brain and the core ways we organize experience. The protein receptors of every cell membrane of the body receive signals about the environment from the brain, informed by the mind, which then activates growth or withdrawal responses (Lipton, 2005). The brain's mind monitors and integrates somatic markers in every experience of consciousness (Damasio, 1999). Perceptions of the world such as "life is a fight and you have to be ready to win at all times" or "life is a wonder to be enjoyed" mobilize the body in different ways that are congruent with these differing life experiences. The mind-body interface can be used in both directions: studying what mental-emotional material is evoked through body-centered interventions, or noticing how the body organizes in response to some mental-emotional input (Fisher, 2002).

Ogden and colleagues (2006) note that it is necessary to incorporate the body, titrating sensation and doing bottom-up processing when there has been trauma. Traumatic events can trigger the primitive fight, flight, or freeze mechanisms that will lead clients to dissociate if standard, mental-emotional top-down processing reactivates the memories through inappropriate timing and preparation. Many chapters in this volume expand on possibilities for using the body in psychotherapy, which is different from using bodywork as an adjunct to psychotherapy (Aposhyan, 2004).

Mindfulness

Though fine tuning one's metabolism to support physical energy is important, Bateson would say that what we were getting at by employing the mind-body interface is his fourth proposition, namely that energy is collateral or secondary in living organic systems characterized by mind. What is of primary importance is the way a system processes information. An atom bomb or a raging rhinoceros has a lot of energy, but not much creativity in terms of processing information. With a relatively small amount of energy, the human body-mind-spirit can figure out a way to write Shakespeare and go to the moon (Baeyer, 2004; Johanson, 2009b).

Think of what happens when a young toddler believes he has lost his mother in a department store. That belief sets off a reaction of uncontrollable fear, crying, disorientation, inconsolable isolation, and panic. No one around the child can comfort him. A second later, when the information registers that mother is returning from around the corner of the jewelry counter to pick him up, there is an instant transformation to joy, calm, easy breathing, relaxation of muscles, and a sense of peace and reconnection. A little information goes a long way to control a lot of energetic processes. Siegel (1999) thinks of this as an example of the nonlinear qualities of a system, where a small input can lead to a large response in which the limbic system fosters a cascade of responses that affect heart rate, a sense of panic, and so forth.

That leads to Bateson's fifth proposition that information is coded, which is a way of saying we organize our experience. Experience does not come to us packaged. We process stimuli from within and without. As Suzanne Langer (1962) suggests, we symbolically transform or encode "the given" of various stimuli to make it available to consciousness. "We do not merely live in the world, we live in the world as we view it, construct it, or interpret it" (Brown, Ryan, & Creswell, 2007, p. 213). Those in the constructivist school of psychology honor and employ this insight (Mahoney, 2003). For Bateson, the way information is organized always goes back to the context of relationships that influence its "form, order, and pattern" (Bateson, 1979, p. 40).

A sixth and final Bateson proposition that we consider here is that information is coded or organized into a hierarchy of levels of organization (Deacon, 2003; Emmeche et al., 1997). In psychotherapy, we are especially interested in high-level encoding—the basic faith or philosophy found in our core organizing beliefs that control both our perception and our behavior, before we have any awareness of perceiving or responding (Kurtz, 1990a; Nowak & Vallacher, 1998). For instance, the core belief "I have to perform to get people's love and approval" encodes and controls a lot of behavior: the way we perceive school and sports, the way we hold our bodies, the expectations we bring to relationships, and more.

In the experience of Hakomi therapy, mindfulness is the most effective tool with which we can study the organization of our experience (Kurtz, 1990a) and begin to relate to it in healing ways (Baer, 2003; Johanson & Taylor, 1988; Siegel, 2007; Weiss, 2008). Mindfulness is a core principle, method, and practice in Hakomi therapy. As Nowak and Vallacher express it: "What really sets the human mind apart from other systems in nature . . . is its ability to reflect on its own operations and output" (1998, p. 4). "The self-evaluation afforded by self-awareness . . . can provide the impetus for people to modify their own psychological structure and thereby change their internal bases for action" (p. 5).

Present experience is always the focus of mindful therapy because that is what is currently organized by core narrative beliefs, and immediately manifests them in sensations, feelings, thoughts, memories, attitudes, relational ways of being, dreams, posture, breathing, movements, and so forth (Borkovec, 2002; Brown & Ryan, 2003; Johanson, 2015; Olendzki, 2005; Roy, 2007). Morgan reminds us that neurologically, "because emotional memory is always in the now, the old perceptions, feelings, and behaviors become blended with the current situation" (2006, p. 15). The chapter on transference in Stolorow, Brandchaft, and Atwood's (1987) work on psychoanalytic intersubjective theory is titled "The Organization of Experience," indicating that transference is revealed in how one has made meaning of one's world, including significant others—something that is present every moment in every situation.

Cultivating mindfulness of something the mind has created (Nyanaponika, 1972) allows clients to get beyond the limitations of ordinary consciousness based on habitual reactions (Bargh & Chartrand, 1999; Watzlawick, Weakland, & Fish, 1974) to observe implicit memory at work (Schacter, 1992, 1996) in the actual, present-moment organization of experience, thus allowing access to the creative core organizers. Mindfulness functions as "a quality of consciousness . . . [that can relate] to the contents of consciousness" (Brown et al., 2007, p. 213).

Mindfulness includes an array of states of consciousness including witnessing, bare attention, and loving presence (Johanson, 2006). In Hakomi therapy, mindfulness is used in two central ways. First, the therapist enters mindfulness and loving awareness (Chodron, 2003; Germer, 2006; Kurtz, 2008) before each session and remains in it, making the client the focus of his meditation. Second, the therapist invites the client into a state of mindful self-reflection as early in the process as is feasible, and helps the client return to mindfulness as appropriate throughout the session. Outside of the therapy context, mindfulness, or a contemplative way of living, can be encouraged as an ongoing practice or way of being (Hayes, 2005). The bare attention of mindfulness combined with the quality of loving presence is important for attending to both interpersonal and intrapersonal attachment security issues that are present (Brown & Ryan, 2004; Shaver et al., 2007).

The therapist's mindfulness is a present-moment enactment of the other Hakomi principles. Using Wilber's model, the all-quadrant-all-level model, aspects of the unity principle acknowledge the social embeddedness of mindfulness, and place "the capacity for mindfulness into a broader conception of social, cognitive, and developmental processes" (Shaver et al., 2007, p. 265). Mindfulness also supports awareness of unity as the therapist remains conscious of her own breath, body, feelings, and thoughts, as well as those of the client. In this state, the therapist can gather significant information about how clients organize their experience (Feinstein, 1990). Mindfulness allows therapists to gather information on dispositions of their clients from all four of the quadrants in Wilber's (1995) model.

Once limiting core beliefs become apparent, they can be changed (see Chapter 20) through mindful, compassionate attention to new possibilities and their accompanying barriers to change (Hayes & Feldman, 2004). Since the limiting core beliefs operate at a very deep level of the client's organization, a small, core-level change can result in a large and lasting change in operant beliefs, feelings, habits, and behaviors—including increased compassion for self and others (Allen & Knight, 2005; Brown & Kasser, 2005; Beitel, Ferrer, & Cecero, 2005; Carson, Carson, Gil, & Baucom, 2004; Shapiro, Brown, & Biegel, 2007; Shapiro, Schwartz, & Bonner, 1998).

Mindfulness interacts with mind-body holism in many ways. Thich Nhat Hanh (1987) defines mindfulness as the state where mind and body become one. Being mindful, the therapist and client can pick up clues about the mind from the body's posture, position, tension, movement, and habits. As we have seen in Chapter 4, the body functions as a royal road to the unconscious. In Hakomi, experiments in mindfulness evoke core patterns through triggering habitual reactions that can then be studied (see Chapter 16). The client thereby finds the psychic distance to have habitual reactions as opposed to simply being the reactions (Baumeister & Sommer 1997; Brown et al., 2007; Teasdale, Segal, & Williams, 1995). In Kegan's (1982) terms, what was once subject now differentiates to become object, as the system is brought under observation.

In practical terms, working in mindfulness guides the therapist to introduce the idea of an internal observer and direct her client toward this style of self-observation. In the process, she monitors the client's state of consciousness and contacts his experience in ways that support the internal observer. She carefully tracks whether the client becomes highly fused, blended, or identified with, let's say, a feeling state, and has a number of ways to help the client back into a more observing state (see Chapter 14). This process can be understood as the coregulation of attention processes by an "external interactive regulator" (Schore, 1994; Weiss, 2008).

In addition to its function in studying and deepening therapeutically into the way we organize our experience, mindfulness functions in myriad ways outlined in the various chapters of this book and referenced in the bibliography on mindfulness and therapy found on the Hakomi Institute website (www.hakomiinstitute.com).

Though mindfulness is a natural, easily accessible state, it needs to be invited and supported in most people (Johanson, 2006). The most common barrier to mindfulness is fear associated with experiences of not feeling safe. This leads us to the Hakomi embrace of nonviolence.

Nonviolence

The fifth and last principle of Hakomi therapy—the one tied most closely to Lao-tzu and Taoism in general—is the principle of nonviolence, which is a variation on nondoing (Johanson & Kurtz, 1991; Sorajjakool, 2009). It is the foundational principle without which the process will not work. This is because to be mindful and turn our awareness inward toward felt, present experience in order to study the organization of our experience, we need to feel safe. There are "conceptual and empirical connections between mindfulness and security" (Shaver et al., 2007, p. 265). Boundaries must be clear and inviolate (Whitehead, 1994, 1995). If we think a therapist or someone else around us is not safe, is up to something, has a judgment or agenda to put over on us, we will resist automatically. We can't keep one eye focused outward, figuratively or literally, and one eye inward. It is like being asked to fall asleep standing up. Lao-tzu is exquisitely clear about this:

> Whoever relies on the Tao in governing men doesn't try to force issues or defeat enemies by force of arms. For every force, there is a counterforce. Violence, even well intentioned, always rebounds upon oneself. (Johanson & Kurtz, 1991, p. 42)

In Taoism, this is called the principle of mutual arising. For every force, there will be a counterforce. Porges's (2001) polyvagal theory outlines how neurologically primed we are to scan for danger, and how inter- or intrapersonal social engagement is only possible through perceived safety. Of course, no therapist or therapy considers itself violent. But when it comes to the question of resistance—the experience therapists have of clients not moving along in the process of therapy—the *Tao Te Ching* poses a question:

> Can you love people and lead them without imposing your will? Can you deal with the most vital matters by letting events take their course? (Johanson & Kurtz, 1991, p. 40)

Most of us in the West cannot. We have been educated to do something, and as therapists, we are tempted to force things "for the client's own good." In many cases, we do so because we simply are not aware of other choices (Sorajjakool, 2001). In the *Tao Te Ching*, Lao-tzu offers alternatives:

> To yield is to be preserved whole. To be bent is to become straight. . . . Do the Non-Ado. Strive for the effortless. . . . Less and less do you need to force things, until finally you arrive at non-action. (Johanson & Kurtz, 1991, p. 43)

The suggestion here, whose worth is borne out in clinical practice, is that resistance be supported in the state in which it naturally arises. Paradoxically, the process can go forward by retreating and actually supporting defenses.

> If you want to shrink something, you must first allow it to expand. If you want to take something, you must first allow it to be given. This is called the subtle perception of the way things are. . . . Tao invariably takes no action, and yet there is nothing left undone. . . . The Tao nourishes by not forcing. By not dominating, the Master leads. . . . Thus the Sage supports all things in their natural state, but does not take any action. (Johanson & Kurtz, 1991, pp. 43, 46, 137)

What is crucial here is the attitude of therapists toward both their clients and themselves (Leary, Adams, & Tate, 2006). Are we sane in Lao-tzu's sense of accepting the world whole, or are we trying to re-create it, to make ourselves into someone we are not? Do we, in fact, respect and honor the organic, inner wisdom of ourselves, others, and nature itself? In the therapy context, do we understand resistance as a natural, organic expression of the system's inner organization that is present for some good reason—whether that is immediately obvious or not—especially if the opposition appears to be counterproductive and self-defeating? Embodying this attitude is crucial for allowing mindfulness to promote affect regulation of negative emotional states (Broderick, 2005; Feldman, Gross, Christensen, & Benvenuto, 2001).

> When you are content to be simply yourself and don't compare or compete, everybody will respect you. (Johanson & Kurtz, 1991, p. 37)

When nonviolence, mindfulness, and compassion meet to create a healing space, a certain economy of therapy arises. There is a sense of ease as the unconscious takes the nondefensive opening to unfold, and both client and therapist effortlessly follow organic signals that lead into what needs healing and reorganization. Unnecessary confrontation and struggle yield, as defenses are respected for the organic wisdom they embody, and are supported as they arise (Johanson & Kurtz, 1991). This opens the possibility of curiously inquiring into the nature of the resistance (Johanson, 1988), rather than trying to push through it. Verbal and nonverbal taking-over techniques (see Chapter 16)—doing for someone what they are already doing for themselves—empower clients to study their experience more safely and mindfully while finding nothing in the therapist to resist (Kurtz, 1990a).

The safe, mindful, nonresistant, seemingly lazy stance of the therapist does not lead to comfortable chitchat and a lack of issues to explore for the client. Paradoxically, the safety and nourishment fostered by nonviolence promotes the courage and support to access core organizing issues quite deeply and quickly (Fosha, 2000). Earlier psychodynamic theory cautioned against being overtly friendly, safe, or nourishing because gratifying patients might take away the psychic energy for them to project the transference of their unmet needs onto the therapist where they could be worked through (Wyss, 1973).

As suggested above, Hakomi sees transference through the lens of systems theory as dealing with the organization of experience (Baeyer, 2004; Stolorow et al., 1987). This is a strong view of transference that asserts it is present in all situations at all times. It cannot be hurt or changed by a therapist being either outwardly friendly or intentionally reserved. In this view, gratification, or more precisely, how clients are unable to be gratified, is seen in terms of what the client has organized out of his experience; what might be missing experiences he has yet to integrate. Again, to be organically self-organizing and self-correcting, all the parts must be incorporated and connected within the whole.

When compassion and nonviolence provide the necessary therapeutic context of perceived safety, it becomes possible in Hakomi therapy to invite a mindful state of consciousness where the precise kind of gratification the patient has ruled out can be introduced through an experiment in awareness (see Chapter 16). For instance, in the case of clients who manifest indicators that they are self-reliant—having organized out the possibility of support—various verbal and nonverbal experiments can be done that incorporate the message, "It is okay to let people support you."

If the indicators have been properly read, these experiments in mindful, theoretically positive gratification would be expected to evoke spontaneous, automatic fears, anxieties, tensions, and such, that put up instantaneous barriers to the possibility of support. Thus, Hakomi therapists paradoxically function as safe, gentle, nonviolent provocateurs using the overtly secure, caring therapeutic relationship to help clients face their deepest fears. In the process, sessions can appear quite quiet, respectful, and contemplative. They can also manifest with considerable emotion and action. It is, of course, a clinical art to be able to keep clients within their windows of tolerance, keeping things neither too safe nor too overwhelming (Ogden et al., 2006), or on the learning edge between order and chaos (Kauffman, 1995).

In terms of systems theory, transformation occurs when clients, in this nonviolent setting, are enabled to organize into their experience some aspect of life (support, in the example above) that they have previously organized out (Johanson, 2015).

Nonviolence is an attitude of trust in the creation. It is a commitment not to interfere with the processes of life, but to celebrate their spontaneous, organic intelligence. Nonviolence promotes a respect for the subtle, almost imperceptible movements of mind, body, and spirit, and gives rise to a yielding or softness that follows and nourishes these movements rather than correcting or conquering them (Johanson & Kurtz, 1991).

Nonlinear Science

As suggested above, Bateson's propositions and Hakomi principles place psychotherapy firmly within the realm of nonlinear science. Bateson was adamant about following scientific principles adequate to describing minds as opposed to material, physical systems. For instance, the concept of homeostasis, stability through constancy, which can well describe a thermostat that returns temperature to a given set point, has been applied inappropriately to the human body, individuals, families, and organizations, as Bertalanffy (1968) cautioned years ago. More recently, Gottman, Murray, Swanson, Tyson, and Swanson have concurred that "when applied to the study of interacting systems such as a couple . . . the concept of homeostasis is highly inadequate" (2005, p. 166). A concept better able to accommodate the features of living organic systems is Sterling's theory of "allostasis" or stability through change. The system is seen as making predictions to adjust parameters to best function in the situation at hand, as opposed to maintaining some mythical, normal set point—for instance, blood pressure fluctuates in an adaptive way depending on the next anticipated activity (Sterling, 2004). Morgan notes that interpersonal neurobiology sees the brain in an allostatic way "as an anticipatory machine" (2006, p. 15). As noted above, Prigogine's concept of negentropy in the organic world of self-healing holons corrects and complements the concept of entropy in the physical world.

In general, we know our clients are not like machines, even information-processing ones, where one input will result in a predictable, deterministic output. Morgan suggests that understanding the brain and mind in terms of "linear thinking involving cause and effect is inadequate. The brain is the most complex structure known in the universe. The human being is way too complex for simple logic. We need to turn to complexity theory for a better understanding" (2006, p. 14). While Bateson (1979) talked of living organic systems, others term this science "the study of dynamic, synergetic, dissipative, nonlinear, self-organizing, or chaotic systems" (Thelen & Smith, 2002, p. 50). John Holland (1995), in line with the work of the Santa Fe Institute, uses the term "complex adaptive systems" (CAS; in Morowitz & Singer, 1995). Laszlo (2004) speaks of adaptive self-regulating systems, and Varela, Thompson, and Rosch (1991) of dynamical systems.

Nowak and Vallacher agree that the brain is composed of

> 100 billion neurons, each of which influences and is influenced by approximately 1,000 other neurons. . . . The range of potential mental states is unimaginably large . . . [and] the same variable can . . . act as a "cause" one moment and an "effect" the next. This feedback process is at odds with traditional notions of causality that assume asymmetrical, one-directional relationships between cause and effect. (1998, pp. 3, 32)

Earlier theories of maturationism, environmentalism, or interactionism between genes and environment have proved inadequate to account for "problems of emergent order and complexity" (Thelen & Smith, 2002, p. xiii), namely how new structures, patterns, or core narratives arise. These older theories basically note the eventual outcome or product of where people end up, but "take no account of process . . . the route by which the organism moves from an earlier state to a more mature state" (p. xvi). To put it another way, development is much messier than our logical, reconstructive theories would have us believe.

As we turn up the magnification of our microscope, we see that our visions of linearity, uniformity, inevitable sequencing, and even irreversibility break down. What looks like a cohesive, orchestrated process from afar takes on the flavor of a more exploratory, opportunistic, syncretic, and function-driven process in its instantiation (Thelen & Smith, 2002).

Our most recent scientific inquiries argue that determinism, or predictive power, is an insufficient and inadequate guiding principle. "We never know, and never can know exactly what any holon will do tomorrow (we might know broad outlines and probabilities, based on past observations, but self-transcendent emergence always means, to some degree: surprise!)" (Wilber, 1995, p. 48).

The good news for psychotherapy is that nonlinear systems are adaptive. They demonstrate the capacity for self-transcendence, symmetry breaks, creativity, or emergent transformation into new wholes or holons with new forms of agency and communion (Clayton, 2004; Clayton & Davies, 2006; Emmeche et al., 1997; Wilber, 1995). The tricky part is that self-organizing systems begin with many parts with large degrees of initial freedom that may then be "compressed to produce more patterned behavior" (Thelen & Smith, 2002, p. 51). "In self-organization, the system selects or is attracted to one preferred configuration out of many possible states, but behavioral variability is an essential precursor" (Thelen & Smith, 2002, p. 55). Nonlinear means order out of chaos (Gleick, 1988; Krippner, 1994; Robertson & Combs, 1995).

Central to understanding chaos in Hakomi therapy is assuming a personality characterized by multiplicity (Rowan & Cooper, 1999; Turner, 2008), or what Schwartz (1995) terms an inner ecology of parts. It is a common observation that a single client can manifest fear, a disposition to withdraw, an offer of help, the face of defensive anger, a dance of joy, and much more. Which might it be? Persons can also show variable forms of attachment in relation to different persons (Siegel, 1999). "The concept that a system can assume different collective states through the action of a quite nonspecific control parameter [external variables that influence behavior] is a powerful challenge to more accepted machine and computer metaphors of biological order" (Thelen & Smith, 2002, p. 62).

Which part-pattern of a client emerges depends on the interactions of her internal parts, and their perception of what is happening in the external world. Neurologically, the activation of one pattern normally corresponds to the inhibition of another, a process known as "soft-assembly" (Thelen & Smith, 2002, p. 60). What provide stability in a living organic system that balances the flexibility of variable soft-assembly possibilities are *attractors*. Laszlo (1987, p. 70) maintains that "the principal features of dynamic systems are the attractors; they characterize the long-run behavior of the systems." Static attractors govern evolution when system states are relatively at rest; periodic attractors govern those systems that go through periodic repetitions of the same cycle; and chaotic attractors influence the organization of seemingly irregular, random, unpredictable systems (Barton, 1994; Gallistel, 1980; Nowak & Vallacher, 1998; Vallacher & Nowak, 1994b).

As Siegel notes, it is when the emotional responses associated with core narrative beliefs become ingrained patterns of neural firing that they come to function as attractor states, which "help the system organize itself and achieve stability. Attractor states lend a degree of continuity to the infinitely possible options for activation profiles" (1999, p. 218).

In systems terminology, core organizing beliefs are referred to as order parameters, or the internal variables or attractors that organize behavior. Thelen and Smith write that "when systems self-organize under the influence of an order parameter, they 'settle into' one or a few modes of behavior [attractor states] that the system prefers over all the possible modes" (2002, p. 56).

Attractors can have varying degrees of stability and instability, continuity and flexibility depending on the reinforcement of learned response schemas to anticipated events. Siegel (1999) notes that neural nets that fire together tend to wire together. Schwartz's ecology of inner parts can be understood in terms of a CAS having "two or more attractors with different basins of attraction coexisting, . . . *multistable modes* which are discrete areas in the state space" (Thelen & Smith, 2002, p. 61). Again, a person can act in varying ways, depending on the context, though Freud's repetition compulsion (Johanson, 1999) speaks to the relative stability of an inner ecology (Johanson, 2009a).

Emergent attractors, order parameters, or core organizing beliefs are considered constraints in systems theory, in that they eliminate "some possibilities by realizing others" (Graves, 2008, p. 94). The freedom of potentiality of "a couple of dollars worth of chemicals in a puddle of water" is reduced when it emerges through structural levels to become a human instead of a raccoon, but the freedom of possibility is opened to more inclusive states of consciousness and relatedness (Graves, 2008). "The arrangement of constraints defines the structure of dynamic form" (Graves, 2008, p. 50), which in Hakomi is related to character theory (Chapters 8 and 23).

While "reality is inherently relational . . . [and] all meaningful relationships constrain reality" (Graves, 2008, p. 45), Hakomi therapy regularly attends to indicators of constraints or core organizing beliefs that limit realistic possibilities for how one is able to relate in the world. The therapy can enable a client to mindfully integrate missing experiences (not just insights) that transform by adding to the complexity and availability of new relational possibilities. In line with Freud and Piaget, a goal of therapy is for a person, as a CAS, to accommodate a new experience as new, as opposed to assimilating it into old order parameters (Brown et al., 2007; Horner, 1974; Piaget & Inhelder, 1969).

What moves a relatively stable client, as a CAS disposed to habitually constrained ways of experiencing and responding, to seek characterological-level therapy and the possibility of a nonlinear phase shift or phase transition is fluctuation (Thelen & Smith, 2002, p. 62). Such fluctuations "are the source of new forms in behavior and development that account for the nonlinearity of much of the natural world" (p. 63). "Change or transformation is the transition from one stable state or attractor to another" (p. 63). To explain it in CAS terminology, transformational changes are fostered when "inherent fluctuations act like continuous perturbations in the form of noise on the collective behavior of the system. Within ranges of the control parameter, the system maintains its preferred behavioral pattern despite the noise" (p. 63). However, when the internal and/or external perturbations sufficiently shake the system's ability to operate satisfyingly out of old order parameters, it can come to a critical or bifurcation point where transformation to new attractor states becomes possible.

So the impetus to seek help is often some crisis, or a long line of noisy perturbations, such as a spouse or friends confronting the client, saying certain behaviors are enough to threaten the relationship; bosses saying addictions are getting out of hand; unhappiness growing through an inability to get beyond predictable, unsatisfying interactions; longings for more meaning than what is being met through work or possessions; children being born or leaving the home; one's once-solid pension being reduced or a decent-paying job being outsourced; a new relationship evoking an internal conflict between longing for nurture versus need for self-reliance; and so forth (Johanson, 2009a).

Conclusion: Hakomi Principles Engaging Nonlinear Processes of Transformation

It is crucial for therapists to maintain the distinction between self-healing holons, that is, nonlinear living systems, and mechanical systems. For instance, we always remain "involved participants" as opposed to "alienated observers" (Berman, 1989, p. 277). We seek to avoid harmful reductionisms (LeShan & Margenau, 1982; Seybold, 2007).

Hakomi principles help engage clients as CASs in appropriate ways. Organicity and nonviolence help create the conditions for psychological transformation, namely organizing into a client's system something like support, intimacy, or freedom to act that has been, to a significant degree, organized out (Johanson, 2015). This reorganization is a matter of experience and not just insight—though insight accompanies the incorporation of a "missing experience" (Chapter 20). The unity principle and negentropy suggest that there is an impulse to heal or move toward wholeness and increased relational complexity that is always consciously or unconsciously present. However, when the system does not feel safe, when it perceives on some level that it is under attack, it automatically reverts to protective attractor states that put enough noise in the system to mask signals for growth and distract the cooperation of the unconscious.

When fluctuations and perturbations strain the adequacy of normal order parameters or core beliefs, and lead clients to seek therapy, mindfulness functions in many ways to relate to the complex, nonlinear situation. Simply inviting mindfulness of present felt experience places a client's consciousness in an open, exploratory, experiential mode that accesses a different level of information than ordinary, conversational consciousness (Schanzer, 1990) in an objective, empirical, scientific manner (Marcel, 2003). Mindfulness and organicity together move both therapist and client to maintain a collaborative and radically nondirective experimental openness to the often mysterious, spontaneous signs (felt sense, sensations, tensions, images, gestures, movements, memories, impulses, and so forth) that reveal the cooperation of the unconscious disposing the way toward desired healing. Unhelpful ego investments in particular results are minimized (Johanson & Kurtz, 1991; Ryan & Brown, 2003). Nonviolence respects, supports, and/or takes over resistance or defenses when they arise, taking further noise out of the system and allowing awareness to go to deeper levels.

When the indicators of missing (organized out) experiences appear, these too can be introduced in mindful, experimental ways that pay exquisite attention to how the system organizes around these new possible attractor states. The curious, experimental aspects of mindfulness are especially maintained when organic barriers to new experiences appear.

Respecting the organic wisdom of these barriers is what leads to the possibility, at crucial bifurcation points, of receiving new experiences leading to new order parameters or attractor states.

While mindfulness enables the healing of a fragmented ego, it also encourages a new way of being or self-state that rests in what witnesses our experiences, as opposed to being identified with or caught up in them (Eisman, 2006; Marlock & Weiss, 2001), thus bridging Hakomi therapy into transcendent levels of the system (Coffey, 2008; Graves, 2008). "When no longer ego-involved, a more fundamental 'I' that is grounded in awareness has room to emerge and guide experience and behavior" (Deikman, 1996, in Brown et al., 2007, p. 227).

CHAPTER 6

Assisted Self-Study: Unfolding the Organization of Experience

T. Flint Sparks

The goal of this new therapy is to contact and understand the events which create and maintain the flow of experience itself.

RON KURTZ, *Body Centered Psychotherapy,* 1991

To study the Buddha Way is to study the self.
To study the self is to forget the self.
To forget the self is to be actualized by the myriad things.

EIHEI DOGEN, *Treasury of the Eye of the True Dharma,* 1223–1227

THE ESSENCE OF the Hakomi method is assisted self-study done in a state of mindfulness. The method specifically assists the client in discovering and opening to unconscious beliefs and organizing principles that are expressed in habitual patterns of thought, feelings, sensations, somatic habits, and behaviors. Once made conscious, early decisions can be changed, long-held emotions can be released, somatic patterns can shift, and new forms of nourishment can be taken in. The method can help us see more clearly how we continually construct both our ongoing experience and our sense of a solid, individual self.

The Hakomi method is not simply a new way to use a special state of consciousness (mindfulness) in order to uncover the psychological structures or realities of the individual— although this is one of its unique features. Germer, Siegel, and Fulton (2005) reviewed these more traditional clinical applications, but at that time did not yet understand the critical and important difference in the Hakomi method. This method helps clients see how they actually construct their realities by the ways in which they organize their experience. By adopting an experimental attitude, the client and therapist collaborate in the unfolding investigation of experience. In the process of this assisted form of mindfulness-based self-study, the client can become more conscious of what is automatic and habitual. Through the nonviolent evocation of experience employed in the Hakomi method, clients have the possibility of cultivating a witness to the organization of experience and, therefore, have a better chance of waking up from the trance of conditioning.

The unique possibility inherent in the Hakomi method is the ability it offers the client to work at two fully embodied levels—psychological and spiritual. The use of mindfulness allows us to gently open to and investigate the complex tapestry of conditioning carried in our bodymind. We begin to see how this moves in and through us, how it all gains a feeling of solidity and reality, and, finally, how it directs the ways in which we navigate the world we have unconsciously constructed, rather than the world we actually live in. Seeing all of this and becoming intimate with the habits of consciousness can be quite liberating. At the same time, we can also begin to witness the ground in which all of this arises. Traditional psychotherapeutic methods tend to emphasize the careful uncovering of the contents of consciousness and its expression in behavior and relationships. The Hakomi method offers the additional possibility of opening to the spaciousness of awareness itself, through the cultivation of mindful attention. The loosening of identification that arises with this awareness offers the opportunity to begin to see through the apparent solidity of the self and gain additional freedom and peace.

Wes Nisker, in reflecting on his more traditional experience of psychotherapy, puts it this way: "While psychotherapy had shown me how to see the origins of my personality, I had been given no clue how to see through it. I had been taught how to gain some freedom for myself, but never how to gain freedom *from* myself" (1998, p. 2). The ability "to contact and understand the events which create and maintain the flow of experience itself" (Kurtz, 1990a, p. 10) can be seen as a kind of scientific approach to understanding reality. By adopting an experimental attitude and investigating small bits of experience evoked in mindfulness, one can gain enormous insight into the structure of the self and the causes of personal suffering. There is great potential for freedom at this level. In addition, the Hakomi method can be thought of as a form of assisted meditation, in which mindfulness is utilized to witness both the contents of awareness and the actual spaciousness of awareness itself. Thirteenth-century Zen master Eihei Dogen invites us not only "to study the self" but suggests that in this form of study we are able to "forget the self," or to see through and beyond the apparent solidity of ongoing experience. Kidder Smith, in commenting on the Buddhist approach to psychology taught by the late Chogyam Trungpa, says:

> Both psychology and meditation have a particular way of working with mind. Skillfully practiced, psychotherapy releases the elaborate disguises we have put upon our thoughts and feelings, revealing ancient gripes that seize them as their proxies. As these patterns come into sunlight, they become transparent—we can see through them, and treat them thus with a slightly distant courtesy.
>
> Meditation introduces us to deeper and deeper registers of mind. At first, it may be sufficient just to see we have a mind, that we are a mind. But gradually, and in a moment's flash, we realize that we are not exactly the thoughts and feelings that constantly occupy us, that had seemed to define us. There is space around them; better, we are this space, and thoughts and feelings occur here as our guests. Actually, though, that space is wisdom itself, and our thoughts and feelings its manifest intelligence. We can relax into this vibrant emptiness. That is the whole path, that relaxation, that falling into basic sanity. (2005, p. xv)

That "basic sanity" into which we can relax is actually the foundation on which all of the Hakomi principles rest (see Chapter 5) and is the core organizing principle of the Hakomi therapist's attitude. It is the path to the relief of suffering.

Organization of Experience

All experience is organized (Stolorow et al., 1987) and yet most of the complex patterns of organization that form our experience are out of our everyday conscious awareness. The Hakomi method offers a way to study, in some detail, the ways in which we create and sustain suffering. Kurtz (2003) summarizes the Hakomi method's basic approach to the organization of experience in the following sequence:

1. Experience is organized.
2. Experience is organized in habitual ways. The habits that organize experience, like all habits, operate outside of awareness. Some of these habits are beliefs. Some habits involve emotional memories.
3. Some beliefs (called core beliefs) influence the organization of nearly all experiences.
4. To work with core beliefs experientially, we must first make them conscious. The method we use to make core beliefs conscious is the method of evoked experience in mindfulness.
5. Core beliefs can be changed once they have been made conscious. New beliefs can be established and stabilized and old beliefs can loosen their influence.

This sequence is a clear map for the assisted form of mindfulness-based self-study inherent in the Hakomi method. A number of contemporary constructivist therapies lend support to this approach (Hoyt, 1998; Mahoney, 2003), although their techniques are often quite different (for example, narrative). A few of them do work in special states of consciousness, but these are almost all forms of hypnosis, especially Ericksonian approaches. Many of the somatic therapies work from the same fundamental series of assumptions and do include the use of mindfulness. A detailed overview of the organization of experience with specific emphasis on somatic therapies is available in a more extensive essay by Greg Johanson (2015). Nauriyal, Drummond, and Lal (2006) have published an excellent collection of articles by leaders in the fields of Buddhist-informed social sciences, psychotherapy, and studies in human consciousness. This volume, *Buddhist Thought and Applied Psychological Research*, posits mindfulness at the center of their reviews of consciousness studies and psychotherapy. Unno's (2006) edited volume *Buddhism and Psychotherapy* offers a cross-cultural perspective on these issues. The essence of all of these approaches and research is to help the individual apprehend, directly and experientially, the constructed nature of the self.

The Hakomi method, in effect, offers us a way to become creative and curious scientists, using ourselves as the subject. It is completely experiential. It is as if there are implicit rules that govern experience, which the individual may be entirely unaware of, but which can be discovered and brought to light. Bringing these rules into consciousness, investigating the habit patterns that the rules generate, and naming the core beliefs that undergird the entire structure begins to loosen the grip of this inner habit pattern. By investigating what is automatic and habitual in our body and mind, we open a window onto these rules and habits. Once made conscious, we have an increased capacity to change what we wish to change, let go what is unwanted, and take in what is needed.

Mindfulness

If we were curious and willing to follow the sequence of investigative patterns set out in the Hakomi method, it would seem to be beneficial to cultivate the ability to stay with present experience and notice what is actually happening in the present moment. This is the function of mindfulness. There are many definitions and characteristics of mindfulness, but they all point to a quality of nonjudgmental observation. Mindfulness is not "thinking about" something. It is not analytical, nor is it a form of concentration. In many ways, it is the open space in which awareness arises, and it has a purely reflective quality. In fact, the Venerable Henepola Gunaratana, an esteemed Sri Lankan vipassana teacher, says, "Mindfulness is mirror-thought. It reflects only what is presently happening and in exactly the way it is happening. There are no biases" (1991, p. 151).

Interestingly, in his recommendations to his trainee analysts, Freud (1912) suggested that they attend to their patients with "an evenly hovering attention," a state of mind with "a minimum of constraints and preconceptions . . . [which] encourages the optimal emergence of the patient's characteristic patterns of seeing and relating to him or herself and others as well as the analyst's capacity for creative listening" (Rubin, 1996, pp. 24–25). This description sounds a lot like the recommendation to utilize mindfulness as a key attitude in listening to the patient who, in turn, might be invited to utilize the same state of mind to begin noting "characteristic patterns" that we would describe as habits or automatic patterns of behavior.

In the Hakomi method, we begin by using mindfulness in rather small doses, usually less than a minute, as we evoke experiences for self-study. However, even in these relatively brief moments of mindful awareness, a radical shift is taking place. The client gains the opportunity to study, maybe for the first time, rather small bits of automatic and habitual experience with curiosity and openness. This is very different from talking about experience, or analyzing experience in an attempt to figure something out. These moments of mindful investigation can be illuminative and transformative in many ways and can set the stage for the development of this increased capacity for studying present experience.

This increased capacity for studying present experience in small doses of mindfulness may ultimately allow deeper and more prolonged experiences of mindful self-study to unfold. In this way, the client may become a more steady and spacious container for experience. This capacity is similar to the cultivation of a witnessing function, very much like that which emerges in traditional meditation training. Mindfulness then serves as a skillful bridge, connecting the gentle unfolding of awareness in psychotherapy with the spacious witnessing capacity of meditation.

When asked to describe the mind of enlightenment, Zen master Dogen replied, "Intimacy with all things." It is this ability to meet each thing as it is, without manipulation and without the addition of judgment or bias, which the mirrorlike quality of mindfulness allows. Along with the more conventional, experimental sequence outlined by Ron Kurtz, there are also contemplative ways of coming to understand the organization of experience that emerge from Eastern wisdom traditions. Reflecting on the centrality of mindfulness in supporting the ability to be intimate with experience, the psychiatrist and Buddhist teacher Mark Epstein has said, "As psychotherapy and meditation begin to come together, it is this function of mindfulness that will prove pivotal, because mindfulness permits continual surrender into our direct experience, from which we have all become experts at keeping ourselves at bay" (1995, p. 147). Through the investigation of evoked experience in mindfulness, we learn about the ways in which we have become unconsciously expert at hiding in habit patterns. Cultivating this capacity is one function of meditation practice as well.

One of the oldest systems for understanding the organization of experience, and which actually forms the basis for the use of mindfulness in the Hakomi method, is the four foundations of mindfulness. These four foundations come from the *Satipatthana Sutra*, considered the core of the Buddha's meditation teaching. In this teaching, the Buddha systematically outlines the ways in which we can come to understand the reality of conditioned existence by looking carefully and systematically at how ordinary experience comes into being. The four foundations are basically as follows:

1. Mindfulness of the body as the body, generally begun with a focus on the breath
2. Mindfulness of sensations or sense impressions—pleasant, unpleasant, and neutral
3. Mindfulness of feelings and states of mind, sometimes referred to as emotion-thought

4. Mindfulness of the objects of the mind itself, or the actual production of the mind states

The complete teachings associated with these four foundations are beyond the scope of this chapter, but suffice it to say that basic meditation practices themselves greatly increase the subject's ability to stay with and observe present experience. This ability supports the cultivation of the witness, a state of consciousness that can then be used to study the organization of all conditioned phenomena. In this way, people gain a perspective that is rare in the conventional world. They are allowed to actually witness themselves and their experience without getting lost in the storyline or the emotional undertow. They can begin to step outside the flow of the experience and yet witness the experience fully. They can cultivate the mind that is "intimate with all things."

One example that helps to illustrate this shift in awareness from being entranced in ordinary experience to waking as the witness is being in a movie theater. Most everyone has had the experience of watching a movie, becoming totally engrossed in the story, and feeling strong emotions as they relate to the characters and their stories. This is similar to the automatic nature of everyday experience. When our internal rules are operating outside of our awareness, we are lost in what seems like a solid, seamless reality. Then suppose someone next to us in the movie theater asks for popcorn or interrupts our reverie to leave to go to the bathroom. We suddenly wake up to the fact that there is a light source in the back of the theater generating a flickering image on a flat surface in front of us, which we have been involved with as if it were real. The witness is that state of consciousness that wakes up from the trance and sees what is actually happening, without bias or judgment. It just observes without being identified with, or as, what is being seen. It also does not reject the experience. It just sees fully what is.

The four foundations of mindfulness help us unpack this solid sense of experience, just as the small experiments in mindfulness in the Hakomi method help us begin to free ourselves from the automatic patterns of conditioning. In the first foundation of mindfulness we enter into a simple intimacy with the body itself, using the observation of our breathing as a focus of awareness. In Hakomi, the body—its movements, gestures, and expressions—is a primary source of data that can reveal underlying habits of mind, core beliefs, or organizing principles for our construction of reality. Since the Hakomi method is a body-centered psychotherapy, this ability to stay with the body is a key skill and is supported in a number of the core exercises in the method.

The second foundation supports our ability to be aware of the flux of sensations in this body in which we find ourselves. This is a subtle lesson, in which we learn to pay careful attention to the ever-shifting bodily energies—positive, negative, or neutral. Here we may begin to notice unconscious habits in the way we experience ourselves. We might become aware of a habitual tendency to feel aversion or clinging, to move toward or away from experiences. We can notice patterns of numbness or deadness.

It is not until the third foundation that we become mindful of the way that these energies collect into actual feelings and thoughts. In the third foundation, we observe the arising of thoughts and feelings together and come to know their interdependent nature. We get to know their meaning, and we observe their impermanent nature, as we watch them come and go. It is here that we also begin to see the repetitive nature of some of our mental states, feelings, and beliefs. Core beliefs are found here, and our ability to witness them, bring them into consciousness, and disidentify as them brings us some freedom from the suffering they may cause.

In the fourth foundation, we learn to turn the mind back on itself and witness how the whole spectrum of consciousness, sensations, reactions, emotions, and thinking all arise and interact with each other. We meditate on mind objects, as they are called—the actual contents of our minds. The four foundations of mindfulness offer us a systematic, contemplative path to do exactly what the Hakomi method is designed to assist in its scientific, experimental manner—the careful study of the creation of the self; how it comes into being, sustains itself in habitual and automatic ways, and can be released and seen through. This is a path to basic sanity.

The Self in Buddhism and Psychotherapy

In both psychotherapy and meditation, the position of the self or the I seems to be central. What is this self that we are investigating? If mindfulness offers us the key to the path, and the core skills and principles of the Hakomi method provide the tools for this exploration, what do we actually discover? In an early essay, Jack Engler reflects on both the Western and Eastern approaches to understanding the self:

> In both psychologies then, the sense of "I," of personal unity and continuity, of being the same "self" in time, in place, and across stages of consciousness, is conceived as something which is not innate in personality, not inherent in our psychological or spiritual makeup, but is evolving developmentally out of our experience of objects and the kinds of interactions we have with them. In other words, the "self" is literally constructed out of our experience with the object world. . . . The self that is being is viewed in both psychologies is a representation, which is actually being constructed anew from moment to moment. . . . Both systems also agree that the self is not ordinarily experienced this way. (1986, p. 22)

This description reflects the same understanding of the self that emerges within the Hakomi method. All experience is organized and is a by-product of ways in which we have interacted with the environment and our histories. This organization tends to form habitual patterns that become automatic and which operate out of awareness. We construct the self, and this construction is ongoing and fluid. These transient patterns can be recognized and explored, bringing self-representations and constructions into consciousness.

In a reexamination of the earlier work mentioned above, Engler (2003) furthers our understanding of the capacities and self-structure that is required for deep exploration, whether through therapeutic investigation or meditation. Note the characteristics he describes in light of what the Hakomi method cultivates and supports explicitly for the client:

> Some minimum degree of structuralization is certainly required: the capacity for moment-to-moment observation of thoughts, feelings, and body sensations; the ability to gradually attend to experience without censorship and selection; the capacity to tolerate aversive affect; some capacity to tolerate primary process material; the ability to suspend or mitigate self-judgment and maintain a benign attitude toward one's experience; the capacity for moral discrimination and evaluation of one's own behavior; and the capacity to mourn. . . . The more intensively mindfulness is practiced, the more important these capacities become and the more capacity is required. (p. 48)

This list could have been written to describe the capacities embodied by the mature Hakomi therapist working in loving presence. The list also reflects the capacities that are supported by the principles of the Hakomi method and which, then, become abilities available to clients in their psychological and spiritual work. These capacities undergird the unfolding of development that John Welwood skillfully describes as "making implicit felt meaning explicit. . . . When we can tap into and speak *from* a diffusely felt sense, rather than just pouring out our thoughts *about* it, this allows a fresh articulation of what is true for us, which was not accessible or expressible before" (2002, p. 90). This truth includes both the contents of our awareness and the space within which that awareness arises—our psychological sense of self, which is ongoing and steady, as well as the spacious mind in which we find no substantial or independent self as an object. With this ability to turn our awareness toward what is evoked, meet intimately what we encounter, and uncover meaning through this contact, we find freedom from the automatic, the habitual, and the unconscious.

Conclusion

In the Hakomi method, we intend to skillfully support self-discovery. We do this through the use of mindfulness and an experimental attitude, which encourages the client to attend to small moments of present experience without judgment or bias. In this process, we become increasingly skilled at noting indicators of what is automatic or habitual. Sometimes we act as scientists, observing with curiosity the patterns we uncover. Sometimes we act as contemplatives, deepening our capacity to attend to the unfolding of moment-to-moment experience. Through both the psychological and spiritual strands of the Hakomi method, we unravel the causes of suffering. Waking up and growing up move together with the release of what was unconscious, automatic, and habitual—and this release becomes a lifelong practice for our clients and ourselves.

CHAPTER 7

The Role of Core Organizing Beliefs in Hakomi Therapy

Anne Fischer

"CORE ORGANIZING BELIEFS" (Kurtz, 1990a) can be defined as the fundamental beliefs that structure a person's experiences of himself in relation to the world and vice versa. A defining characteristic of these beliefs is that they are generally unconscious; people usually are not aware of the core beliefs they hold, how these beliefs have come into existence, or the role they play in organizing present experience. In Hakomi, a therapist's role is to provide an environment that offers opportunities for clients to become aware of, reflect upon, and mindfully explore their core organizing beliefs, so that more nourishing life choices can be made.

Some examples of potential core organizing beliefs include these: "The world is a safe place," "It is better not to trust anybody," or "I'm only worth something when I'm doing something for someone else." These kinds of beliefs organize perception, experience, thinking, and action, and contribute decisively to the formation of embodied personality. Kurtz differentiates between a person's conscious and the unconscious awareness of her beliefs in this way:

> There is always another, a deeper layer of organizing material, like core beliefs, of which the storyteller is unaware. This deeper layer is having a direct influence on the storyteller, the telling of it and on the relationship of the storyteller

and the listeners. . . . In the effort to understand people and to help them change, it is crucial that we become aware of this layer of organizing material. (2000, p. 2)

Often, people become aware of their core beliefs only when they notice that others react to similar situations with different perceptions and behavior. A person who responds to new, unfamiliar situations with skepticism or feelings of vulnerability, for example, may come to notice that others remain grounded, or are even pleased with the opportunities and challenges provided by new situations. A person who consciously "knows" that elevators are safe comes to view his own fear as excessive, even if he cannot control the panic he feels when faced with riding in an elevator.

In interpersonal relationships, a person may recognize that her reactions seem to be uncontrollably out of proportion with the situations at hand—perhaps fearing the loss of a partner when differences in opinion or interests arise. In this case, the underlying belief could be: "I must comply with others in order to be loved." A person with this belief and its accompanying fear may have trouble perceiving her own sensations and may encounter even greater difficulty in expressing her own opinions. Having to do so creates internal turmoil. The risk involved will seem enormous, even if the person's partner appears unambiguously friendly and inviting.

These examples demonstrate why Hakomi therapy is centered on working with core beliefs. These beliefs can dramatically restrict people's lives, limiting their perceived ability to express themselves, make good choices, and realize their potential. When willful effort is not enough to break out of stuck patterns, it is the experience of these kinds of limitations and impediments with their corresponding suffering that often leads people to seek therapeutic help.

Many people already have a clear idea of what needs to be changed. One person might formulate his goal straightforwardly: "I just need to have more confidence in myself." Others might add that they recognize that there are actually good reasons for having better self-confidence: "I really don't understand why I have such a low self-esteem. I've actually accomplished quite a bit in my life already." This example reflects the recognition that a personality can contain multiple beliefs that are not necessarily congruent, as well as the recognition that there are different kinds of knowledge: the explicit, declarative knowledge of rational consciousness that works logically, expresses itself linguistically, and whose processes are primarily located in the neocortex of the left hemisphere of the brain; and procedural knowledge, knowledge that often becomes manifest in the form of emotions, and is primarily stored in the brain's right hemisphere and the limbic system (Damasio, 1994, 2003; Lewis et al., 2000; Schacter, 1996).

Procedural knowledge refers to (now) automatically occurring patterns that have become unconscious, as well as to prelinguistic somatic and affective impressions that have formed themselves into frameworks (also known as schemas; see below) and always have been unconscious. An example of the power of this kind of framework can be found in an anorexic 15-year-old's conviction that she needs to lose weight—regardless of any objective argument to the contrary—even given her intellectual understanding that she is running the risk of starving herself to death. She cannot perceive herself as anything other than too fat.

Beliefs and the Body

With the Hakomi method, Ron Kurtz developed a way to directly access core organizing beliefs through mindfulness and self-observation. Performing experiments in a mindful state provides clients with an opportunity to observe, examine, and dehabitualize their automatic tendencies, and to create connections between spontaneous behavior patterns and their underlying meanings. At the same time, Kurtz has demonstrated how substantially the body is involved in this process, and placed an emphasis on attending to the inseparable unity of mind and body.

In keeping with this holistic view, Damasio (1999) states that the human mind and self-consciousness are not only expressed through the body, but also have their roots in the unconscious processes of the body. He refers to these processes as "somatic markers." Just as emotional states become physically expressed—a person who is angry, for example, may wrinkle his forehead and tighten his jaw while his hormone levels change accordingly, his heart races, breathing changes, and so forth—enduring core beliefs and their corresponding internal reactions also become manifest on the bodily level in more lasting ways, reflected through the body's gestures, movements, muscle tension, posture, or psychosomatic symptoms.

With this knowledge, it isn't difficult to imagine typical categories or patterns of experience, as well as typical ways of expression and action—what Hakomi calls character strategies (see Chapters 8 and 23). Although each person develops his own distinctive style—with unique personality being informed by dispositions and temperament in relation to life experience—similar experiences as well as similar ways to process and respond to them will be found across people. Someone who is convinced that human relationships are about power, and that it is important not to be weak, for example, will be likely to have a slightly tense body, a posture expanded upward, and a breathing pattern that emphasizes the chest and upper body. This type of person may look intimidating, and will do his best not to let his eyes betray any longing that he may be experiencing.

Character theories have long claimed a connection between certain patterns of physical embodiment and qualities of a person's character. Some of these claims have been deterministic. Kurtz (Kurtz & Prestera, 1976) and other pioneers of body-oriented psychotherapy, such as Reich (1949), Lowen (1958, 1967, 1975), Pierrakos (1990), and Keleman (1986), for example, have provided more detailed investigations of the connections between externally identifiable bodily manifestations (tension, relaxation, motor impulses, facial mimicry, and changes in the vegetative nervous system) and subjective feelings, emotions, and attributed meaning. These pioneers' works provide a greater understanding of the patterns involved in the complicated process of the formation of a person's self-organization while simultaneously demonstrating how each person comes to have a personality that is uniquely her own. Their work also calls attention to the fact that the body is the means of expression for both the unconscious and conscious aspects of the personality. The body contains and expresses that which is not conscious, but which is of central organizing importance to a person.

Gaining Access to the Beliefs

Given this understanding of the embodied self—of human beings' bodies revealing information not consciously available in the declarative mind—it seems reasonable to encourage the client to enlist his body in the quest to recover the fullness of his experience. As Marcel Proust so wonderfully portrayed in his novel *Remembrance of Things Past*, our conscious memories of certain events, people, or facts are only a very small part of the whole of the experiential memories storied in our bodies. As noted above, in addition to explicit memory (referred to as declarative memory because it is possible to formulate its contents into language), there is also implicit memory, where conditioned reflexes, learned interaction sequences and skills, and subliminal perceptions are stored (Grawe, 2004; Schacter & Scarry, 2000).

The impossibility of a person concretely and consciously remembering things that happened in early childhood, that is, before developing the capability to use language, can also be understood from within this framework. In these contexts, there is no linguistic framework in which memories can be woven and put into relationship. The scientific community has come to a general agreement around the idea that, although these early experiences are not consciously remembered, information about these experiences, including the person's relevant sensory-motor reactions to them, is stored in the implicit memory, and contributes substantially to the forming of core organizing beliefs and the organization of the self.

The organization of one's self-experience is based on subjective reactions from one's subjective framework of core organizing beliefs. Further, each core belief makes sense when viewed within the context in which it was formed. (Neurolinguistic programming, developed by Bandler and Grinder in 1976 after they observed master therapists like Milton Erickson and Virginia Satir, is another approach to therapy based on this understanding.) This statement remains true for those patterns that have come to be consciously seen and experienced by the person in question as dysfunctional. It is important to remember that these reactions also were initially born in the service of meaningfully addressing the situational needs of a particular context. A symptom like chronic neck and shoulder tension, for example, can originate from a posture that the body takes on to protect a frequently hurt heart.

The whole point of Hakomi's mindful exploration of consciousness-raising experiments is to access the level of meaning, to understand the context for old patterns, and to explore and anchor new, alternative action patterns within the frame of these experiences. Inviting clients to slow down and mindfully attend to patterns of experience and action interrupts processes that would normally progress automatically. It creates the space to attend to and examine the client's own spontaneous gestures, such as a typical posture or the flow of the breath at a certain moment. Other techniques that can be of aid during these experiments include exploring the impact of consciously amplifying or reducing an element of the experience, slowly repeating an experience, and asking clients to stay with their experiences longer. Hakomi experiments often evoke germane feelings and images, and will often result in gaining access to a pattern's underlying original contexts, as well as the beliefs that developed out of these experiences, and a person's corresponding protective mechanisms.

Case Example

A client, Tina, falls in love again and again with unattainable men, a pattern that brings her great suffering. She already "knows" that this probably has to do with the early loss of her dearly loved father, who died suddenly when she was 10 years old. Tina judges herself harshly and feels "stupid" for not being able to get out of this pattern. In addition, she suffers from neurodermatitis, the symptoms of which appear only on her hands.

At first, she indignantly resists the suggestion of the therapist to turn her attention to her hands while pondering the words, "They are being particularly stupid now because of all the stress I'm under." Then, however, despite lingering doubts, she lets herself engage in this exploration and notices that an experience that she ordinarily perceives as an itch, an experience that she typically responds to with scratching, is actually a kind of restlessness throughout her hands. While mindfully examining this, and doing some small experiments, memory images emerge in which Tina, as a young girl, is sitting behind her father on a motor scooter and holding onto him with her hands. She becomes very sad, sobs, and discovers that, in the end, her hands have been expressing the conflict between a longing to hold on and a previously unconscious decision to never again let herself get so involved with another person.

Tina came to realize that she had organized herself and her life around the core belief, "I can't rely on others. I can only depend on myself." After coming to these realizations, she was able to slowly, carefully, and mindfully explore what it was like to reach out toward, touch, and, for a moment, to really hold the female therapist's hands. Tina was able to experience firsthand how difficult this was for her, how vulnerable she felt, how much fear she had that the hand would leave again, and, through these experiences, came to develop a more conciliatory and accepting stance toward the pattern in which she was stuck. She began to take steps toward a new way of being.

The difference between rational explanations of certain events and the experience of a sensory connection in one's own body—an experience linked with feelings, pictures, and memories—is tremendous. The latter permits the client to look for new, small impulses that enable her to go beyond the previous limitations. Body, emotions, memories, and meaning patterns are closely interwoven with each other.

For Kurtz, this is the point that makes change possible: If change is to take place, a person's core beliefs must be engaged. If a person is to be genuinely open to new experience and able to let new experiences have an impact on her life, she must go through the process of reengaging with aspects of her experience that have previously been filtered out, and differentiate or change meanings that she has actively, though unconsciously, constructed in relation to these experiences.

Tina's belief that she couldn't rely on others could, with some new experiences—not simply new insights—modulate into an alternative, more inclusive belief: "While some people cannot be relied upon, I can explore the possibility of trusting certain others." With this belief, she would be enabled to approach others with a new openness and curiosity, and not just selectively attend to experiences that would reconfirm her previously unquestioned core beliefs.

Core Organizing Beliefs and Recent Research

Research on development and neurobiology has produced results that support the notion of connections between early experience and meaning making. Stern (1985) and Dornes (1993, 2000) observed infants and toddlers in interaction with their mothers and made note of the bidirectional nature of the relationship. From the very first minute of the mother-child relationship, "the competent infant" (Dornes, 1993) is an active contributor. Babies will turn away from people that engage in behavior they find overstimulating. They will try to reconnect with their mother when noting that she has suddenly frozen her facial expressions (Brazelton, Koslowski, & Main, 1974).

Differences between babies' relational behaviors are found even at this early age—differences that are linked to the capacity of the relating person to accurately attune to and respond to the needs of the child. It seems that a fine-tuned synchronization is taking place between caregiver and child. Our understanding of the processes by which this occurs has greatly benefited from today's comprehension of physiological data and computer-aided data analysis. Much of this data suggests that the formation of affective-motor patterns occurs quite early (Downing, 1996; Wehowsky, 2015). These patterns can be seen as the basis of representations that later come to be symbolized with prelinguistic and linguistic content, and can be conceptually brought into close connection with the concept of beliefs.

Schemas, as defined by Piaget (1926), are frameworks that organize the developmental process and successful interactions with the environment. To simplify the point, one could say that schemas bring order to the incalculable flood of stimuli the organism is continually faced with in order to make meaningful interactions and learning possible, enabling us to prepare for the future with the benefit of past experience.

In the language of complex adaptive systems (Waldrop, 1992), this phenomenon is referred to as anticipating the future (Holland, 1995). To the degree possible, experiences are organized into already existing schemas (assimilated). When existing schemas are no longer able to accurately incorporate the experience in question, an adaptation process at the level of the organizing frameworks becomes necessary (accommodation). This usually represents a differentiation. In other words, the schemas become more complex.

What is new in this use of the concept of schemas is that it is used as a description for the recording of relationship patterns, and that this use provides an image of a hierarchically organized, developmental progression from early physical sensory and affective-motor reactions, to the first symbolizations of image, to cognitive-intellectual representations.

An example of an early mother-child interaction that leads to an affective-motor pattern could be when the pleasurable sensation and feeling of satiation that result from breast-feeding come to be associated with the rhythm of muscular tension and release, the mirroring gaze of the mother, the sound of her voice, and the warm feeling and the tactile experience of being held. This sensual-physical experience of relating is stored in the so-called procedural memory long before the ability to symbolize through language is developed, and yet still serves to prepare the ground for the arranging and meaning making of future experiences, as well as the experience of the self.

In this example, an infant who has had the positive experience of his mother turning toward him lovingly will tend to turn to his next interactions with his mother with positive expectations; whereas an infant who has received contradictory or rejecting signals will tend to withdraw into himself and either wait for positive signals or try to avoid the contact.

Bowlby (1969, 1973) and Ainsworth, Blehar, Waters, and Wall (1978) have documented how early the attachment patterns of small children come to be formed by their experiences with the first persons to whom they relate. Early experiences serve to shape later ones by producing mental frameworks that lead a child to more readily notice those experiences that are compatible, to process these perceptions in similar ways, and to thereby strengthen already extant schemas (Schore, 1994).

It is with the above in mind that body-oriented psychotherapy emphasizes the meaning of experiences stored in the memory of the body. These memories—which are not accessible through the explicit memory systems' concrete recollections—usually have a highly significant influence on a person's organization. Therapeutic techniques that encourage mindful attention to experiences within which a client can explore new possibilities across multiple modalities (for example, sensory, motor, mental, and so on), are much more effective than methods that appeal predominantly to the cognitive level. The superior impact of experience-oriented methods has been demonstrated through research (Grawe, 2002, 2004) and has come to be embraced by many therapeutic orientations.

In keeping with the above, the Hakomi method targets experience in the present moment. Here in the now, old limiting beliefs can be discovered and new, freeing experiences can be incorporated and become the foundation for the transformation of beliefs (see Chapter 20). Mindful, curious turning of attention toward the processes of perception and experience strengthens and deepens experiential intensity. It makes room for the awareness of the relevant contents of the hierarchically ordered modalities of experience.

The purpose of this is to become conscious of unconscious beliefs, and to gain access to the level of consciousness where meaning is created. Hakomi therapists are guided by this goal in everything they do, whether this means simply waiting and making room for the client whose process is becoming richer and deeper through his own work, or suggesting an experiment aimed at gaining access to meaning-making consciousness. Throughout this work, the therapist looks for indicators that may suggest the presence of core organizing beliefs that may be limiting the client. The therapist looks for these signs in his own reactions to the client as well as in the client's presentation. Through this process of increasing mindfulness, clients are enabled to see how they have come to organize their experience, and to see how this organization makes sense based upon their life experiences.

Gaining access to these underlying meanings also leaves the client with an unambiguous sense of subjective truth, or what Petzold (1977) refers to as the "vital evidence." In these moments, the client often comes into contact with impulses that previously had to be suppressed or restrained in favor of habitual management strategies. The client can then become open to exploring these impulses, or to following suggestions of the therapist for doing experiments aimed at integrating new, more inclusive experiences.

In the above-mentioned example of Tina, this experience was found in the moment when Tina was willing to move her hands toward the outstretched hands of the therapist, and let her hands touch those of the therapist without closing up internally. This experience helped her begin to accept the pain of losing her father for the first time and to recognize that it is good to connect—that she didn't always have to protect herself from the threat of loss. Beyond that, she was also able to access concomitant beliefs about her own self-worth, and about the necessary degree of loyalty toward her father. She was able to do all this without resorting to intellectual speculation. Instead, these shifts were each intimately connected to her experience. These kinds of events are healing precisely because they enable the organization of self-experiences to form new schemas and alter existing beliefs, thereby simultaneously restructuring future being in the world. While a single connection of a client with his "missing experience" (Kurtz, 1990a) is not likely to dislodge a long-standing pattern, it brings new options and opportunities to life.

Connection to Other Theoretical Concepts

The psychodynamic view that the shape of a personality is largely based upon the influence of early experiences is directly mirrored in the implications of the concept of core organizing beliefs (Gabbard, 1994). Developmentally informed basic human needs (to be securely accepted, held, and fed; to have autonomy; to be valued and recognized) form the context for these beliefs. Core organizing beliefs are formed from a person's experiences in relation to the environment's response to his basic needs. It is these beliefs that lead to the creation of character strategies (see Chapter 8). Psychoanalytic object relations theory's description of the process by which relationship structures become internalized (Horner, 1974; Winnicott 1965, 1971) has also contributed a great deal to the comprehension of the meaning of early interaction patterns, and provides theoretical insight into therapeutic relationships. In keeping with the psychoanalytic idea of transference, a client will form his relationship with a therapist based on his beliefs (Stolorow et al., 1987). The therapist will personally experience the impact of a client's beliefs (Gill, 1983) and can draw attention to and invite the client to explore this (Feinstein, 1990).

Case Example

A client, Mark, almost never arrives on time for his appointments. While excusing his lateness, he often smiles. When invited to explore what is behind the smile, he recognizes that he becomes aware of his physical size in connection with the smile, and that he is glad about this. "I feel elated, victorious." He also comes to realize that he feels like he is winning a power struggle every time he's late—that being late is an expression of his decision to refuse to submit to any externally imposed rules. Further, he remembers how as a little boy, his big brothers and sisters did not have to follow the rules that he was expected to keep; that he had experienced this as humiliating, and he still experiences the observance of rules as humiliating. Only with this discovery was he able to open to the reality that rules do not apply only to little kids. They also serve to facilitate adults' coexistence as well. Their observance does not always reflect submission, but may be instead an expression of mutual respect. His old belief, "Others think I'm little, but I won't let this happen anymore," was now able to move toward a new belief: "I am respected, and can also respect others."

The Hakomi concept of core beliefs, of convictions that organize our perception, experience, and behavior by processes of selection (we tend to perceive that which fits with our convictions and confirms them, as long as divergent information is not attached to an especially strong stimulus) is also almost identical to the schema as defined in cognitive psychology. However, an essential difference lies in the fact that in behavior therapy, cognitive schemas are understood mentally, whereas for body-oriented psychotherapies like the Hakomi method, the affect-motor schemas are of central importance. In other words, Hakomi focuses on unconscious patterns formed at the body-and-feeling levels that are represented mentally only under certain circumstances (Downing, 1996). Actually, third-wave cognitive-behavioral therapies are increasingly embracing this position (Hayes, Follette, & Linehan, 2004). In general, the process of becoming conscious—with the attendant possibility of broadening the client's schemas—is a principal task of psychotherapy.

From the systemic perspective—a perspective that views the person as a living organic system—beliefs can be understood as a system's organizing structure. Systems develop from simpler to more complex forms, and each developmental progression always integrates the previous one (Wilber, 1995). (This process of development is described in terms of schemas above.) A system also acts and organizes itself as a whole based upon communication between its parts (Bateson, 1979; Maturana & Varela, 1992; and, well summarized in reference to psychotherapy, in Johanson, 2008). As such, beliefs are comparable to the concept of internal models of reality (Holland, 1995; Waldrop, 1992). Successful interactions with the environment depend on the fact that the organizing structure and internal communications remain fluid, developing and accommodating themselves in response to changes in the environment (Bateson, 1979).

Currently a great number of efforts are underway in the service of integrating psychotherapeutic insights. Struggles between theoretical orientations have thankfully begun to wane. Instead, increasing efforts are being made to create a common language that examines common factors. Efforts along these lines have been particularly prevalent in neuroscience and psychotherapy research in relation to the origins of beliefs, how they develop, and how change in belief takes place. This research has resulted in further validation of the importance of the role of core beliefs and, with this, has corroborated one of the central concepts of the Hakomi method.

CHAPTER 8

Hakomi Character Theory

Jon Eisman

AS ALREADY DESCRIBED, Hakomi focuses on the way somatic, emotional, and cognitive experiences form from deeply held beliefs, which in turn generate habituated behavior and perceptual patterns. These behaviors and perceptions may then be processed utilizing mindfulness and the careful study of present experience to uncover the underlying formative "core material" (Kurtz, 1990a, p. 115). These operational precepts of the body —mindfulness, present experience, and neurologically held belief patterns—form the cornerstones of the Hakomi method.

While each Hakomi session seeks to embrace and reveal the individual nuances of these belief systems, it is also true that there are great similarities and consistencies among clients' experiential patterns. Because of this, Hakomi employs a variety of psychostructural maps to frame, articulate, and facilitate the terrain across which clients travel. Central among these maps is character theory.

Hakomi's original character map is an evolution of the theories of Wilhelm Reich (1949), Alexander Lowen (1958, 1975), David Shapiro (1965), and John Pierrakos (1990). Character in general seeks to describe the learning tasks of child development; the internal and external factors that contribute to that process; the successes, omissions, and wounding that occur during that learning; and the various, specific, strategic adaptations that people create to compensate for the gaps and impediments they encounter in their search to become integrated and fully resourced.

Since this learning takes place in relationship to others, character at its root is a description of relational processes. As Frank Lake describes it, "The various reaction patterns of personality are shown to represent reactions of loss, or the threat of loss, of various aspects of the normal dynamic cycle of loving dependent relationships in infancy" (1966, p. xvii). Character, however, also articulates the internal personal frameworks (habitual perceptual, experiential, and behavioral patterns) that develop as a result of these relational experiences: thoughts, beliefs, perceptions, somatic responses and defenses, emotions, moods, and so forth. Vygotsky generalizes by stating, "Every function in the child's cultural development appears twice: first, on the social level, and later, on the individual level; first, between people (interpsychological) and then inside the child (intrapsychological)" (1978, p. 57). This applies, of course, to both healthy learning and adaptive, characterological fixation.

An element of character theory that distinguishes it from numerous other personality maps is its focus on somatic processes (Kurtz & Prestera, 1976)—the ways in which the physical body both holds and expresses the psychological identity. Reich (1949) referred to this somatic component as "armoring," the total chronic bodily tension of the person that protects him from others and his own suppressed impulses. "The character of the individual as it is manifested in his typical pattern of behavior," wrote Lowen, "is also portrayed on the somatic level by the form and movement of the body. . . . The body expression is the somatic view of the typical emotional expression, which is seen on the psychic level as 'character'" (1975, p. 115).

The theories named above from which Hakomi derives its character model were all authoritarian and classically medical in their orientation. That is, they viewed strategic adaptations to developmental wounding (in Hakomi called "character strategies") as signs of pathology—as unhealthy, neurotic disorders that required the diagnosis and intervention of an authoritative healer to remedy (Dychtwald, 1987). Hakomi takes a gentler and more systemic view. We see character not as a pathological digression, but as a creative attempt to assert one's organicity—to find personal empowerment in an untenable situation. Thus, character is not a measure of what's wrong with a person. For the Hakomi practitioner, character theory allows us to identify and attend to the habitual, neural-based, conditioned perceptions, responses, and personas that arose in the child's developmental experience, which ultimately overshadowed the hypothetically free-functioning development of the client. We are not looking to "type" our clients, but to recognize universal categories of wounding and strategy, and to use this recognition as a vehicle for mindfully exploring the specifics of a particular person's inner organization.

Neurologically, experiences happen because a specific collection of brain cells (neurons) fires together, activating thoughts, emotions, bodily events, and so on. When they fire, a link develops among them, creating a network. Even after the firing ceases, this link, like a kind of channel dug between the cells, remains. The more this network is activated, the stronger the link becomes. In this way, neural patterns are "use dependent." Use a pattern a lot, and the tendency for that pattern to fire again becomes more entrenched. Disuse leads to such links fading away (Perry, Pollard, Blakeley, Baker, & Vigilante, 1996).

Furthermore, the more ingrained a pattern becomes, the less it takes to activate that pattern. This is called sensitization. "Once sensitized, the same neural activation can be elicited by decreasingly intense external stimuli. . . . The result is that full-blown response patterns . . . can be elicited by apparently minor stressors" (Perry et al., 1996, p. 275).

In this way, habits are created. As children, we learn how and what to feel in specific situations, how to respond, which aspects of our humanness to embody, how to perceive events, and so on. As experiences repeat themselves (our parents being calm and available or not, our bellies being full or empty, feeling safe and welcome or threatened and anxious), our neural patterns become habituated. As adults, characterological responses arise in us when some present event activates the old, habituated neural pattern. Thus, character is the practical description of the neural patterns we form in response to what we have learned about living. It reflects the way we manage our experience.

A general neurobiological sequence can be outlined for the development of character:

1. The child is well regulated or not. Strong, affirmative, limbic resonance and secure attachment allow the child to thrive (Ainsworth et al., 1978; Bowlby, 1973). Harsh resonance and poor attachment, on the other hand, not only instill limiting, social neural patterns, but also cause the child to operate from a threatened, survival mode, activating the more reptilian survival defenses of flight, fight, and freeze (Karen, 1998; Lewis et al., 2000). The first levels of character formation, then, are marked by the reversion of the child's psyche from the emotional stability of strong limbic resonance to the more reptilian world of life and death.

2. In any case, limbic feeling states arise in response to developmental success or stress. Emotions arise, and somatic responses erupt.

3. Repetition of the success or stress creates neural patterns that form around these limbic feeling states. That is, an emotional framework, for better or worse, starts to wire in, along with somatic patterns of armoring, expression, and containment.

4. These habituated somatic, emotional, and energetic patterns synergize to create a neural network: a complex aggregate of interactive experiences.

5. This network stimulates the neocortex to provide a rational context for these experiences. Cognitive beliefs, perceptions, and behaviors are generated, which then become part of the network.

6. This entire collective network constitutes a character pattern.

7. Attractors—"ingrained prototypical neural links . . . that influence perception according to past experience . . . and lead us, at times, to see what we expect to see, rather than what is actually present" (Morgan, 2004b, p. 55)—evoke character responses when a life situation triggers some element of the pattern. That is, a single new element of experience (a look, a word, a gesture, and so on) that has a related reference in an existing neural network may activate the entire character pattern, even though the new experience is not actually challenging the person's sense of safety or integrity.

8. As a pattern gets stronger, it takes less and less to trigger it (the sensitization process cited above).

9. We can develop numerous such networks, and therefore have different character-ological responses to varying life situations, depending on which neural networks are activated.

When we observe characterological behavior, then, we are seeing the expression of deeply wired, neural patterns in the person's brain and body, which typically misinterpret present experience. Some are lodged originally in the reptilian brain, generating primarily survival- and attachment-related experiences (though as the child develops, more sophisticated experiential content will arise); others are primarily limbic or cortical, manifesting as emotions, attitudes, beliefs, thought patterns, introjected voices, posture, and so on (Eisman, 2005). Overall, however, there is an integration of characterological patterns throughout all levels of the bodymind (Johanson, 2011c; Siegel, 2009).

The Character Map

Hakomi identifies eight basic character patterns, representing the perception of basic developmental learning tasks. Below are brief overviews of these eight basic patterns, presented in chronological (developmental) order. Since everyone goes through all of these stages, and there is almost always some interruption in the learning of the developmental tasks, we generally form a constellation of character patterns. Some people seem to dwell more consistently in one or another, whereas others are more fluid, with various character postures arising in response to different situations, and sometimes more than one pattern within the person arising in the same situation.

Being and Belonging: The Sensitive/Withdrawn Pattern

The sensitive/withdrawn pattern is marked by the person's withdrawal from embracing full human experience. Typically developing from prebirth to about six months, the child, in a global state of consciousness and not yet able to discriminate himself well from the world around him, experiences whatever happens outside as an internal event. Such experiences form the framework for the child's sense of identity. If the events are harsh in nature, the child develops a primarily kinesthetic and limbic sense of being harshness personified. (Positive experiences, of course, would engender positive identifications.)

Attachment and issues of affect regulation are central here. Since the child requires dyadic affect regulation to survive (Schore, 1994), any limitation or interruption to this feeling of a safe container leads the child to revert to reptilian survival mode: fight, flee, or freeze. In this mode, ordinary painful experiences become perceived as life threatening, and the child's defenses are constructed around these survival responses. In Lowen's theory of basic conflicts, the child chooses "existence" over organically satisfying "need."

We, therefore, see the sensitive/withdrawn pattern as exhibiting reptilian defense mechanisms: withdrawal from experience; dissociation; later refuge in fantasy or cognition (flight); chronic hyperarousal, tension, anxiety, and underlying rage (fight); and frozen core tension, armoring, terror, and robotic behavior (freeze).

Since, at this time, the child is coming to terms with being alive, feeling welcome in the world, and experiencing the range of events allowed by having a complicated set of sense organs, the interruption of these learning tasks causes the child to fear existing, to feel unwelcome and invaded by experience, rather than supported by it. The fact of being becomes painful, and the world appears to be a relentlessly harsh place.

Physically helpless, and with an as-yet undeveloped rational and verbal function, the infant's only real defense is to withdraw from experience, and—as he gets older—to live either in a fantasy world of the imagination in which he has control over the creation of experience, or an analytical world of machines and precision in which feelings and needs either don't exist or are mere data entries. In either case, there is retreat, and others are kept out. In short, the strategy is to withdraw from both external and internal actual experience, and to substitute a self-generated facsimile of human experience—acting as if one is human, but without actually knowing and feeling what humanness is like.

On the positive side, this embodiment of fantasy and analysis, coupled with the freedom from following the usual social norms, often allows people engaged in this pattern to be particularly creative artists and thinkers. While the internal world is often quite sensitive and painful, the artistry expressed may be quite brilliant. A good example is the painter Vincent van Gogh. As a refuge from the harshness of this world, the person may also pursue deep spiritual experience. The underlying innocence of the aspiring self often leads people in this pattern to be exquisitely honest and to expect the same from others.

Getting Support: The Dependent/Endearing Pattern

From about six months to a year and a half, the child views the world as the source of his or her unending and essential needs. The child is functionally helpless, and needs and expects sustenance to come from the outside. The provision of such nurturing is expected by the child, and, in fact, the child is wired hormonally and neurologically to engage with a nurturing other while being sustained and regulated (Schore, 1994).

Against this very real backdrop, the child needs to learn that he will be sustained here, and that such sustenance can and will come from others. If successful, he will learn about the continuity of life and the abundance that allows it. If interrupted, the child is taught instead about the possibility of not continuing, about collapse and despair. Instead of abundance, the child will internalize a sense of emptiness, neediness, and abandonment.

It is important to note that such a sense of abandonment may have various origins. The adults responsible for nurturing the child may be ignorant, absent, ill, or stressed. They may be following some theoretical idea of how children should be managed. There may be economic or social factors, like poverty or war. The child's metabolism may be weak or inefficient, resulting in nutritional deprivation.

In any case, the strategy that develops is the continued and undiscriminating pursuit of getting needed support, even though it is continually frustrated. If he is to stay alive and keep from being abandoned, the child must somehow endear himself to others. He must appear helpless and needy, and arouse in the other the motivation to provide.

The dependent/endearing child seeks attention and the demonstration of caring. Of course, locked into a sense of emptiness, the child becomes unable to take in offered support, and the efforts of the provider are wasted. He ends up feeling still unsupported; the impulse to give up and collapse arises again, and the strategy is triggered once more. Just as the sensitive/withdrawn person fails to see the potential for pleasure in experience, the dependent/endearing person fails to accept nourishment. He is, as Kurtz has said, "starving at a banquet."

Adults experience this pattern as an ongoing sense of deprivation and dependency. There is a feeling of being drained, inadequate, or somehow lacking in the right stuff: others have more than they, they just can't seem to get ahead, and life feels unfair. They feel great rage, which they must try to hide in the service of seeming endearing. In terms of basic conflicts, they have chosen to forgo independence until they can secure their unmet needs.

On the positive side, people in this frame may be nonthreatening, affectionate, considerate, and endearing to others, with a strong sense of devotion to group and family. They are typically easy to talk to, and often have a warm, cuddly sweetness to them.

Independence: The Self-Reliant Pattern

From approximately one or one and a half years to about two or two and a half years, children slowly become more independent. They progress from rolling over to sitting up, to crawling, toddling, and now walking. They start to speak, naming their experiences and expressing their needs more precisely. They are delighted to be more self-sufficient, yet they still require constant outside support. At this point children need to learn that they can integrate their physical needs and desires with their newly developing skills, all the while still being sustained by outside support. Along with experiencing "I will be helped," they need to master a sense of "I can do it!"

The parents may be neglectful, too busy to help, or may expect the child to fend for herself. Thus, the child learns, "Others will not help. I have to do it myself. If it's going to get done, I'll have to do it." Finally, if she can successfully attend to her own needs, she develops the belief, "I can handle it myself."

Because this child is able, she responds to her sense of abandonment and dependency not by becoming endearing, but by becoming self-reliant. Lowen (1975) referred to this character pattern as "compensated oral." The strategy is to rise to the challenge of independence in order to avoid collapse through the failure of others to provide support.

The person with this pattern will see everything as a challenge to her ability to handle situations, and will then mobilize to handle it. All of this is done both because there is no other apparent choice, and also, at a deeper level, to avoid the disappointment of not having been helped. Because others will not be helpful and life is about dealing with challenges and stresses, as opposed to relaxed relating, the person with the self-reliant strategy has little dependence or use for others. Sometimes people with this disposition will put out a lot in service of others. On the one hand, they are modeling for others what they want for themselves, but on the other, they are not able to receive mutual help when offered. They will tend to operate parallel to the participation of others. When something needs to be done, they will jump in to take care of the situation without even considering others' offers of help. As a result, they might live with an underlying resentment that they do more than their share.

Self-reliance is very prevalent in our culture, and, in fact, is often held as a virtue. While having the ability to be self-reliant is, of course, a valuable skill, the automatic interpretations that others are irrelevant and that situations are challenges to one's ability to survive are quite limiting.

Such self-reliance leads to great resiliency, and often a large measure of competency, especially around material concerns. Organized around survival, people in this pattern are indeed skilled at getting by and getting things done. They can be quite decisive, and are usually very dependable in accomplishing a variety of tasks.

Interdependence and Intimacy:
Tough/Generous and Charming/Seductive Patterns

As the child continues to learn, hopefully, that he will be helped with his needs, he is gaining a greater and greater sense of individual accomplishment. Less and less dependent on others for mastery of the physical world, the child begins to feel independent, a necessary step in becoming a wholly individuated being.

At the same time, the child now begins to see himself in the context of the world. The surrounding environment is no longer just a source of mechanical need satisfaction. The world and people become a source of human, relational interest. The child, in short, moves from a self-centered search for needs and pleasure to an engagement with others that includes the desire for mutual satisfaction. The child needs to learn about interdependence, and desires equally independence and intimacy.

A conflict between independence and intimacy arises when the child's search for or expression of his own wish or needs in relationship is met with manipulation, ridicule, teasing, criticism, bargaining, disinterest, dismissal, or other such limitations on the free acceptance of his will in the service of the other person's will. The problem is relational, and the issue is not "I can" or "I can't," but "I will" and "Will you also?"

If the child is not met with respect for his will, but instead encounters opposition or ridicule for the benefit of the other, his sense of mutuality will be violated. The child, typically, feels deeply offended, minimized, or even crushed and betrayed. These feelings may lead to further criticism or humiliation by others. The primitive camaraderie of parallel independence becomes a competitive struggle for dominance, with the child having to adopt the position of either supporting his own will at the expense of the others, or surrendering his own sense of individuality at the expense of himself. Everything in his world becomes colored by the issue of power.

He will then adopt a dual strategy of hiding his own vulnerability and neediness (for these are what evoked the offending response in the other) while seeking to dominate others, both to minimize their threat by not giving them leverage and to assert his own power. Adopting this strategy will see to it that the person appears carefree, competent, authoritative, and generous, with a bit of danger about him that will keep people respectful, but distant enough so that they will not try to be intimate and thereby a potential threat. Of course, this charade of invulnerability must also apply to the person himself, so that he often does not feel the need to act on his own needs, and can actually be less sensitive to pain than the average person. This can serve as a point of pride.

Out of touch with his own sensitivity and cut off from intimacy, the tough/generous strategy keeps the person in a world of competitive, illusory power and security, without the hope for true intimacy and with only indirect opportunities for nourishment. Those embodying this strategy might attempt to curry favor and care from a position of power such as buying things for another, protecting, or helping them out somehow.

In a similar way, if the child is not so much ridiculed, minimized, or constrained in her attempts at independence as coerced, manipulated, or taken advantage of, then she may learn not so much to dominate but to evade. Here the issue is not about being confronted or crushed, but about being manipulated or tricked. The other is seen not as an opponent in a win-or-lose battle for autonomy, but rather as an inconvenient obstacle on the path of self-satisfaction. Because the other was supposed to be helpful but is now in the way, the child feels more betrayed than offended. Rather than rising above to invulnerability and competing with the other for supremacy, the child may learn to charm and countermanipulate the situation or the other in order to get her own way.

The selfish but charming lover or the solicitous con man are both stereotypes of this strategy. The strategy creates an apparent, but false, intimacy while underneath using this illusory closeness to achieve a much more self-centered goal. The person gets the indirect benefits of the pretend relationship, but not the depth of direct, vulnerable intimacy.

Resources and strengths of people with these patterns include the ability to recognize and exploit opportunities, and the ability to disregard their own needs and feelings for the sake of others or for the cause they have committed to or are leading. The impulse to dominate provides a foundation to initiate, command, and lead with a decisiveness that often does not seek or need the input of others. It can help these people be successful in acting, since they are not hampered by stage fright or afraid of making a fool of themselves like others might be. In relationships, people with these patterns are often, quite successfully, the caretaker, protector, or benefactor. They can sustain relationships where they enlist an attitude of "it's us against the world," again a power theme. Their resistance to being controlled or manipulated can lead them to operate outside the rules, and they can be creative outlaws, rebels, and innovators, originating their own vision or path, and often inspiring and leading others. These gifts can also be employed in matching wits with offenders as officers of the law.

Freedom: The Burdened/Enduring Pattern

Assuming the child has attained a sense of independence, she next needs to learn about the application of her independence in a relational world. She must learn the balance between freedom and responsibility, between autonomy and consequence.

We can make a distinction between independence and freedom in this way: independence is the sense of being functionally separate, whole unto oneself, whereas freedom is the ability to be that separate self within the context of other independent selves. Though the child learns about independence in the context of others, and is impacted by their response to her efforts, the learning task of independence itself is not about the relationship. It is about one's own ability and self-image. It only becomes about relationship if it is interrupted. We might say that during the development of independence, the child needs the support of others but has no wish yet to be influenced by their parallel needs.

During the next learning stage, the pursuit of freedom, the child is trying to strike a balance between his own needs and wishes, and the needs and wishes of others. For the child in the independence/interdependence phase above, such a project is an aberration of his natural timing; through collapse, self-reliance, invulnerability, or manipulation, such a child is forced to include the needs of others before he is ready to, and so must come to view the needs of others as antagonistic, threatening, or inconvenient.

The freedom-learning child, however, willingly seeks such engagement, especially if secure in his own sense of independence. Mutuality is a state whose time has come, and the child, moving from a sense of "I" to the beginnings of "we," hopes to master it.

At first, the child explores freedom by asserting it as absolute, testing how much autonomy is truly acceptable in the relational context. This is when children learn the word "No" and use it as a mantra: "Do you want a bath?" "NO!" "Do you want a spanking?" "NO!" "Are you my little boy?" "NO!" If they are opposed in their freedom—say, forbidden to explore that mysterious cabinet below the sink—they may be insistent, even rude, in their responses. If unable to prevail, they may express their rage in a temper tantrum.

Over time, the child is trying to learn what the actual rules and boundaries are, where the compromise is between self-indulgence and pleasing those around them. It is important to emphasize that both of these concerns—the assertion of personal will and the generation of pleasure in significant others—are simultaneously at the forefront of the child's interest. He wants both to happen and is trying to learn how to accomplish this juggling act. Children want to learn both freedom and responsibility—freedom for themselves, responsibility to the needs of others.

If during this stage the child is forced to choose between these two concerns, he may tumble into an impossible double bind. If, for example, the child is constantly told that his drum banging gives Mommy a headache, the child must either sacrifice Mommy's well-being to support his own musical explorations, or he must deny his own impulse to play the drum in order to protect Mommy. It is a lose-lose situation, in which he must surrender either his own freedom or Mommy's pleasure. Either way, he fails at accomplishing the dual task of freedom and accommodating the other. He can hurt himself or he can hurt the one he loves. He is stuck. There is no good choice, and the child becomes burdened by the weight of this impasse.

Outwardly, the child solves what Lowen calls the conflict between freedom and closeness by voting for the closeness he craves at the expense of the freedom to be himself, a terribly painful bargain of resigning to the tyranny of feeling loved or accepted conditionally. Especially if the child's expression, individuality, or negativity have been severely dealt with and disallowed, the child learns that such organic expression will surely lead to being cut off from the desired closeness, which is likewise intolerable. Depending on how volatile or close to the surface the never-ending bind is, the person might demonstrate more or less passive-aggressive behavior, and more or less judgment toward others who display the freedom to not toe the line.

To resolve the continuing inward bind, the child develops a strategy that attempts to include all needs, though, of course, he cannot truly succeed. On the surface, the child will accede to the other's need, for he feels blamed and guilty that his own need hurts the other and does not want to damage the precious bond of intimacy. He represses his impulse to freely express and indulge himself (in our example, no more drumming). At the same time, the impulse is an authentic part of who he is, so it leaks out in the safe but private form of internal grumbling and tension against the contraction. Since he is violating his natural impulse to be expressive, his love for the other becomes tinged with underlying resentment. In addition to the intimacy, he also feels shame at violating himself, as well as a bittersweet superiority toward the other (based on his choice to take care of her at his expense, which she did not do for him). All of these emotions together—the love, the intimacy, the guilt, the resentment, and the superiority—form a very tense and compact little world that the child must manage and endure.

To relieve the pressure, the child will see to it that, while not in any way directly confronting the other on the bind she has put him in, he will nevertheless get back at her by somehow undermining her needs. He may lose a shoe just as she's hurrying to leave the house for an appointment. He may bump into her special vase while innocently playing. He may poke her in the eye while reaching to hug her. Again, none of this would be consciously planned—the child might feel quite surprised and innocent doing these things. But, underneath, there is a kind of smirking glee at having found some situational power by sabotaging the one who burdened him with such an impossible bind.

A low-grade depression is always near because of the deep unmet need to have someone take delight in him as he is. The depression can evaporate quickly when someone does express interest and invites him to join in. However, hopes of unconditional friendship or contact are inevitably dashed as the child projects not only onto the primary caretaker but onto every significant person he meets that the other is simply the latest in a long line of people who only accept him if he accommodates to their needs and wants, as opposed to his own. If there is a choice of what movie to see, he knows ahead of time that he will go to the one the other wants, or end up going to his own first choice alone.

Because of this lose-lose bind, the person with this strategy becomes uncomfortable with choosing. Since his perception is that any choice will lead to pain, either for himself or another about whom he cares, he will steer as far from decisions as he can. Knowing that there's a tiger behind either door, the person with the burdened/enduring disposition prefers to delay and defer. He ends up having serious difficulty actually knowing what his choice would be, since so much energy has been spent wondering what choice the other wants. "How do *I* like my eggs?"

This strategy, while not as well regarded in our culture today as it was in the 1950s, nevertheless includes a great percentage of our population. Caught between decency and impulse, duty and resentment, civilization and anarchy, most of us in one way or another sacrifice our true autonomy in service to getting along, pleasing the boss or our families, making the payments, loyally showing up for work, being good citizens.

To be sure, much of this is noble and productive—remember, supporting the relational context is a highly desired goal for this person—and loyalty, concern, endurance, and a sense of justice are strengths of this pattern. A person organized this way is often able to remain patient, stable, and unmoved in difficult conditions. She may find satisfaction being able to continue with unpleasant tasks that others can't stay with. Caring and devoted, people in this pattern seek to enjoy family and friends as deeply as possible.

Acceptance and Equality: The Industrious/Overfocused and Expressive/Clinging Patterns

By the time the child is about five or six years old, he has hopefully accomplished a sense of safety and sustenance in the world, and an independent and autonomous self, which can both recognize personal boundaries and interact easily with others. The creation of a self as a distinct entity should have taken place, but another step remains: for the self to take its place in the community as a contributing member. If the self were a car, we might say that it has been fully assembled and is now ready to learn how to travel on the highway of life with other cars.

At this time, the child's focus, while still firmly embedded in the dynamics of the family, expands to include an eager awareness of the world at large. The child's sense of self not only is now influenced by what goes on at home, but in a deliberate way, seeks also to learn directly from experience in the community.

The goal of this phase of development is to end up feeling like an equal member of society (both the one at home and the global one), with equal rights, recognition of one's presence, and acknowledgment of one's own accomplishments. The child needs to know she has arrived, is included, that she is somehow complete enough to take her place among the community's membership, and to contribute.

This sense of recognition can be interrupted in various ways: one or more parents or significant outside others may compete with the child and overwhelm her abilities; a parent might be withdrawn, demanding, or critical; because of their own need to appear successful, the parents may pressure the child to overachieve; the parents may have unfair standards or expectations; or circumstances may require the child to take an adult role in the family. In any case, the child's innate sense of worthiness for being a valued part of things gets ignored, and the child must strive to attain the recognition and inclusion she needs.

As a strategic response, then, the child adopts a policy of industrious, highly focused behavior and constant self-critical assessments that drive her to endeavor even harder— because of a nagging belief that she is not yet quite good enough to be fully included. If she gets an A at school, she'll dwell on how she could have gotten an A-plus. If she scores two goals in soccer, she will go home wondering about the third that didn't happen, or how she let her opponent score two goals. These children live in a world of achievements that are never quite good enough, measuring their worth not by who they are (as they had naturally wished) but by what they do or, more accurately, what they didn't do yet, and whether those efforts will be acknowledged.

Such constant effort requires them to focus on tasks rather than pleasure or feelings, and generates an overall tension of readiness and mobilization. When this strategy is evoked, the person experiences herself as being always at the starting blocks, waiting for the gun to go off, to try, one more time, to win the race and gain the acclaim that should have been hers in the first place, just because she exists.

During this developmental stage, another kind of wounding and strategy can happen as well. In this situation, rather than striving to excel and prove her worthiness, the child becomes ambivalent about growing up and taking her place as an equal in society. Typically, the child comes to feel that to embrace fully the transition to equality will mean the loss of the closeness that being immature allows, as well as the delights of being little and less responsible. Maturity seems to come at the expense of caring and affection. A typical scenario might be that the child is now regarded as too old to be cuddled; or the child might be seen as being old or mature enough now not to need much parental support. Instead of playing freely, the child may now be required to do chores.

In any case, the child ends up feeling rejected in her essence, and valued now only for her emerging more mature self. The full range of her being—the maturity and the vulnerability, the competence and the neediness—is not validated, and the child struggles to have these elements of her being recognized.

Strategically, then, the child may both achieve and also regress to a more helpless state, alternately producing some creative marvel and begging for help with the simplest tasks. She will try not to achieve recognition (as with the industrious strategy above), but to get attention. She desires to be included like the industrious child, but one of her thoughts is that the reason she is not embraced as before is not that she is not yet good enough, but not quite interesting enough. To counter her fear of rejection, the child will develop a dramatic flair—expressing great emotions or having serial problems or crises. The person with this pattern will remember how she was so adored or protected or held close when she was younger, helpless, and interesting enough to be delighted in, and will cling to this image and behavior from the past, unwilling to grow all the way up.

Such a dramatic orientation will show up in adults as the need for attention and the amplification of small things into epic events ("Oh my God!" "What is it?" "We're out of mayonnaise!"). Because the strategy is adept at seeking or capturing attention, others may often feel attracted to the drama generated, and to the person generating it. After a while, however, the drama becomes routine. When interest from others subsides, the person again feels rejected, and so begins another cycle of hurt and drama.

Both industrious/overfocused and expressive/clinging persons express great energy. Both patterns tend to be well socialized and functional, with opposite digressions: the industrious becoming overfocused and the expressive becoming diffuse.

On the resource side, people in these patterns are often competent, high achievers with good social skills who accomplish a great deal. Responsible, grounded people, they tend to interact maturely with others, are attractive with high energy, are generally very cooperative and dependable, and are often admired by others for their functionality. Their respective strategies lead them to have good initiative, to be action or people oriented, and to be good at problem solving. They are typically easy to inspire and mobilize, and can be good leaders who proceed with determination, or team players who perform well under pressure.

Comparison Chart of Characterological Terminologies

Table 8.1 is provided to compare a few characterological languages among many for those interested in how the various systems go together, even when they are not precise match-ups. Many clinicians deal with the *Diagnostic and Statistical Manual of Mental Disorders* (*DSM*). Notice that the *DSM* does not even have a categorical equivalent to rigid, conscientious, industrious/overfocused dispositions because unrelenting doing and achieving are valued as virtues in American culture. A good deal of research is related to Loevinger's (1976) characterology. Like Kurtz, Loevinger chooses to use words descriptive of a particular predicament, as opposed to pathological labels. She also has a couple of characterological dispositions that go beyond character as normally understood.

In the theory behind the presentation of Table 8.1, the starred (*) conditions are thought to be disorders of self-leadership. Instead of having the consistency and stability to take a position on a particular end of a basic conflict, such as Kurtz's sensitive/withdrawn people

Table 8.1 Character Terminology

Lowen Basic Conflicts	Lowen Terms	Kurtz Terms	Loevinger Terms	*DSM-IV* Terms
Existence versus need	Schizoid	Sensitive/withdrawn	Presocial Symbiotic	Schizotypal avoidant Schizoid or paranoid (Borderline*)
Need versus independence	Oral Compensated oral	Dependent/endearing Self-reliant	Impulsive	Dependent (Narcissistic*)
Independence versus closeness	Psychopath	Tough/ generous Charming/seductive	Self-protective	Antisocial
Closeness versus freedom	Masochist	Burdened/enduring	Conformist	Passive-aggressive (Compulsive*)
Freedom versus surrender	Rigid	Industrious/overfocused Expressive/clinging	Conscientious (Autonomous) (Integrated)	Histrionic

*Conditions thought to be disorders of self-leadership.

choosing existence over need, they flip-flop between positions. The borderline disposition may be seen as flip-flopping back and forth between withdrawal and longing-dependent needs, not settling on one particular solution. Narcissism can be understood as flip-flopping between the longing needs of the dependent position and self-protective independence. Those who present as compulsives seem to shuttle between the conforming of the burdened/enduring position and the conscientiousness of the industrious/overfocused.

Character in the Real World

In Western culture, almost everyone has at least some of these various patterns, hurts, and strategies, simply because we all have gone through the same basic developmental stages. We've all had more or less success with the particular learning tasks of our era, and therefore rely on and exhibit varying degrees of these strategies. The presentation of those raised in different cultures would certainly vary among many variables (Paniagua & Yamada, 2013).

At different times, depending on the demands of a situation, different neural patterns may be triggered, and we will shift into a certain habitually wired, experiential network to respond to that particular moment. We may then shift out of the strategy when the situation is resolved, and later be triggered into some other wound that generates a second, third, or tenth kind of strategic response. As complex adaptive systems, we embody a multiplicity of attractor states that organize us in a variety of ways given our immediate circumstances (see Chapter 5).

Furthermore, as we grow and learn, we discover that we can blend strategies, adapting certain ones in new ways to support different kinds of needs. For example, we may learn that we are more successful in confrontations of power when we withdraw slightly, rather than when we try to dominate. Or to protect a sense of not belonging, we may find that staying busy and focused—industriousness—keeps us safer than withdrawing.

As a result, we develop all sorts of hybrid wound and strategy arrangements: tough/withdrawn, sensitive/overfocused, dependent/seductive, and so forth. Like a tradesman with his box of tools, the malleable self has assessed the particular nuances of a problem and has learned to choose the strategies that best seem to address the momentary need. Also, most standard characterologies deal with one's early years of development, while Erikson (1963) has taught us that human development embraces stages throughout life. What happens when we send someone who has had a decent childhood off to a messy, ambiguous war at age 18 and in the stage of identity consolidation? While a disposition to withdraw classically happens during the early tactile time of development, it can also be evoked at 32 when one becomes a refugee or prisoner of war.

Clinically, then, we need to remain open to the specifics of the client's unique, internal organization and not be coerced by the linear descriptions of the character patterns. We need to respond moment by moment to the actual experiences of the client, allowing the character map to serve as a consulting framework for the possible meanings of the various presenting elements of the client's body, perceptions, and behaviors. In this way, the

Hakomi practitioner remains congruent with his or her highest mandate—to allow the client's inner wisdom to unfold.

It is always acceptable for practitioners to have a hunch about what is going on and propose an intervention based on that hunch informed by character theory (see Chapter 23), but as with all Hakomi interventions, the Chinese proverb remains true that the way is easy for those who go forward with no preferences. Practitioners must not be attached to their hunches. Perhaps the character-based intuition is that someone is not going forward in his life because he is afraid of falling on his face and being embarrassed for incompetence. But then it turns out that the person has been in military service and has embodied a fear based on experience that if he leads the way, someone might literally be killed.

Both Lowen and Kurtz, in their later years, claimed to no longer use character theory in their work, but simply contacted and followed the unique experience of every client (Greg Johanson, personal communication). This was a bit disingenuous, since they had both integrated the lessons of character work so deeply that they could afford to not think about them, but concentrate instead on fine-tuned variations. The Hakomi Institute faculty still consider learning the character basics of commonly negotiated, developmental conflicts like learning the scales on a keyboard so that later one can do jazz variations. Every practitioner does not need to reinvent the wheel and ignore the hard-earned wisdom of those who have gone before. It does remain paramount, of course, to resist the temptation to consider any person pathologically as an "it," a "type," a "character," ignoring the person's creativity, organic wisdom, capacity for emergent properties, and ability to relate from a larger self-state (Almaas, 1988; Eisman, 2006; Monda, 2000; Schwartz, 1995).

Methodology and Therapeutic Strategy

CHAPTER 9

The Therapeutic Relationship in Hakomi Therapy

Julie Murphy

The basic work of health professionals in general, and of psychotherapists in particular, is to become full human beings and to inspire full human-beingness in other people who feel starved about their lives.

CHOGYAM TRUNGPA, Becoming a Full Human Being, 1980

The Therapeutic Relationship

THERAPY NORMALLY REQUIRES a living, conscious, trusting relationship. As each therapist-client relationship is unique and creates a particular outcome (Cozolino, 2010), it is the therapeutic relationship that provides the container in which healing takes place. Kurtz (1990a) has maintained that the therapist's first job is to create and sustain the healing relationship. For him, the client's sense of safety, the "cooperation of the unconscious," and the general unfolding of the therapeutic process all depend on the alliance between therapist and client no matter what method the therapist follows.

Researchers describe the personhood of the therapist as more central to the success of the therapy than any particular technique or theoretical background (Cozolino, 2002; Lambert & Ogles, 2013; Mahoney, 1991; Orlinsky & Howard, 1986). As interpersonal neurobiology becomes better understood, so does its role in the therapeutic process. When a limbic episode establishes itself within a neural pattern, it takes a limbic occurrence to reverse it (Lewis et al., 2000). "A *safe and empathic relationship* establishes an emotional and neurobiological context conducive to the work of neural reorganization" (Cozolino, 2002, p. 291). Thus, the attitudes and qualities of the therapist are vital to the success of therapy.

Different approaches and theories emphasize different relational styles and modes of participation for the therapist. In order to elucidate the Hakomi understanding of how the therapeutic relationship is built, it is useful to compare it to other, more traditional psychodynamic approaches. Traditionally, the psychoanalytic therapist was a "blank slate" and the emphasis rested solely on the inner drives and conflicts of the patient. As the field has developed, so has the role of the therapist and the therapeutic relationship.

Classical Analysis

In traditional psychoanalytic theory, the analyst participates in a relationship focused on the client's inner structures. She purposely tries to give as few hints about herself as possible for the sake of the client's unadulterated projections. Because she views the psychopathology of the client as the result of inner conflicts and tensions (Stark, 1999), making the unconscious known becomes her work. The analyst makes interpretations, particularly of the transference, providing insight into the client's motives and the understanding of his internal structures to promote his healing.

In contrast, rather than offering interpretations, the Hakomi therapist might employ analytic theories and interpretations to understand the client, and then use those intuitions to create little experiments in mindfulness that enable the client to study his experience (Marks-Tarlow, 2012). However, she would not base the relationship on this dynamic or lead the exchange with her client in an analytic mode, agreeing with others that silence is not a neutral act (Stolorow et al., 1987). In Hakomi, insight is never enough. An insight cannot counteract transference based on experience. It takes an experience to moderate another experience (Greenberg et al., 1998).

Self-Psychology

The self-psychology therapist seeks to provide the client an experience of goodness that was lacking in the client's early childhood by empathically validating the client's experience. Healing comes through the client's experience of this goodness and his growing ability to come to terms with the imperfection and fallibility of the therapist (Stark, 1999). The therapist focuses on the affective, present experience of the client, not on making interpretations of the client's internal structures or the actual relationship between the therapist and client. Self-psychology emphasizes the client's experience of goodness in the face of disappointment and the therapist's empathic recognition of the client's experience. When the client has accepted the initial goodness and mastered the frustration and grief resulting from inevitable disappointment in the therapist, then the goodness has been internalized.

These transmuting internalizations (Kohut, 1966) theoretically build the internal structures (archaic, validating, self-object ties) that were missing in the client, and the client successfully learns to deal with the impossibility of perfection in self or others. While the Hakomi therapist may address early deficit reflected in a client's present experience, he looks for the opportunity to do so as a collaborative experiment within the actual relationship between therapist and client. He also seeks to engage the compassionate witness of the client in relation to the internal organization of experience, so there are both intrapsychic and parallel interpersonal aspects to the therapy (Germer, 2006).

Object Relations

The object relations therapist also engages in the therapeutic relationship in order to fill early childhood deficits. The id's needs for instinctual gratification can be frustrated, whereas the ego's needs for connection and understanding cannot (Winnicott, 1965). Using the present relationship (with the therapist), the therapist gives the client the goodness that was missing and assists him to feel his rage at early frustrations. Because the therapist creates space and understanding for the client's experience, the client can feel the therapist respond. He can have the corrective experience of feeling important in the context of an actual connection. The therapist's active participation is critical—she is the object (that is, good mother) that fills the deficit.

While the Hakomi therapist may deal with the provision of needs or missing experiences, she does not consider her role as defined or limited by such. Certainly, the discernment between authentic needs and instinctual wants would become a joint venture of study, rather than an interpretive activity of the therapist. In addition—as stated above—encouraging a supportive internal relationship between the client and his organic self (Eisman, 2006) that brings compassionate awareness to bear on hurting parts is as crucial to overall growth as a nourishing therapist-client relationship.

Though Hakomi recognizes the importance of historical object relations on the fragmentation of the ego (Eisman, 1989; Schmidt, 1994), it does not accept that poor object relations leads to a poor self in terms of the human capacity to be mindful and compassionate (Fosha, 2000, 2005; Panksepp & Northoff, 2008; Russell & Fosha, 2008; Schwartz, 1995). In object relations and self-psychology schools, the object is nearly absolutized and the subject minimized—implying pathology, a lack of responsibility, and a possibly interminable therapeutic process.

In terms of reformulating the psychodynamic theory of building an egoic level self through introjecting "self-object ties" from interpersonal relationships, Bons-Storm suggests alternatively that the basic building blocks of personality might be thought of as "self-narratives using stories about experienced events" (1996, p. 47). This is a more satisfying formulation for Hakomi therapy. It suggests that what is introjected is not blind, random units of pleasure or pain, but intelligible, intellectual-emotional events—events that the imagination transforms in meaningful ways according to core organizing beliefs, and then integrates into one's ongoing story according to Piaget's processes of assimilation and accommodation (Gendlin, 1992; Horner, 1974).

Contemporary Relational Psychoanalysis

The relational therapist engages in an authentic two-way relationship with the client. Unlike client-centered empathy, the analyst stays centered in herself, and responds to the concrete relational dynamics that the client actually plays out in the therapeutic relationship (Stark, 1999). Both therapist and client actively participate, moment by moment, and cocreate all meaning and experience. The therapist is mutually impacted by the relationship.

This approach to therapeutic relationships is more akin to Hakomi. The client experiences the therapist through the lens of his past (subjective transference) as well as his real-time interactions with the therapist (objective transference) (Stark, 1999). The client heals through understanding these dynamics and through participating in the relationship. While the relational therapist still relies on interpretations, she engages in the intersubjective field as fully as the client does (Stolorow et al., 1987). The mutual sharing of impact between client and therapist has a profound healing influence. The client must know that just as the therapist changes him, he changes the therapist (Stark, 1999).

Depending on the stage of the therapeutic process, the Hakomi therapist uses a range of therapeutic relationships. If the therapist encourages the client to mindfully study the organization of her experience (the essence of working the transference, according to Stolorow et al., 1987), this would be one-person therapy in Stark's (1999) schema, since the therapist is leading the client into a deeper relationship with himself. If the client is taking in a new missing experience from the therapist, it would be one-and-a-half-person therapy for Stark because the therapist is bringing her best or ideal self to the interchange. When the client is in the integrative stage of working a new element into the organization of his experience, the process may move into two-person therapy, where both client and therapist are fully present in an intersubjective way.

It should be noted that relational psychoanalysis has recently moved to encompass the body more fully in its work—something significant for Hakomi since it, too, encompasses a somatic dimension. Aron (1998a, p. xx) argues that "our self is first and foremost a body-as-experienced-being-handled-and-held-by-other-self, in other words, our self is an intersubjective-bodily self." He likewise says, "I believe that research into and clinical study of self-reflexivity [mindfulness] (and especially the relationship among self-reflexivity, intersubjectivity, embodiment, and trauma) is among the most promising areas of psychological research and psychoanalytic investigation taking place today" (p. 4).

Intersubjective School

Stolorow (Stolorow et al., 1987) coined the term "intersubjectivity" to describe the therapeutic field as one that involves two subjects (therapist and client) as an attempt to move away from a one-way therapeutic relationship between self-object (therapist) and subject (client), and toward a more authentic relationship that includes both (Stark, 1999).

The old days are over in which it could be assumed that the therapist sees things as they are because she has been "analyzed" while the client sees things subjectively because he has not, and will only be cured when he sees in the same manner as the therapist. Both therapist and client always and only perceive things subjectively. Thus, when the Hakomi therapist perceives that the world of the client is too narrowly organized to include all that life offers, the perception must be held lightly as it is checked out collaboratively and experimentally with the life world of the client (Duncan, 2010). Since Hakomi therapy deals with transference in terms of the organization of experience in an intersubjective, collaborative manner, it is a psychodynamic form of psychotherapy.

> Transference in its essence refers neither to regression, displacement, projection, nor distortion, but rather to the assimilation of the analytic relationship into the thematic structures of the patient's personal subjective world. Thus conceived, transference is an expression of the universal psychological striving to organize experience and create meanings. This broad conceptualization of transference holds numerous advantages over earlier ones. . . . It clarified the contributions of both analyst and patient in shaping the patient's experience of the therapeutic relationship. . . . Most important of all, the concept of transference as organizing activity, by encouraging an unwavering inquiry into the patient's subjective frame of reference, opens a clear and unobstructed window to the patient's psychological world, and to its expansion, evolution, and enrichment. (Stolorow et al., 1987, pp. 45–46)

This intersubjective field is continuous and mutual (Beebe & Lachmann, 2002). Advances in both psychology and neuroscience give credence to the notion of intersubjectivity and expand its relevance to all relationships. Studies of the function of mirror neurons, contagion, and right hemisphere processes delineate their roles in our ability to affect another's brain activity and emotional state, intuit others' possible intentions, feel empathically what another is experiencing, and our innate capacity to know another's mind (Damasio, 2003; Gallese, 2001; Lewis et al., 2000; Schore, 2003; Siegel, 1999, 2006; Stern, 2004; Watt, 2005). Infant research sheds much light on the ways infants and adults relate and share experience as well as the role of attachment in adult relationships (Aitkins & Trevarthen, 1997; Beebe & Lachmann, 1998, 2002; Stern, 1985).

We live life in an intersubjective matrix—a matrix where we live, breathe, and move knowing from the inside what other people are doing and feeling. Distinct boundaries exist between self and other, but remain permeable (Whitehead, 1994, 1995). We can no longer view our existence as completely independent and separate. We resonate with each other; we coordinate our actions with each other; and we synchronize our experiences. These "moments of meeting" are of relatively short duration, but recur reliably (Stern, 2004). Stern (2004) considers intersubjectivity a condition of humaneness and, as such, a motivational system, like attachment or sex. It contributes to the survival of the species by promoting group formation, enhancing group functioning, and ensuring group cohesion through the development of morality.

These findings necessitate a new view of the therapeutic relationship.

> Intersubjectivity in the clinical situation can no longer be considered only as a useful tool or one of many ways of being with another that comes and goes as needed. Rather, the therapeutic process will be viewed as occurring in an ongoing intersubjective matrix. (Stern, 2004, p. 78)

It is this matrix, then, that informs the therapist of relational dynamics and allows moment-to-moment, relational-corrective experiences to occur. These dyadic interchanges form the basis of the client's healing and affect the therapist as well in the unique rhythm of the relationship of the pair (Beebe & Lachmann, 1998, 2002). "Internal processes and relational processes are inextricably coordinated, and are organized concurrently" (Beebe & Lachmann, 1998, p. 488).

This coordination is formed in the resonant emotional field, and the perception of facial expressions and resultant brain activation (Beebe & Lachmann, 1998). Wounding that occurs in relationship must heal in relationship (Lewis et al., 2000), both interpersonal and intrapsychic. "Self-regulatory behaviors of patient and analyst, such as subtle head and gaze aversions, postural orientations, and varieties of self touching, add invaluable information to the treatment when they are recognized, acknowledged, and their place in the ongoing interaction is understood" (Beebe & Lachmann, 1998, p. 505). When applied to psychotherapy, as in the Hakomi method, intersubjectivity as a motivational system yields two important consequences: (1) therapy is necessarily a cocreated process; and (2) "it is clinically helpful to view the desire to be known and achieve intersubjective contact as a major motive in driving psychotherapy forward" (Stern, 2004, p. 148).

Rogers

Rogers's (1951, 1961, 1980) "person-centered approach," described as the capacity each individual has for self-understanding and reorganizing attitudes, beliefs, and behaviors, has a close, though less than defining (see Chapter 12), kinship with Hakomi. The qualities required to promote this self-directed growth apply to personal growth in therapy, as well as in group leadership and teaching relationships. They are described in these basic attitudes of the therapist: genuineness, "unconditional positive regard," and empathic understanding (Rogers, 1961, 1980).

> If therapy were optimal . . . it would mean that the therapist feels this client to be a person of unconditional self-worth: of value no matter what his condition, his behavior, or his feelings. It would mean that the therapist is genuine, hiding behind no defensive façade, but meeting the client with the feelings which organically he is experiencing. It would mean that the therapist is able to let himself go in understanding this client; that no inner barriers keep him from sensing what it feels like to be the client at each moment of the relationship; and that he can convey something of his empathic understanding to the client. It means that the therapist has been comfortable in entering this relationship fully, without knowing cognitively where it will lead, satisfied with providing a climate which will permit the client the utmost freedom to become himself. (Rogers, 1961, pp. 184–185)

Rogers foreshadowed the focus on empathic attunement in object relations and intersubjective forms of psychotherapy by emphasizing congruence between therapist and client (Cozolino, 2002). Rogers (1961) also describes the individual's growth as a process of becoming, not a fixed state. He continued to develop his ideas on viewing the propensity of individuals to develop in a nurturing environment toward positive and constructive directions, not as a chance event, but rather as a

> tendency which permeates all of organic life—a tendency to become all the complexity of which the organism is capable. . . . We are tuning in to a potent creative tendency which has formed our universe . . . and perhaps we are touching the cutting edge of our ability to transcend ourselves, to create new and more spiritual directions in human evolution. (Rogers, 1980, p. 134)

Hakomi shares a spiritual trajectory with Rogers (Coffey, 2008; Kurtz, 2008) as well as a focus on the full and authentic person-to-person exchange between client and therapist.

Fosha

In recent years, Diana Fosha (2009a, 2009b) has presented at a number of Hakomi events and demonstrated a very Hakomi-like dynamic way of bringing a psychoanalytic background to doing safe, compassionate, accelerated experiential work with affect within the context of a highly attuned, dyadically regulated relationship. Here positive emotions such as love, gratitude, joy, accomplishment, and strengths are not considered the end products of successful therapy, but essential components of the change process. Through tracking and contacting these positive affective experiences that arise as an integral part of healing, what Fosha terms "metatherapeutic processing," they become the sustained focus of experiential exploration. A cascade of transformation is often released that culminates in a core state of being, a positive affective state of calm and centeredness in which integration and consolidation of change takes place and a coherent self comes to the fore. Once in a core state, empathy and self-empathy, wisdom, clarity about one's truth, and generosity become the currency of the realm, something akin to what Eisman (2006) refers to as an Organic Self place.

The Hakomi Method

In Hakomi therapy, the therapeutic relationship is the necessary context in which self-study occurs. In whatever way the therapist offers nourishment to the client, it happens in genuine and authentic relating between two human beings. Mastery of technique comes slowly in this method, not because the techniques are in themselves difficult or complex, but because being oneself in the role of therapist using this method requires noteworthy practice. Learning to relax and be oneself, without following old habits or enacting limiting beliefs, and cultivating an ongoing state of mindfulness and loving presence requires the Hakomi therapist to practice and grow. To this end, Kurtz and the Hakomi Institute have developed numerous exercises and practices that help the therapist to identify and cultivate the self-state outlined below. Finding and developing this capacity are the very core of every Hakomi training.

Attitude of the Therapist

The healing relationship and attitude of the therapist in Hakomi are in service to the client's self-discovery and reorganization. The therapist engages in the intersubjective field with an attitude of loving presence. Empathically, he aims to join with the client in her experience and at the same time, create a warm, open space for the client to deepen, discover, and explore her habitual responses, core beliefs, and unconscious material. The therapist is not viewed as an expert that knows best, but rather as a facilitator that leads by following (Johanson, 2009b). The client remains the expert on her experience, and an equal participant in the process (Kurtz, 1990a). The relationship between therapist and client is based on the attitude of collaboration and cocreation (Duncan, 2010). The therapist uses his own insight to shepherd the client's awareness toward her deeper experience, not through interpretation that causes anxiety (Stark, 1999), but by tracking the client's present-moment experience, contacting what is tracked, and creating experiments in mindfulness to help the client access and work with her core material. The client experiences the warmth and emotional understanding of the therapist, which supports her own discovery and growth (Fosha, 2009a; Kurtz, 1990a). Because the therapist leads by following and joins with the client's authentic curiosity (Johanson, 1988), general resistance to the growth process is lessened as the cooperation of the unconscious increases (Kurtz, 1990a).

Attunement, Resonance, and Use of Insight

A therapist must be open in order to attune with the client. All notions of certainty must be held lightly. To attune to another, the therapist must be able to let go of her expectations and allow herself to rest in the mystery and uncertainty (Johanson & Kurtz, 1991) that comes with being awash with present experience (D. Siegel, 2010). Once attuned, the two can resonate with each other, making a functional whole of the two autonomous entities that is larger than the sum of its individual parts (D. Siegel, 2010). The client can feel the positive regard of the therapist; the therapist can sense and feel the inner experience of the client. Therefore, the Hakomi therapist pays attention to her own experience while simultaneously tracking the client to attune and resonate with him, moment by moment. In this way, the therapist endeavors to maintain the allostatic attunement (Sterling, 2004) with the client without disruption.

When the therapeutic alliance is resonating in place, the therapist invites the client through this attunement to study the organization of his experience (Piers, Muller, & Brent, 2007). This approach uses insight, experience, and relationship (Stark, 1999), but not interpretations or interventions by the therapist that would disrupt the client's experience, the empathy of the therapist, or the intersubjective field. As Morgan (2013) expresses it:

> Attunement and empathy is an essential foundation to therapeutic change. Hakomi therapists become skilled in tracking. This is essential for the contingent communication that activates resonating brain states and corticolimbic connections. Therapists need to be adept at tracking their own body processes, as these are vital in connecting deeply with another. Therapists need to be willing to compassionately repair empathy lapses as these repairs pave the way to self-regulation in the client. Attuning to and managing shame states allows for new growth in limbocortical pathways. (p. 55)

The Hakomi therapist seeks to lower the noise in the relational system by not giving the client anything to resist, so that the client can concentrate on how he organizes his experience and allow new possibilities to emerge (Kurtz, 1990a). This relationship is based on the therapist's belief in the inherent wholeness and goodness of the client and his natural ability to reorganize toward increasing wholeness (Monda, 2000). However, since barriers to reorganization are normally habitual, implicit, and unconscious, the therapist tracks and contacts potential barriers, shepherding them into the client's awareness where they can be dealt with. Thus, the therapist demonstrates trust in the client, in their relationship, and in the process itself, including fears and obstacles. The therapist is not caught between empathy and interruption, or the client's need to be understood versus the need to understand, nor between being a good object versus being a real subject (Stark, 1999). All of these purposes are joined together in the therapeutic relationship and the full, conscious participation of the therapist.

Creating the Bubble

In the Hakomi method, the therapist constantly tends to the therapeutic relationship through the techniques of contact, tracking, and creating the bubble. The bubble is a metaphor for a palpable connection between client and therapist that is infused with warmth, presence, awareness, and attention. This is the particular flavor of the intersubjective field that the therapist fosters that is open to whatever quality is needed in relation to the kind of attachment needs the client brings (Eisman, 2005; Fonagy & Target, 1997; Fosha, 2003; Morgan, 2013). The therapist's ability to be present, to attune, and to resonate with the client allows the client to feel "felt" (D. Siegel, 2010).

"Good therapy has a feel to it" (Kurtz, 1990a, p. 59). The therapist uses all of her faculties—cognition, intuition, awareness, emotions, and so on—to deepen her understanding and stay in authentic contact and connection with her client. While the therapist may have a strong empathic response, as well as other subjective reactions, she does not completely believe them, but continues to be open to confirming, disconfirming, nuanced, or new forms of information. Her goal is to join in the experience with the client in order to create a therapeutic alliance of perceived safety, which inspires the curiosity of the client to study his own experience (Kurtz, 1990a). In addition to not giving the client anything to resist, safety means supporting a spaciousness that allows the client room to explore—once he is convinced the therapist is in the bubble with him, helping him to go where his inner wisdom wants to take him at the deepest levels.

Loving Presence

Loving presence is defined by Kurtz as a state of being—a state of consciousness. In this state, a person experiences an embodied sense of well-being and positive affect (Fredrickson, 2001; Fredrickson & Losada, 2005; Johnson, 2009). Loving presence implies an awareness of self and other and the interconnectedness between them. It requires a connection with one's own sense of goodness, as well as the goodness of the other, and the goodness of life in general. Warmth and friendliness emerge with this state. Everything is welcome without bias. Such presence adds another dimension to therapy (Fosha, 1992, 2004). The therapeutic "relationship transcends itself and becomes part of something larger. Profound growth and healing and energy are present" (Rogers, 1980, p. 129).

The Hakomi therapist actively uses mindfulness to work with his own state of mind as he strives to cultivate loving presence. While great effort may sometimes be required in the practice of loving presence, ultimately it is a state of willingness rather than willfulness (May, 1982), of being rather than doing.

When a therapist is in a state of loving presence, he feels calm and open (Eisman, 2006). He can receive the client's whole experience in an embodied way (Marlock & Weiss, 2001). This includes whatever the client is consciously presenting, as well as that which is present and unconscious or nonconscious. A limbic resonance (Lewis et al., 2000) develops between the two. This attitude on the part of the therapist is "crucial and is not easy. It requires a deep understanding of one's self as well as the client. It must be part of the emotional makeup of the therapist, not something one simulates as part of one's role" (Kurtz, 1990a, p. 60). The loving presence of the therapist also helps the client develop this inner attitude of warmth and friendliness through modeling (Rogers, 1961).

The authentic curiosity of the therapist in this state prevents his own agendas or thought process from taking over the therapy. If the therapist engages in the intersubjective field from a more subjective orientation, then he risks allowing his own beliefs, interpretations, and needs (conscious and unconscious) to dominate in the exchange, thereby compromising the client's process. The therapist can be aware of his needs (for example, to know, to understand, to be right, to be helpful, to be liked, to be with or avoid strong emotions, chaos, confusion, and so on) in a state of mindfulness, with a powerful internal observer present, and with loving presence. This way he can both manage them appropriately and gauge their impact on the client. The practice of loving presence creates space for the therapist to know his experience and draw from it by choice (Prenn, 2009).

Empathy and Understanding

Loving presence includes empathy and authenticity (Decety & Jackson, 2004; Paivio & Laurent, 2001). Authenticity reflects the therapist's experience directly, including her countertransference and personal bias. In being empathic, the therapist leaves aside her own thoughts and feelings and joins with the client in his world. "Empathy enables the creation of 'intersubjectivity' and the increasingly social and shared nature of much of the content of human consciousness, in which individuals can have deeply shared emotional spaces, with this becoming a critical aspect of all long-term attachments" (Watt, 2005, p. 205). Along with resonance with another's pain (perceived or inferred), empathy indicates an associated desire to mitigate his suffering. According to Watt (2005), empathy is possibly the most critical outcome variable from the therapist's side in the therapeutic interaction.

The selflessness of empathy and the reactivity of authenticity are both tempered by mindfulness and compassion (Davidson & Harrington, 2002; Fehr, Sprecher, & Underwood, 2009; Gilbert, 2005). Like two reins held together, the therapist can both locate in the client's experience without losing herself, and she can observe her own experience while distinguishing between reaction and response. Loving presence takes the therapist out of the duality of empathy versus authenticity into a larger arena that includes both. In this way, loving presence creates safety by allowing the process to unfold in accordance with the client's needs and integrity.

Even when moments of empathic failure occur, the therapist can come back to loving presence and authentic truth sharing. Empathic failure can be useful in therapy. At those moments, the pain is present in the moment, as is the possibility of repair when the therapist is truthful about what has occurred and actively moves to mend the break (Meares, 2005). The failure affirms the distinction between the inner world and the outer. In such moments, the client comes to realize the therapist is human, not omniscient and omnipotent (Meares, 2005). Tronick (1998, 2007, 2009) considers the working-through process in therapy to be a dyadic venture of interactive repair. The therapist's ability to navigate relationship repair depends very much on the therapist's ability to recognize and regulate the negative affect within herself (Schore, 2003), transcending shame and pride in the service of connection.

The process is fostered by the Hakomi attitude of proceeding experimentally, never being attached to a particular result, along with being prepared for the process to self-correct through the direction of the client's organic wisdom. It is especially important for Hakomi therapists to monitor the parallel interpersonal process to the client's intrapsychic one (Lamagna & Gleiser, 2007). For instance, if a therapist were not able to tolerate anger in the client's relationship with her when the client is working on a new core organizing belief that anger is okay in relationships, the result would be a characterological disaster confirming the client's worst fears, if the therapist were not to recognize it and make repair.

To these ends, the therapist allows real intimacy in the relationship. That is, she allows herself to be fully touched by the client's experience and she uses her own experience with the client as a basis for an authentic response (Natterson, 1991; Prenn, 2009; Rogers, 1951, 1961, 1980), as well as a means of gathering information about the client (objective countertransference) and what is happening in the moment. The therapist is a witnessing participant (Hirsch, 1987) and, in cultivating mindfulness with her client, encourages the client to also become a witnessing participant (Weiss, 2008).

Such reception precedes any intervention so that the therapist's responses and interventions are based on and embodied in the unique, authentic, dyadic relationship rather than cognitive processing. By being receptive to the client, the therapist can attune to the pace of the client and his unconscious needs, thereby increasing the general safety.

Listening to the Storyteller

The therapist demonstrates his understanding of the client not only by what he says but also by what he does and how he relates to the client. This understanding encompasses not only the "story" the client is telling, but also the storyteller. It is too easy to become lost in a client's story and its thousand variations, and lose sight of the core narrative beliefs that generate the basic themes of the storyteller. In a state of loving presence, the therapist gathers the deepest levels of information from the nonverbal presence and expression of the client. The client's use of language, her tone and rhythm of speech, and her gestures and overall body state are conveyed to the therapist, who listens for beliefs and assumptions, and connects present behaviors and beliefs with possible childhood situations or experiences (Fisher, 2011; Kurtz, 1990a).

When the therapist cultivates a state of loving presence, he can bear witness to the experiences and parts of the self the client avoids or represses with the utmost warmth and friendliness. He can pay constant attention to what the client neither tells nor remembers, but what is enacted or communicated in the session in extraverbal forms—allowing the prosody to pierce his countertransferential skin more than the semantic content of the client's narrative (Mancia, 2006).

The therapist resolves to not lose himself in his role; he desires to remain relaxed and attentive to the client's experiences without reacting to the storyteller's story from a place of egoistic fear. Nothing is viewed as a problem or difficult. Everything is a reflection of how experience is managed. Loving presence allows for strengths and beauty to be experienced in the midst of pain, confusion, or strong emotion. Whatever emerges can be met with loving-kindness, thereby enhancing the safety in the relationship and the trust in the process. Loving presence anchors the process in the here and now and generates flexibility. It invites the guiding wisdom and signals of the unconscious to become more and more present, and assists the client in moving toward her innate sense of wholeness, through the possibility of organizing in elements of the core narrative (contact, support, intimacy, freedom, ease, and so on) that were previously organized out (Johanson, 2015). The practice of loving presence cultivates the optimal conditions for human growth and change (Bridges, 2006).

Safety

Each client experiences safety uniquely. A therapist has to tend to each client individually, addressing both conscious and unconscious needs for safety. Safety is always defined by the way a client perceives a situation, whether it is "objectively" safe or not. Porges (2011) notes that neuroception—a person constantly scanning for safety—is ever present. If the therapeutic process slows or stops, it is inevitably a safety issue on some level. The attitude of loving presence, the therapist's abilities for attunement, empathy, and understanding as well as her ability to actively demonstrate them, all add to the client's felt sense of safety.

Just as infant-caregiver relationships are recognized as unique dyads with an inherent rhythm of relationship, so each client-therapist pair engages in a rhythm all its own (Beebe & Lachmann, 1998, 2002). As adults, clients may have an aversion to care and compassion, so the therapist must be able to track and contact that aversion without taking it personally. The therapist who can be authentically and naturally present with the client in a way that joins a particular client's need for closeness and/or distance has all of her resources available for the client's safety.

Tracking the moment-to-moment relationship provides the therapist with invaluable data regarding the safety status of the client, what relaxes him, and what activates him. How relaxed the client is, how open and forthcoming, the amount and quality of eye contact, all give clues to the client's safety in the relationship and with the psychological material emerging. The more the therapist stays in contact with the client, not caretaking, but providing authentic safety, the more the client is available for self-study. In this way, following the client's lead and pace, staying on equal ground (not becoming the expert or in any way removed from the client), and allowing the client to follow his own insights and curiosity all add to the safety in the relationship.

The therapist's genuine warmth and caring are essential ingredients for the client to allow difficult unconscious material to emerge. Any harsh judgment, perceived by the client or not, will interfere with the therapeutic process. The skillfulness of the therapist, as well as her openness and confidence, add to the safety of the client. Porges's (2009) polyvagal theory demonstrates that everyone scans for safety before being able to engage socially. Cozolino asserts that the warmth, enthusiasm, and encouragement of the therapist optimize the biochemical conditions for learning—the "enhanced production of dopamine, serotonin, norepinephrine and other endogenous endorphins . . . support neural growth and plasticity" (2002, p. 300). Engaging in the therapeutic relationship provides safety moment by moment as well as enhancing the overall safety and well-being of the client.

Cooperation of the Unconscious

The therapeutic relationship impacts the "cooperation of the unconscious" quite directly. Kurtz (1990a) used this term to describe the goal and primary outcome of a well-working therapeutic relationship. When the client feels safe, the process moves along, there is cooperation of the client's unconscious, and previously repressed or dissociated material emerges. When resistance arises, it is because the dyad is misattuned or some need of the client has gone unattended. Perhaps the therapist misunderstood the client or shifted out of mindfulness and loving presence. Perhaps he sped up when the client needed to slow down. Resistance always has emotional intelligence at work—it has a good reason to be there. When even a slight resistance is tracked, contacted, and honored, the cooperation of the unconscious can be established or regained, and whatever interaction interfered with the client's feeling of safety can be studied in mindfulness. It becomes a constructive moment of repair.

Signs for the cooperation of the unconscious in the client include a focused attention to the moment-by-moment interaction; thoughtful consideration and responses to the therapist's questions and suggestions; the inclusion of the therapist in the client's interactions; and genuine participation (Kurtz, 1990a). A therapist needs to be able to read the signs of the unconscious and adjust to the client's needs and interests in order to earn her cooperation. If the therapist fails to do this, the client will demonstrate signs of resistance: disregarding the therapist's input, proceeding without connecting with the therapist, taking off in a different direction, not considering the therapist's interventions or suggestions, and so forth. "When the unconscious cooperates, significant material emerges" (Kurtz, 1990a, p. 59).

The safety of the relationship and the cooperation of the unconscious are not dependent on whether or not the therapist correctly interprets the information gathered from the client. Because insight is used to create little experiments in mindfulness rather than as interpretations in and of themselves (Feinstein, 1990), the client's defenses are befriended rather than challenged. Because interpretation is not necessary to the implementation or success of the process, a Hakomi therapist has no investment in being an expert or being right. Consequently, little resistance to self-study is created. Whatever insight is required for change to occur arises primarily from the implicit experiences of the client. Together, therapist and client discover the meaning throughout the stages of the Hakomi process. It is this kind of continual involvement of cognitive and emotional processing that is essential for positive change (Cozolino, 2010).

To be creative and intuitive, to participate fully in the healing relationship, the therapist must cultivate the cooperation of his own unconscious (Kurtz, 1990a). Thus, the therapist must be able to hold himself with the attitude of loving-kindness and be connected to his own experience (Cooper, 1999; Eisman, 2006). When everything is accepted, when nothing is a genuine problem, when all experience is welcome, the feel of the interaction is very open and even playful. Playful exploration of experiences, amplification of the client's awareness, and the sense that the experiences are the client's own reflect the proper role of the therapist (not demonstrating the therapist's brilliance) (Meares, 2005). Both client and therapist feel the genuine goodness that accompanies self-discovery and loving presence.

Summary and Conclusion

The therapeutic relationship is the container in which all healing takes place in psychotherapy. It is crucial not only to the success of the therapy, but also to the overall positive experience of the client. This relationship works on many levels, both conscious and unconscious. It requires great attention on the part of the therapist and wholehearted effort to cultivate the attitudes that promote healing: loving presence, warmth, empathy, authenticity within intersubjectivity, openness, clarity, self-awareness, acceptance, discernment, and trust in the client's unfolding process. Such ongoing practice not only benefits clients but also deepens the therapist's inner experience and wholeness. As the therapeutic relationship creates safety for the client, it promotes full cooperation of the unconscious, which in turn provides the organic impulses and signals toward the healing needed. This kind of exchange occurs in an intersubjective field of real contact between two human beings. The resonance between therapist and client works both inside and outside of consciousness. The path of self-discovery and healing is not traversed alone. The love and connection inherent in this human bond become part of the reorganization of the client on every level.

CHAPTER 10

Mindfulness as a Psychotherapeutic Tool

John Perrin

It is your mind that creates the world.

The Dhammapada

Cognition is not a representation of an independently existing world, but rather a continuing bringing forth of a world through the process of living.

Francisco Varela and Humberto Maturana,
The Tree of Knowledge, 1992

Mindfulness is the aware, balanced acceptance of the present experience. It isn't more complicated than that. It is opening to or receiving the present moment, pleasant or unpleasant, just as it is, without either clinging to it or rejecting it.

Sylvia Boorstein, *It's Easier Than You Think*, 1997

THE VALUE OF mindfulness is finding widespread acceptance within mainstream psychology, four decades since Hakomi founder Ron Kurtz pioneered its use in psychodynamic therapy—and over 2,500 years since its healing properties were first recognized and its practice codified by Eastern wisdom teachers. Today, a strong movement is developing toward the use of mindfulness in both the psychodynamic traditions (Germer et al., 2005) and the cognitive-behavioral traditions (Hayes et al., 2004; Johanson 2006; Mace, 2008; Segal et al., 2002), while Zen Buddhist training has influenced Jon Kabat-Zinn's mindfulness-based stress reduction programs and Marsha Linehan's dialectical behavior therapy.

The Act of Just Noticing

Mindfulness can be understood as a special state of consciousness, characterized by "receiving the present moment, pleasant or unpleasant, just as it is, without either clinging to it nor rejecting it" (Boorstein, 1997, p. 60). Typically, attention is focused on internal experiences, either on the inner world in general or on specific features of this landscape. The attitude is open, receptive, and curious—without acting on any impulse to change, judge, or prove a theory about what is being observed. It brings bare attention in a being, noneffortful mode. The pace is slower than ordinary consciousness, and one can lose a sense of time and space, like a child lost in play. This is in contrast to ordinary consciousness that is often in an active, fast-paced, goal-directed, habitual, unreflective doing mode that is effortful, with a narrow focus and external orientation toward dealing with some kind of problem to be solved. Mindfulness is also known as witnessing, open attention, or open awareness.

Although mindfulness is a natural state of consciousness, it typically has to be learned and cultivated in an ongoing process of deepening skill—and isn't always easy (Faucheaux & Weiss, 1995). Traditionally, mindfulness has been achieved by dedicated practices such as daily sitting or walking meditation, yoga, tai chi, and so forth. The cultivation of mindfulness is a form of meditation, but the two terms are not strictly interchangeable. Meditation practices pursue a variety of goals, such as calming the mind, increasing concentration, expanding awareness, and promoting equanimity and compassion, which might or might not be in line with the immediate unfolding needs of psychotherapy.

For meditation purposes, a range of techniques is employed. The meditation student may at first simply concentrate on an object in present experience. For example, a foundational exercise is to count one's breaths from one to ten, without losing focus. (Easier said than done, as it turns out.) Alternatively, one may immerse the mind in a mantra or a chant, or exhaust one's enthusiasm for logical thought by contemplating a Zen koan. There are a number of established variations. It may involve the practice of pure open attention, such as the Shikantaza (just sitting) practice observed by Zen Buddhists of the Soto school, or the systematic sweeping of attention through the body and the active differentiation of mental processes that characterize vipassana (insight meditation) practice. There are analogous meditation forms in other worldwide traditions.

Often, meditation is practiced in a peaceful setting, where external distractions can fade. As the mind settles, it becomes possible to observe mental activities as they arise within the field of awareness. This process is often likened to dropping a stone into a still pond and watching the ripples that are automatically and effortlessly created.

Regular meditation can improve focus, calmness, self-regulation, and expansiveness, sometimes in profound and lasting ways. It improves with practice, and experienced practitioners can develop highly refined states of awareness. Skilled meditators show interesting changes, such as the effective dissolution of the startle reflex (Goleman, 2003).

Mindfulness in Psychotherapy

Mindfulness practice can be a lifelong path, leading perhaps to the deeply absorbed states achieved by experienced meditators—called samadhi in the Buddhist and Hindu traditions—and maybe even ultimately to a state of enlightenment. In psychotherapy, we can employ mindfulness for more modest aims. Even fleeting glimpses of deeper awareness can be immensely useful in therapy.

The practice of mindfulness utilizes the internal observer or witness—an aspect of the mind that is inherently detached or disidentified from the objects of which it is aware, constituting a different neural net than the parts of one's ego with object relations histories (Kershaw & Wade, 2011). There have been analogous concepts in psychotherapy. Psychoanalysts talk about employing the reflexive ego. The externalization techniques of Gestalt and other modalities put clients in the position of observing inner dynamics, as opposed to being blended or fused with them. Cognitive-behavioral therapists have realized the importance of distancing to many of their techniques (Beck et al., 1979; Hayes, 2004; Hayes et al., 2004). As Kegan (1982) suggests in his approach to therapy, it is important that what was subjective is made objective for a person to have freedom to grow.

Mindfulness can be used to promote greater detachment from thoughts and feelings. For example, instead of trying to distract from or argue with an unpleasant thought, mindfulness simply makes the thought less important by being able to witness it as one aspect of experience among many. When mindful, individuals are able to observe the panoply of sensations, feelings, thoughts, images, and memories that typically bypass conscious awareness. This bare attention has great power. By "decentering" from the contents of mental phenomena, clients are able to tolerate distressing thoughts and feelings without avoiding or "acting out" (Fulton & Siegel, 2005). Moreover, mindfulness also allows an automatic response to "recognize itself" before it is carried out (Myllerup, 2004). Studies indicate that even though the intention to act is formulated in the brain before we are aware of it, people have veto power over motor activity when they are mindful (Libet, 1999 in Germer, 2005, p. 23). Mindfulness thus modifies automatic habits by putting distance between one's feelings and impulses and by making unconscious impulses conscious. Consequently, mindfulness has become an accepted practice in the treatment of depression, anxiety, obsessive-compulsive disorder, borderline personality disorder (Baer, 2003), and other disorders.

Even a modest practice of mindfulness can produce a range of benefits, including improved immune function; improved response flexibility and the capacity to understand someone else's mind (Siegel & Hartzell, 2003); improved self-regulation (the ability to modulate emotional reactions); greater self-awareness; and a capacity to develop distance from impulses, beliefs, or feelings as they arise (disidentification).

Becoming mindful generally expands the field of awareness through locating one's consciousness in a serene, poised mental state that can release itself to a wider spectrum of experience. Over time, the chatter of thoughts tends to recede, displaced by the more immediate sense of aliveness that arises from the constantly changing waves of sensation and sense experiences that are the foundations of the self (Damasio, 2000). With sufficient practice, mindfulness can produce clear and lasting shifts in consciousness that make it easier to connect and center oneself in its qualities of awareness and compassion (Hanson with Mendius, 2009).

Repairing Disconnections

Change is founded on the capacity for self-observation. Eugene Gendlin (1982) observed that the capacity of a person to remain focused on present experience is a trustworthy indicator of good outcomes in psychotherapy. Moshe Feldenkrais understood the vital role of awareness in achieving change, and was known for saying that until you know what you are doing, you cannot do what you want.

Mindfulness increases coherence between various mental functions, weaving together thinking and feeling, connecting the left and right brains, and improving communication between, and awareness of, various ego states or subpersonalities (Siegel, 2007).

By making the mind space bigger, mindfulness allows for a higher-order understanding of mental processes. This has been likened to zooming out a camera lens. We begin to see the forest and not just the trees. We are identified with the seer, not fused or blended in what is seen. As the field of awareness is expanded, disconnected aspects of experience can be integrated into a more complex whole. This is in accord with Wilber's (1979) suggestion that therapy can be conceived of as healing disconnects or splits. Perhaps one part of the mind (anger or sadness) is split from another (care or independence). The mind might be disconnected from the sensations, feelings, and muscle tensions of the body. The mind-body self might not sense its connection to the environment around it. Kabat-Zinn concurs with this perspective: "With regard to disease and dis-ease, we might say that most fundamental dis-ease stemming from disattention and disconnection, and from mis-perception and mis-attribution, is the anguish of the human condition itself, of the full catastrophe unmet and unexamined" (2005, p. 124).

Lost in Thought

Mindfulness promotes experiential knowledge over conceptual understanding. This reverses a form of disconnection that can be broadly characterized as a split between thoughts and direct experience (Johanson, 1996; Johnson, 1985). The mind has an automatic tendency to reify experience—to substitute symbolic representations (thoughts, ideas, images, and so on) for experience itself. When we are swimming in an ocean of concepts, mistaking them for reality, we are not "grounded" but rather cut off from the aspects of our intelligence that arise from the direct experience of sensations and feelings (LeDoux, 1996). Charles Tart suggests this is an especially contemporary ailment: "Believing that we fully know a thing just because we can give it a verbal name and associate other intellectual knowledge to it is one of the greatest failures of modern culture" (1987, p. 190). While modern culture may indeed encourage us to become lost in thought, this tendency has been recognized for centuries. Not to mistake the pointing finger for the moon to which it is pointing is a counsel of ancient Buddhism.

Falling Asleep

The human mind naturally tunes out, or disconnects, from painful or unwelcome aspects of experience. This censoring leads to a range of dissociated states, some which have been likened to being partially asleep (Cozolino, 2010).

"Dissociation" is a loose term that describes a vast and complex range of mental phenomena. Fragmentation of experience may occur for short episodes or may be effectively permanent. We can check out anywhere along the continuum of ordinary human experience that ranges from thought to feeling. At the thought end of this spectrum, we may become ungrounded—disconnected from the immediate somatic experiences that give us the sense of embodiment. In such a state, we lose access to the felt sense of our emotional intelligence. Folk wisdom has long recognized this phenomenon. Popular parlance reflects the value of "coming to our senses." At the other extreme, we may become flooded (Gottman, 1998) in strong feeling states without much capacity for thought, self-awareness, or self-regulation. Disconnection may arise between the building blocks of experience (thoughts, memories, images, feelings, bodily sensations, impulses, and sense experiences) or between higher orders of psychological organization, such as between different subpersonalities or ego states (Watkins & Watkins, 1997).

While dissociative responses are usually understood to be self-limiting, they can also be seen as functional attempts to deal with internal conflicts when more effective resources are not available. Gestalt therapist Joseph Zinker says,

> This sleepy wakefulness, this creative adaptation to the pain in the world, is . . . resistance to contact and resistance to awareness. In this way, resistance . . . allows the avoidance of one type of contact in favor of maintaining contact with something other than the immediate experience; unawareness becomes for the organism the "lesser of two evils." (1994, p. 117)

Optimal psychological organization broadly involves a combination of thinking and feeling, a connection between what Gilligan (1997) has termed the autobiographical self and the somatic self. But adapting to emotional insults may bring a kind of psychological fragmentation, as certain aspects of experience become split off or dissociated.

The end result of this process has been termed "self-negation." Although it is an intelligent attempt to adapt to a particular environment, there is a cost to such a strategy. A part of the person has been shut down or kept out of awareness. As Almaas explains, "But something happens when we build a shell and hide inside it, which is the source of most human complaints. When we cover up our vulnerability so we're not open to hurt and pain, fear and influence, we also become insensitive to joy, love, happiness, pleasure, and aliveness" (1990, p. 196). This splitting off creates the kind of disconnection that mindfulness can eventually integrate or repair. Mindfulness is great medicine for almost all forms of dissociation.

A special case of dissociation, of course, relates to those dealing with post-traumatic stress disorder, which includes lower brain activation stemming from fearing one's life is in danger. Mindfulness is crucial to healing such conditions, but the therapist must switch to mindfulness of sensation and bottom-up processing so that retraumatization is avoided (Ogden et al., 2006; see Chapter 24 on trauma).

Disidentification

Entering into mindfulness can radically change our notions of who we are. While we may embrace the ego's conceit that it is the author of our experience, our sense of identity is in fact an artifact of mental processes, and not the source of them. Brain studies have shown that our experience is constantly being generated before we become aware of it. In the 1970s, Benjamin Libet, a psychologist at the University of California, San Francisco, found that brain signals associated with voluntary actions occurred half a second before the subject was conscious of deciding to make them.

Not only is our ego identity haplessly astride an experience-making vehicle over which it has no real control, but further investigation also reveals that there is not even one single, reliable I. For this reason, the koan "Who are you?" has long been employed for its powers to loosen the grip of the autobiographical self. To likewise loosen up one's sense of solidness, Kurtz invented an exercise in which one person would ask another some basic questions, one at a time, such as, "How old are you?" "Are you male or female?" "How many children do you have?" The one questioned would sit with his or her response until able to say, "I don't know."

In contrast to the myth of a monolithic self, many schools of therapy (such as Gestalt, transactional analysis, psychosynthesis, and so on) have recognized that human psychology is organized into a repertoire or multiplicity (Rowan & Cooper, 1999) of distinct personality patterns, which can be thought of as "parts" (Schwartz, 1995) or "trance identities" (Wolinsky, 1991).

Typically, we are not aware that we contain multitudes. The mind conceals an automatic procession of characters by creating an overarching sense of "I-dentity" that endorses each state in turn as "This is who I am." Without mindfulness, the transition from one part to the next happens unconsciously and automatically, as the costume of one player is seamlessly exchanged for that of the next. However, through the use of mindfulness, we can cultivate a witness that is able to watch this inner pageant from a detached yet compassionate perspective. When we can observe our experiences as they arise, we begin to directly discern automatic responses, to understand them and to free ourselves from their grasp. As we become disidentified from what would otherwise be automatic patterns of perception and behavior, we become more self-aware. Daniel Goleman (1996) has called this the cornerstone of emotional intelligence. This is immensely useful in individual psychotherapy and it is also of tremendous value when working with couples or groups, where mindfulness can disrupt the inevitably cyclical interplay of such automatic patterns (Fisher, 2002).

Mindfulness in Hakomi Therapy

Hakomi therapy employs mindfulness in that most traditional of psychotherapeutic pursuits: the making conscious of what is unconscious. Thus, like the spiritual traditions it has borrowed from, Hakomi employs mindfulness with the aim of helping people to wake up—to become conscious. The use of mindfulness is deeply integrated into the methodology and process of Hakomi. This is in contrast to therapeutic approaches that employ mindfulness simply as part of a tool kit, where clients are taught elements of mindfulness as an adjunct to traditional treatment protocols.

Talk therapies seek to reveal the hidden layers of the mind through techniques such as free association or self-reflection. This kind of inquiry often brings a certain calmness that comes simply from deeper understanding. But mindfulness can take us far deeper than mere introspection. It can also provide access to the deep psychic structures that directly shape what we like to think of as reality. The human mind relies heavily on stored models of the world, which are generalized from previous formative experiences. Most of these patterns are useful, but some contain inherent limitations because they are historical in nature and therefore not necessarily a very good fit with the present moment. Elements that were wisely shut out of one's life—such as support, intimacy, or self-assertion—because it made survival sense at earlier times continue beyond the time when they could be realistically reintroduced.

Ron Kurtz has called these mental maps the "organizers of experience." "These core organizers are definitions and blueprints of the most basic issues about our being in the world. They are our reference points, our measures of the self and others, with which we set our expectations, goals, and limits" (Kurtz, 1990a, p. 14). They are part of our universal need to make meaning out of the life we experience (Stolorow et al., 1987).

These mental maps are encoded in what is known as nonverbal (implicit) memory. In contrast to verbal (explicit) memory, when implicit memory is retrieved, it lacks the internal sensation that something is being recalled. Thus, emotions, behaviors, bodily sensations, perceptual interpretations, and the bias of particular nonconscious mental models may influence our present experience (both perception and behavior) without our having any realization that we are being shaped by the past (Bennett-Goleman, 2001; Siegel & Hartzell, 2003). In this fashion, human psychology is greatly determined by automatically arising patterns of experience. As creatures, we are most typically on autopilot.

The normal narrowing, shrinking, or fixating of attention of everyday consciousness has been characterized as a kind of trance (Wolinsky, 1991). While such trances are a natural (and often functionally necessary) aspect of the mind, some in particular can prove troublesome, because they are strongly regressive and, at the same time, profoundly compelling. They bring issues and emotions from long ago into what Hakomi founding trainer Dyrian Benz has termed the "past-infused present." To the extent that we are not aware of these patterns, we are at their mercy. But with consciousness, we can free ourselves from their grasp.

It is possible to reach the underlying material that shapes our trance states by paying mindful attention to aspects of present experience shaped or organized by the core narrative beliefs.

> When you work in therapy to study how a gesture, a feeling, or whatever, is automatically made part of experience, you eventually come to memories, images, and beliefs about who we are, what's possible for us, what type of world it is, what it wants from us, and what it will give and take. (Kurtz, 1990a, p. 14)

Observing the automatic nature of self-organization is a central undertaking for Hakomi therapists. On one hand is the stream of automatic, somatic, emotional, and mental self-organization. On the other hand is the observing mind. This observing mind, what is often called the internal observer or the witness, is the Hakomi method's vehicle toward conscious awareness. Mindfulness is the premier tool for empowering one to study the organization of one's experience and get some freedom from its automaticity at the same time (Bargh & Chartrand, 1999; Eisman, 2006; Kershaw & Wade, 2011).

Through the observation of emotions, sensations, impulses, and other automatic reactions to stimuli, we can begin to become conscious of automatic reactions as they arise. Thich Nhat Hanh notes,

> Bare attention identifies and pursues the single threads of that closely interwoven tissue of our habits. . . . Bare attention lays open the minute crevices in the seemingly impenetrable structure of unquestioned mental processes. . . . If the inner connections between the single parts of a seemingly compact whole become intelligible, then it ceases to be inaccessible. . . . If the facts and details of the conditioned nature become known, there is a chance of effecting fundamental changes in it. (1976, pp. 10–11)

It is this capacity to directly observe experience, rather than simply engage in introspection or mental reflection, that makes mindfulness such a potent instrument in therapy.

Present experience is the royal road to implicit memory. Implicit memory networks shape our present experience directly. Thus, by mindfully paying attention to present experience, we can reverse engineer our way to the underlying patterns themselves. As implicit memory networks are lit up, profound and unexpected information, insights, and new possibilities often come to the surface. The emergence of these potent and often unexpected new experiences is a distinctive feature of Hakomi therapy.

Since Hakomi therapists pay disciplined attention to when the unconscious is using a mindful thread of inquiry to lead to what Perls called "unfinished business"—as opposed to simply allowing everything that enters consciousness to float by like a cloud, the method is more precisely considered "mindfulness of the mind," as suggested by Nyanaponika:

> [Use] your own state of mind as meditation's subject. Such meditation reveals and heals. . . . The sadness (or whatever has caused the pain) can be used as a means of liberation from torment and suffering, like using a thorn to remove a thorn (1972, p. 61)

Opening to one's experiential realm through mindfulness enables the processing of formative experiences. By our shepherding of the client's attention, we deepen into experience (Chapter 15) so that regressive states are accessed—taking care to keep the observer present so that there is no danger of malign regression. Then the therapist, with the help of the mindful client, looks for and introduces new experiences previously organized out as too threatening, to help integrate a fuller organicity to the system (Chapters 18–20)—what is also termed "memory reconsolidation" (Cozolino, 2010). This whole process, from the beginning of accessing to the integration of transformative missing experiences, is wrapped in mindfulness, without which it would be impossible.

Assisted Self-Study: Mindfulness in the Therapeutic Relationship

Unlike traditional mindfulness practice, employing Hakomi's mindfulness of the mind is a kind of collaborative meditation that Kurtz has described as "assisted self-study." The use of mindfulness in relationship enables access to otherwise uncharted territory, partly because the therapist, through providing safety and loving presence, has an opportunity to actively, though nonviolently, influence the focus of a client's awareness. Left to its own devices, a person's experience tends to organize itself along habitual lines. From a therapeutic point of view, this process yields little or no new information and may result in interminable therapy without some active, collaborative (Duncan, 2010), organically informed intervention.

Even prolonged classic meditation practice has its limitations. As Zen teacher Joko Beck has warned, the meditation cushion can become a parking lot. Critical aspects of experience remain unconscious, in a dissociative process John Welwood (2002) has called "spiritual bypassing." Experienced meditators are not immune from such blind spots. Buddhist meditation teacher Jack Kornfield observed, "there were major areas in my life, such as loneliness, intimate relationships, work, childhood wounds, and patterns of fear, that even very deep meditation didn't touch" (1998, p. 38). Therapists can help people remain mindful of how their unconscious is leading them deeply into core organizers that need attention when difficult or chaotic material arises. In his book *A Path With Heart*, Kornfield (1993) recommends Hakomi texts and methods when one's ability to progress with classic meditation is compromised by unconscious emotional barriers.

Regulation of Attention Processes

Through inviting the client's attention processes toward a calm, open, and compassionate attitude, the therapist models an expansive consciousness, repeatedly acknowledging the reality of various parts of the client as they arise, but never losing sight of the bigger picture.

The regulation of the bigger picture in terms of attention processes is a fundamental task for the Hakomi therapist. It requires that the therapist track the client's state of consciousness from moment to moment, specifically to distinguish between reactive, habitual, and automatic (identified) reactions versus those where the internal observer (mindfulness) is present.

Becoming mindful is not always easy. Some people need quite a bit of help to learn how to witness to their own experience. Even experienced meditators may unwittingly move away from painful or difficult psychological experiences. Hakomi therapists, therefore, function to actively shepherd consciousness by gently disrupting and redirecting automatic patterns of experience in favor of felt, present experience. We study when our clients are in the grip of automatic behavior or outdated maps of reality, watching for when they are being reactive, rather than mindful or responsive.

Being reactive shows up in terms of clients identifying with a part or self-state of the ego. They act and talk as if they are sadness. They are anger. They are fused, blended, or hijacked by a part of their inner multiplicity (Goleman, 1996; Schwartz, 1995). This is different from being present to one's experience and able to notice and report on it without losing contact with it: "I notice sensations around my mouth and neck, and they have the quality of sadness . . . no, more like grief." Or, "I notice the muscles in my arms and stomach tensing up, and wanting to strike out. And there is a sense of unfairness coming up, and memories of a second grade teacher that are not quite clear." These reports reveal the person is in a mindful self-state that exhibits the ability to be present to spontaneous experience, but distant enough to be able to bring awareness and curiosity—qualities of mindfulness along with compassion and wisdom. As with training a muscle, the more often clients access these qualities of what can be termed the essential self (the more the neural nets are strengthened through usage) helps clients more easily find their way back to it. It is also a supportive form of resourcing to help clients into this larger self-state as soon as possible in the process so that more stressful ego states are not unnecessarily empowered and reinforced (Eisman, 2006; Fosha, 2009b; Schwartz, 1995). Over time, the essential self or mindful aspect of consciousness becomes more central as historical wounds weaken their influence on present-moment experiencing.

Typically, the process will begin with helping clients to slow down and redirecting the focus of their attention toward present experience. When the client is not mindful, the therapist's job is to intervene in ways that coax forward the client's internal observer and essential self-qualities. While the initial phase of the therapy allows clients to tell their stories, the therapeutic phase moves into the depth area of core narrative beliefs or filters that characterize the storyteller. When deepening into core material, therapists particularly learn to track for indicators—the external, unconscious mannerisms that give us clues about the client's core material (Chapter 3)—including gestures, posture, quality of concentration, gaze, patterns of tension, tone of voice, and so forth. By tracking these cues, it is possible to direct the client's attention to those points in the process where the therapist sees evidence of limiting, formative experiences.

Significant emotional memories are often activated when people become mindful. These patterns, encoded in implicit memory, take longer to light up than their better-known cousins, verbal or explicit memories, with which we are more familiar. For this reason, when we invite a client to mindfully stay with an experience, it may initially seem as though nothing new is emerging. At this stage, we may need to encourage our clients to linger beyond a point where they would not otherwise do so. If we persist in this way, after what may take up to several minutes, we can expect to see them undergo a distinct shift in their state of consciousness, as they settle into a mindful state, with their attention focused in the here and now. The emergency emerges, as Perls used to say, as the normally unconscious disposition toward increased wholeness leads the client deeper into core material, as the safe and mindful state of the therapeutic bubble is stabilized.

A foundational job for the Hakomi therapist is closely tracking and responding to the client in the service of stabilizing this process. This is crucial, because even if one starts with a focus on present experience, the client's attention can rapidly become occupied with associated thoughts that lead away from embodied experience. This can be particularly true for someone who highly values verbal understanding, as Daniel Stern describes:

> Often when the (psychodynamically well-trained) patient starts to tell about a present moment, as soon as he comes upon a sensation, feeling, image, or word that leads to an associative pathway, he is likely to take that path. This means the exploration of the experienced-as-lived gets interrupted by associative work that leads away from the original present moment. (2004, p. 138)

This tendency can short-circuit the deepening of focused attention. The Hakomi therapist can counteract this, if an object seems connected to limiting beliefs, through actively regulating the client's attention, using the technique of staying with and deepening of focused attention (see Chapter 15).

Once mindfulness is stabilized, the client's process tends to unfurl itself. This unfolding is supported by spaciousness on the part of the therapist. In fact, being unobtrusive is part of the art of Hakomi: "when the client is dealing with something new and surprising, and usually emotional, the client needs time to think and feel. This is the time when being silent is the most helpful thing a therapist can do" (Kurtz, 2006, p. 5).

Conclusion

The healing qualities of a mindful state of consciousness have been understood for millennia within Eastern wisdom traditions. Today, mindfulness seems destined to occupy a permanent place of importance in Western psychology as well. The growing interest in its use in therapy may also herald the emergence of a more unified model of psychotherapy, suggests Christopher Germer: "Mindfulness might become a construct that draws clinical theory, research, and practice closer together, and helps integrate the private and professional lives of therapists" (Germer et al., 2005, p. 11).

Aside from its therapeutic value for clients, the practice of mindfulness produces tangible benefits for therapists. "Meditating therapists often report feeling more 'present,' relaxed, and receptive with their patients if they meditate earlier in the day" (Germer et al., 2005, p. 18). There are many ways to integrate mindfulness into therapeutic work. "The meditating therapist can relate mindfully to his or her patients within any theoretical frame of reference, including psychodynamic, cognitive-behavioral, family systems, or narrative psychotherapy" (p. 18). This is a core skill for therapists since working so closely with many different clients tends to evoke many parts in the therapist that serve as valuable countertransference information, but will derail the therapy if the therapist becomes fused or blended with them. Thus, in Hakomi, the mindfulness of the therapist is not simply desirable, but is a fundamental ingredient in the therapeutic process. The emphasis on nonjudging awareness of present experience by both therapist and client informs every aspect of the Hakomi method.

Perhaps this is the distinctive contribution of the Hakomi approach—the use of mindfulness as the very foundation and main tool of the therapeutic encounter, as opposed to an adjunct activity.

CHAPTER 11

The Experimental Attitude in Hakomi Therapy: Curiosity in Action

Maci Daye

HUMAN BEINGS ARE hardwired to explore. Our dogged pursuit of knowledge is fueled by the biological imperative to make sense of ourselves and our world (Johanson, 1988). In psychology, for example, researchers assiduously test theories regarding human behavior, while clinicians wrestle with the vexing question: Can people change, and, if so, how? Ron Kurtz devoted his life to answering this question by conducting experiments in the therapy office instead of the lab. A scientist by trade, Kurtz imported an experimental attitude into his exploration of human change processes. Accordingly, Hakomi involves observing behavior, making guesses about underlying processes, and conducting live experiments to discover a person's most deeply held, limiting beliefs about life. The assumption is that these core organizers of experience may hold repetitive, self-defeating behaviors or experiences in place. Change occurs when core organizers are made conscious and transformed. Kurtz explains:

> The essential process is to create the conditions that will bring normally inaccessible, unconscious beliefs and habits into consciousness, beliefs and habits that are inaccurate in some significant way that causes unnecessary suffering.

For example, an unconscious belief that one is not attractive or worthy. Ordinary people operate on the basis of unconscious beliefs like these. These beliefs act to maintain habits that keep the beliefs alive. Experiments done with the client in mindfulness are what we use to bring those beliefs into consciousness and to evoke the memories and experiences associated with them. (2003, p. 5)

Making Guesses

While scientists are trained to remain objective and emotionally distant from their subjects, Hakomi therapists get up close and personal. They track nuances in affect and behavior, then try these on to determine which unconscious beliefs are likely causing the client to act this way. During sessions, Hakomi therapists ask themselves:

1. What stands out in the client's presentation?
2. How does he or she sit and speak?
3. What facial expressions, gestures, and other movements keep reappearing?

The therapist then wonders:

4. What need is being met by this behavior? (That is, what is this person trying to get or keep away by acting this way?)
5. What life stance or attitude is reflected physically, in the shape and movement of the person's body?
6. What life experiences would engender this attitude? (That is, what didn't this person get enough of as a child? What developmental processes were likely interrupted?)

This process of making precise observations and speculating on the formative events that gave rise to the client's manner is hardly a detached endeavor. Rather, it is an attempt to join with the client by sensing what she is likely experiencing on the inside. This empathy both strengthens the client-therapist alliance and informs the therapeutic strategy.

Entering a person's inner world requires an open mind but, more importantly, an open heart that is free of condemnation. It also requires some literacy with the indicators of unconscious processes, since the unconscious communicates through voice tone, facial expression, gestures, and sensations rather than through words (Kurtz, 2002b). Yet "every person broadcasts information about his inner world. . . . If a listener quiets his neocortical chatter . . . he will catch sight of what the other sees inside that personal world, start to sense what it feels like to live there" (Lewis et al., 2000, p. 169).

Types of Experiments and Therapeutic Rationale

There are well over 30 standard Hakomi experiments, although some of the best experiments are created on the spot. (For a more detailed discussion of the kinds of experiments used in Hakomi therapy, see Chapter 16.) In general, verbal experiments involve offering a potentially nourishing statement ("You're a good person") to the client to see if it is accepted or rejected, as well as taking-over inner voices that serve to keep such statements out ("Yeah, right!"). The therapist may also externalize ruminating thoughts or differing aspects of an internal conflict that create noise in the client's system.

Physical experiments involve making adjustments to the client's posture, shaping the body to represent an attitude or belief, having the client repeat a spontaneous gesture, or taking over a blocked impulse. For example, the therapist may elongate the client's arms in a gesture of reaching out, or hold them back, in effect, taking over whatever mechanism is blocking expression of the impulse. The therapist may also apply pressure to some part of the body, mimicking any tension reported there. This allows the client to study underlying processes more directly, since bodily tension often serves to keep feelings and memories out of awareness.

Regardless of which experiment is used, the intention is to access core material—emotionally charged memories stored in the implicit (emotional, intuitive) memory system of the client's unconscious (Kurtz, 2002b). Specifically, the therapist helps the client become mindful and begins the experiment by asking, "What happens when . . . ?" The experiment is conducted and the client reports on her automatic reactions. Implicit memories and their resultant beliefs presumably condition these reactions. Once these beliefs are brought to light, new experiences are offered that expand limiting, historical ones. According to William James, "Introspective Observation is what we have to rely on first and foremost and always. The word introspection need hardly be defined—it means, of course, the looking into our own minds and reporting what we there discover" (1890, p. 127). Olendzki states, "Meditation has much in common with the scientific enterprise of empirical observation. One is simply regarding as objectively as possible the data of passing phenomenological experience, using the apparatus of direct introspective awareness rather than the microscope or telescope" (2005, p. 244).

Implicit Processes

According to Germer, "Cognitive Psychology is undergoing a 'second cognitive revolution': a new understanding that much of what we think, feel, and do is the consequence of unconscious, 'implicit' processes" (2005, p. 21). For example, Bargh and Chartrand (1999) cite numerous studies indicating that mood states and higher-order processes, such as planning and judging, occur automatically in response to unconscious cues. This is because consciousness, like memory, is a limited-capacity system. It can only attend to one cognitive process at a time. For economy, biologically adaptive shortcuts have evolved to conserve our brainpower. Rather than consciously determining our responses to events, an unconscious appraisal and response process is set in motion by a single visual, auditory, or somatic cue. (Computer buffs will recognize the similarity to a macro, which allows frequently used or repetitive sequences of keystrokes to be performed automatically through the prompt of a single function key.)

For example, we do not need to question if our mental association between "lion" and "predator" is accurate when we are at risk of becoming the lion's lunch. Luckily, the cue "lion" signals the body to run well before the intention to flee registers consciously. Yet when skin color or gender cue behaviors that conform to stereotypic expectations, our associations may be faulty and harmful. Likewise, when individuals chronically respond to neutral—even nourishing—experiences in a defensive and constricted manner, we know that past events are unconsciously influencing the person's automatic appraisal and response system. Moreover, once a correlation is formed, the unconscious system tends to see it where it does not exist, thereby becoming more convinced that the correlation is true (Wilson, 2002).

Clinicians will immediately recognize the relevance of this to clinical practice. Clients often get stuck in limiting and faulty mind-sets that persist despite evidence to the contrary. As Lewis and colleagues explain, "Behind the familiar bright, analytic engine of consciousness is a shadow of silent strength, spinning dazzlingly complicated life into automatic actions, convictions without intellect, and hunches whose reasons follow later or not at all" (2000, p. 112). However, recalcitrant attitudes and beliefs can change, particularly when implicit memories and limiting core beliefs are consciously accessed. For example, the work of Nadel (1994) indicates that when a memory trace is activated, it can be changed before it is recoded (cited in Morgan, 2006; Siegel, 1999). This is good news for therapists who work with core material, for it suggests that once a limiting belief is made conscious, it can be modified. The obvious question is how. Germer believes that mindfulness will eventually be regarded as "*the* technology of access" (2005, p. 21).

Hakomi has always used mindfulness as an "accessing tool." Much of the method involves conducting experiments in mindfulness to make unconscious organizing habits, or implicit processes, conscious (Kurtz, 2002b). Specifically, clients are instructed to turn their awareness inside to study their immediate experience. Attending to body sensations and working directly with present, felt experience increases activity in the right posterior region of the brain. This is where implicit memories or "core organizers" are stored (Myllerup, 2004). Thus, a big part of the Hakomi therapist's job is to "manage consciousness," that is, to stabilize mindfulness. In so doing, multiple regions of the client's brain light up, creating the optimal conditions for accessing and modifying emotional memories and the meanings assigned to these events.

Complex Adaptive Systems

Researchers at the Santa Fe Institute coined the term complex adaptive systems (CAS) to describe systems that maintain an internal coherence without an obvious conductor (Holland, 1995). For example, a city like New York retains its essential character, despite the introduction of hundreds of daily transplants. At the same time, the city accommodates this growth by developing an increasingly complex infrastructure.

Likewise, human beings evolve to higher levels of complexity through the introduction of novel elements and by achieving a balance between stability and change (Kauffman,

1995; Morgan, 2006). Complex adaptive systems also learn through a process called aggregation. We acquire an increasingly large internal database against which novel experiences are matched. Differences are filtered out, so that we selectively attend to what is already familiar (Holland, 1995; Lewis et al., 2000; Siegel, 1999). Thus, our experience is determined by external reality and by our uniquely personal way of converting information through the nervous system into feeling and meaning (Kurtz, 1985).

According to Olendzki, "Ours is a universe of macroconstruction in which the continually arising data of the senses and of miscellaneous internal processing are channeled into structures and organized into schemas that support an entirely synthetic sphere of meaning—a virtual reality" (2005, p. 244). These schemas (called core beliefs in Hakomi) color our perceptions and explain why people respond differently to the same event. For example, one guest has a marvelous time at a party and finds everyone friendly. Another has a miserable time and feels isolated all evening. Such reactions say more about the partygoers than the party. Each has a radically different way of organizing her experience. The former organizes her experience into a virtual heaven, the latter, into a virtual hell. The core beliefs, or implicit realities, that filter out positive experiences are of great interest to Hakomi therapists. Such beliefs are maintained by unconscious habits of perception that are efficient, but distorted (Olendzki, 2005). And "because human beings remember with neurons, we are disposed to see more of what we have already seen, hear anew what we have heard most often, think just what we have always thought" (Lewis et al., 2000, p. 141).

Fortunately, adaptive systems are also self-correcting. A small input can produce a major, predictable change in how information is processed (Holland, 1995; Kauffman, 1995). Capitalizing on this amplifier effect, Hakomi therapists help clients "update their files" by pointing out small distinctions between experience and reality. First, we conduct experiments to make implicit organizing habits explicit. These experiments demonstrate how experience is being organized here and now. Our primary goal is to promote a flexible way of experiencing that is also more accurate and fulfilling.

Trusting Organicity

To study the organization of experience, we must plumb the deeper psychic strata. This makes therapy both more alive and less predictable than working solely at the cognitive level. Consequently, Hakomi practitioners must cultivate a modicum of comfort with uncertainty, since

> just creating a situation that has the potential to evoke previously repressed memories, thoughts, feelings, and desires is an opportunity of immeasurable consequence, both good and bad. No amount of training and research, of statistics gathering and empathy, can offset the unique uncertainty of the encounter. (Phillips, 2006)

While this can be discomfiting at times, our humanistic bias is that "the unconscious is naturally oriented towards growth and wellness rather than regression and pathology" (Felder & Weiss, 1991, p. 2). Consequently, "spontaneous expressions of the unconscious, even in their most primitive form, are not disregarded but are sought out and invited into conscious awareness. They are understood as efforts towards health rather than indicators of pathology" (p. 2).

Many psychotherapists have come to regard pain, fear, and other uncomfortable feelings as normal rather than pathological. In fact, the new "acceptance therapies" recognize what the Buddhists have known all along, namely, that resisting experience tends to exacerbate symptoms, and "suffering is in the reaction not inherent in the raw experience itself" (Fulton & Siegel, 2005, p. 36). This may be why Seligman (1998) urges clinicians to help clients build "buffering strengths," such as perspective taking, optimism, and hope. He contends that "by working in the medical model and looking solely for the salves to heal the wounds, we have misplaced much of our science and much of our training" (p. 2).

Healing

Hakomi practitioners view healing as integration rather than as repair. Accordingly, we don't "fix problems," or break things into parts in search of a "root cause." This medical approach, with its Cartesian underpinnings, violates the mind-body-spirit holism upon which the Hakomi method rests. Instead, we make the inner life transparent so that corrective action can occur organically. "There is a strong underlying faith in the unity and organicity of the person's system that it is self-directing and self-correcting when all the parts are communicating within the whole" (Johanson, 1988, p. 31).

Hakomi therapists support spontaneous behavior because self-organization and the emergence of new, more complex levels of order are features of all living systems (Williams, 1997). This means the therapist must suspend the need to know and allow whatever psychic forces are emerging from within the client to reorganize limiting beliefs without the therapist's interference.

> Because the unconscious is naturally oriented towards growth . . . the therapist's role in the psychotherapy is to be a participant, a catalyst, a midwife in a naturally occurring birthing process of unactuated potential; a process directed by the patient's subjective, unconscious experience rather than by the therapist's objective, conscious perspective. (Felder & Weiss, 1991, p. 8)

In practice, Hakomi therapists engage in a dialectic between doing and being. We actively manage consciousness, by turning the client inward, especially when interpretation and storytelling interrupt mindful self-study. Yet we practice noninterference once the client's unconscious is "online." We actively suggest experiments to try, but willingly change course to honor the emergent properties of the unconscious.

Emergence

A good traveler has no fixed plans
and is not intent upon arriving.
A good artist lets his intuition
lead him wherever it wants.
A good scientist has freed himself of concepts
and keeps his mind open to what is . . . .
He is ready to use all situations
and doesn't waste anything.

LAO-TZU, *Tao Te Ching*

In science, chance events can yield exciting discoveries. For example, penicillin, aspirin, and Velcro were all the result of experimental "mishaps" (Gold, 2004). Likewise, in therapy, we may head in one direction only to find the unconscious takes us in another. When room is made for the unexpected, it garners trust in the mysterious ways that the psyche mends and transforms itself.

Case Example

I was about to use a probe—a classic Hakomi experiment in which a positive, potentially nourishing statement is said aloud while the client is mindful. During the setup, the client opened her eyes and said, "I just need to know—will you always say something positive, because I notice I'm already bracing to hear something really bad." The seasoned practitioner recognizes this question as laden with core material, since "bracing for something bad" most surely has powerful, historical antecedents.

Instead of continuing with the probe, the bracing now becomes the object of exploration. Once the client experiences "bracing for the worst" as a habitual life stance, it opens the door for the neural rewiring made possible when a new experience (for example, relaxing without incurring negative consequences) is filed alongside a historical one.

After taking time to explore the felt experience and meaning of the bracing, we created the probe: "It's not your fault." Upon hearing the statement, the client reported, "I have a dismal, sinking feeling in my chest related to the arbitrariness of life. . . . Nothing is in my control." With that, her face reddened and she quickly went into the "rapids"—Kurtz's metaphoric description of the emotional intensity that makes witnessing one's own experience impossible. Under such conditions, data collection is suspended and the therapist supports emotional expression, or its management, until mindfulness returns.

In a younger voice, she continued, "If it's not my fault, then I can't make it better." This realization triggered another rush of tears. Kurtz says, "a good experiment, done well, results in the client's awareness of a core belief or memory" (2002a, p. 13). *In this case, the experiment revealed a belief, "bad things happen because I'm bad," accompanied by a compensatory strategy to be "really good." The probe, "It's not your fault," is thus automatically resisted because it makes null and void the client's first line of defense. While initially frightening and unpalatable, it also allows for an uncoupling of black-and-white thinking ("bad things happen so I must be bad") from the magical thinking that maintains the strategy ("If I'm really good, I can make good things happen").*

Processing in child consciousness is how Hakomi therapists repair narcissistic injuries of this sort. The therapist helps the woman of today inform the child of the past that, even though bad things happen, she isn't bad. Likewise, the inner child can stop looking for the badness inside her because it was never there to begin with. When this information is experienced as a visceral reality and encoded in mindfulness, new meanings become associated with early emotional events and a more accurate and self-affirming belief takes root in consciousness.

Curiosity

The experimental attitude requires an abiding curiosity in the client's inner world. Both therapist and client must be equally engaged in the process for healing to happen. This means the therapist must regard even exasperating behaviors as indicative of core processes and, therefore, worthy of study. What sustains the therapist's curiosity is the understanding that client and therapist are cohorts on the human journey (the unity principle). It is not enough to simply observe and follow the process; the therapist must actively support the experience that wants to happen, or "take charge," in Hakomi parlance. This allows whichever growth processes were interrupted to move forward again.

To sustain the client's curiosity, the therapist must help the client shift out of the "doing" mode of daily life and into the "being" mode of mindful self-study. She must also honor the client's pace by acknowledging signs of resistance and accepting the client's need to defend as willingly as his need to progress. Finally, the therapist must help the client maintain a level of arousal that's optimal for inner exploration. For example, too little arousal leads to disengagement, whereas too much incites the threat response, resulting in constricted awareness, vigilance of one's surroundings, and loss of curiosity (Johanson, 1988; Ogden & Minton, 2000; Siegel, 1999; Van der Hart, Nijenhuis & Steele, 2000).

Validity and Reliability

Experiments conducted in mindfulness are not subject to the rigorous controls academic researchers labor over. For example, we don't concern ourselves with whether or not an experiment will measure what we hope to measure because the unconscious, like a gyroscope, pulls the observer toward whatever is in need of healing.

Likewise, we have no qualms about the subjective nature of the self-report. We invite clients to author their own experience. We accept discrepancies, partial disclosures, and novel outcomes affably because the psychic landscape is both dynamic and emergent. And while we expect the client's organizing habits to be pervasive and repeating, our reliability standards are equally permissive. We hope these habits will transform over the course of therapy, making the data time limited. To test this assumption, we might offer the same probe at the end of the session that was originally used to access core material. In such instances, we are checking to see if the client can take in nourishment that was initially refused, now that fresh experiences have been integrated.

Conclusion

Hakomi is an experiential psychotherapy designed to access and transform limiting beliefs. During a Hakomi session, the therapist makes guesses about the unconscious habits that organize the client's experience in limiting and painful ways. Often experiments are conducted in mindfulness to evoke experience, since "gathering information directly from present experience is the most . . . reliable way of discovering how meanings are assigned to events" (Kurtz, 1985, p. 7).

The experimental attitude is thus curiosity in action. It is sustained by staying open to outcome and trusting the client's intrinsic ability to heal and grow. In this atmosphere of mutual exploration, unconscious habits are made conscious and corrective experiences that promote transformation are introduced and assimilated.

CHAPTER 12

Following and Leading

Carol Ladas Gaskin and David Cole

*Nonviolence promotes a respect for the subtle almost imperceptible move-
ments of mind, body, and spirit and gives rise to a yielding or softness which
follows and nourishes these movements rather than correcting or conquering
them.*

GREG JOHANSON AND RON KURTZ, *Grace Unfolding*, 1991

Following

IN HAKOMI, AN understanding of the principles of organicity and nonviolence allows us
to follow the natural pathway of a client's own movement toward self-healing. We believe
and trust that there are deep inner signals, sent from a normally unconscious wisdom that
wants to move the system toward increased complexity and wholeness. These signals function in the service of the system being self-organizing, self-directing, and self-correcting
(see Chapter 5). Thus, Hakomi therapists trust that, at the deepest levels, clients are the
world's experts on their own experience.

However, at the surface level where people are talking in ordinary consciousness, habitually organized by unexamined core organizers in implicit memory, we do not trust that
they are the world's expert on what healing is possible (Eisman, 2006). We begin our work
by creating those conditions that will allow the person access to her deep structures and
the quality of consciousness that will enable her to listen deeply to the wisdom of her own

experience, and follow where it might lead her (Weiss, 2008). Empowering the client to follow her own organic unfolding, and gaining the cooperation of her unconscious, is prerequisite to the therapist following the process on the deepest levels.

Since safety, nonviolence, and acceptance are necessary for the client to be able to switch into an exploratory, mindful state of consciousness, we begin by internally contacting our own appreciation for the client, regardless of how the session might go. We notice some way that the client delights and inspires us. In that state of loving presence, and what Kurtz called non-egocentric nourishment, we can rest and be nourished as we pay attention to following the client's inner state with gentle, empathetic awareness. We can calmly and compassionately follow his nonverbal signals that assist us in intuiting core material. We are following by staying with both the client's and our own present-moment experience. By doing so, we model what we want to encourage in the client.

We also encourage working collaboratively (Duncan, 2010). By participating as a team, we support ripening without forcing. We might ask, for instance, "Does it seem like you have shared enough of your story, so that now is a good time to become mindful of the anxiety that's up?" We wait respectfully for the right moment to offer a probe or nourishment. "Is this a good place where we can do an experiment in mindfulness that studies what the anxiety does when it is offered hope?"

By following present-moment experience—that which is presently organized and contains impulses to reorganize or transform—we convey to the client that we trust his own process. By naming what is here and now, we are following, and at the same time encouraging the client to follow her own inner state. "Some emotion arises, huh. . . [?]" "So, your head straightens a bit when you say that. . . [?]" "Some part of you is not so sure. . . [?]" (The [?] is a symbol for a shift in the therapist's voice that suggests the client might want to be curious about this instance of present-moment experience, and explore it more fully while the therapist simply overhears what is going on.) When we say these things as therapists, we are following our own curiosity, but are most interested in engaging the client's curiosity (Johanson, 1988). To paraphrase Winnicott (1971): It does not really matter how much therapists know, as long as they can keep it to themselves.

Hakomi is assisted self-study. The whole process involves trust in the client's search for wholeness (Monda, 2000). It depends on our ability as a therapist to be willing to not be the one who knows, but to unfailingly befriend whatever arises. "Oh, some kind of ocean air smell comes up. . . [?]" Emerging insight comes from this region of not knowing. "Stay with the smell. Let's see if it leads us anywhere." By bringing friendly attention, loving presence, and acceptance, we are freed of an agenda, which then allows us to follow our intuition (Marks-Tarlow, 2012). We don't have to be right. "Oh, so someone is not pushing you. It is more like they are calling to you. . . [?]"

At times in Hakomi, we find that we must retreat from the leading of our intuition. For example, the therapist may offer a contact statement that is not accurate, or a probe that goes nowhere. When this occurs, she does not press onward; she drops back and saves the session from the pitfalls of so-called client resistance. We track when our leading is wrong, contact that truth, and get back on track by following once again. "Uh, huh. It is not sadness so much as grief. Good. Let's let the grief have its voice."

We are following and contacting the body's messages, its living experience of embodiment (Barratt, 2010), which gives us ongoing, immediate feedback about whether we are in a creative, mindful space or not. When there are strong emotions, we assist the client by inviting him to stay with his feelings long enough to explore and discover their meaning. "How about we listen more to the anger, and get clearer about what wrong it feels such a need to make right?" We follow spontaneous unfolding and expression, always with the intent to assist the client in self-discovery of unconscious beliefs and memories. "Notice that your shoulders come up as you anticipate the interview with your boss."

One of the keys to following is knowing when to be silent. As Kurtz often said, there are several instances when silence is essential. When a client is integrating something unexpected that has just emerged in consciousness, we are attentive and quiet, letting the client discover and integrate on her own. When a contact statement has just been made, we wait and notice the client's response in silence, not pushing for any hurried reply. When we offer a probe, we are silent and respectful of the client's timing, which could be more slow or more hasty. By being silent, unhurried, and present, we create an environment that is safe and attuned, which communicates our trust that significant unfolding is happening. The client's adaptive unconscious is leading. Silence allows the client to feel attended to, but not interrupted. It allows the therapist time to take in where the process is going. When the process is unfolding, we follow.

Leading

> *Power is the capacity to have influence. It is the ability to act on behalf of one's self and for others. The challenge of right use of power and influence is one of the most profound and important we face in our professions, in our cultures, and in our personal growth.*
>
> Cedar Barstow, *Right Use of Power*, 2005

> *Lao-tzu affirms the paradox that the sage stays ahead of events by following them. This detachment from self-concern from the self-interest of being regarded a leader allows the sage the freedom to be at one with what is happening.*
>
> Greg Johanson and Ron Kurtz, *Grace Unfolding*, 1991

Even though listening fully and following constitute an essential aspect of Hakomi that provides the broadest context for its practice, leadership has an important role in each session. It is often necessary as opposed to discouraged or devalued. The use of the word "leading," however, is qualified because it is not leading in the traditional Western sense.

In the practice of Hakomi, the intent of taking the lead is not to change the direction or the outcome of the client's ongoing process, but to ensure that it is a mindful, experimental process, not at the mercy of fear-based, unconscious organizers. Thus, taking charge or leading in Hakomi often has to do with managing states of consciousness. When signs of hyper- or hypoactivation are tracked, the therapist takes the lead in bringing the client back within the boundaries of his window of tolerance (Ogden et al., 2006; see Chapter 24). Nor is leading used to impose an agenda upon the content of the session. In this regard, one might call leading in Hakomi a kind of leading within following. It is, therefore, not the kind of leading in which one goes on ahead of the other to light or guide the way. We recognize that, like our clients, we do not really know what lies ahead or where the process should be going.

However, the therapist has an ongoing sensitivity to whether the client's awareness is turned inward toward present, felt experience, and whether the words used resonate with the truth of the embodied experience. If the words seem distant from the experience, the therapist leads the client back into the bodily present moment. "How do you experience this jealousy in your arms?" If the client is deeply immersed in her experience that seems to be circling, the therapist can lure the client toward meaning. "What would that impulse to reach say if it could use words?" If words and experience seem to reverberate with alive resonance, the therapist allows the process to unfold organically (Johanson, 1996).

Leading is the exercise of specific skills that are acquired through training and rehearsal. With practice, they become both automatic and adaptable. The Hakomi approach to leading is comparable to how jazz improvisation is created. One can think of the client playing the solo instrument and beginning the piece or leading with a theme. The therapist listens closely to sense its essence and direction before joining and supporting the soloist's statement. Each time the supporting therapist plays a note or phrase, his intention is to acknowledge, deepen, or develop the possibilities introduced by the soloist. Neither musician knows exactly what is going to happen, but they trust that the music will find its form and the various tensions that are produced will come to a satisfactory and nourishing resolution.

The skills used to lead in Hakomi can be described according to their intention (Cole & Ladas-Gaskin, 2007). Some intentions are realized through the combination of a number of skills. For example, the intention of building relationship with the client is realized through loving presence, tracking, contact statements, and acknowledgments. While some of these skills are more passive than others, they all lead the process within the context of gaining the cooperation of the unconscious that establishes the safety and trust to follow deep impulses toward healing. Actively encouraging the presence of the larger or compassionate witness of the client does not change the essential course of the therapy, but makes it markedly more clear and efficient. The signals of organic wisdom that need to be followed become more apparent, and a process for doing so is fostered.

Leading Within Following

What follows are some brief examples of skills that lead and influence the therapeutic process within the context of following deep movements toward transformation. They are used within the ongoing tension of knowing and not knowing—keeping in mind the intentions mentioned above and the stage of the therapeutic process within a session or course of therapy.

Building Relationship

We don't know exactly what the client needs from us in the therapeutic relationship. We do know it needs to be based on the truth of present-moment experience, so we often lead by contacting that. "So, a little shy, a little cautious. . .[?]"

Evoking and Modeling Mindfulness

We don't know how much a person needs to talk about his story in ordinary consciousness to feel safe. We do know we normally need to lead the process toward a mindful, exploratory consciousness, since this is not where inexperienced clients have a habit of going. "Why don't we hang out with this sense of cautiousness, and maybe it will tell us more about itself."

Slowing the Process Down

We have no idea what is at the root of the cautiousness in the above example, but we do know we need to stay out of the hurried pace of ordinary consciousness to discover it. "We could both make some guesses about where the sense of caution comes from, but why don't we just slow things down and allow it to have its own voice? Maybe we can start by exploring how you experience the caution in your body. . .[?]"

Helping the Client Attend to the Present Moment

We don't know what will gather around this thread of caution, but direct the client to the present-moment experience that is now organized around caution in the service of deepening into its meaning. "So, there is a slight tensing of the arms when you allow the caution to be present. . .[?]" The more experienced a client is with the process, the shorter the therapist's intervention needs to be. "Ah, some tensing in the arms. . . [?]"

Calling Attention to Something That Has Been Out of Awareness

While we could guess at the meaning behind something like caution, we do know that the way clients manage their experience of such things is habitual or chronic—which means mostly out of their awareness—so we take the lead in contacting those nonverbal, unconscious indicators of management. "And your head turns to the right as you tense. . .[?]"

Deepening the Client's Experience of the Present Moment

While we respect our clients' internal wisdom in leading us where it wants to go, we know that the tendency is for clients to come out of a fruitful, mindful state to report their findings, instead of allowing their experience to deepen. Once they begin a mindful exploration (accessing), we act to help them maintain their mindful state (deepening). Sometimes this can be extensive and directive. "See if you can name your experience without having to come out of it to tell me about it. . . [?] What other sensations, thoughts, feelings, muscle tensions, attitudes, or whatever, do you notice gathering around the arms tensing and head turning?" Again, with more experienced clients, we could simply say, "Stay with that" or "Notice anything else."

Accessing Unconscious Material

While we as therapists follow organic signals from the client to where they lead us, we know that most clients who live in a busy, full world are not sensitive to the importance of seemingly insignificant signals, and so we often lead in calling attention to their possible importance. "Oh, some kind of musty smell comes up. . . [?] Can we just stay with that for a moment?"

Accessing and Exploring Memories

We have no idea what a musty smell connotes for the client, but we know that core organizers of present experience often have historical roots in formative memories frozen in time. This is a tricky place, because the therapist must not suggest any particular memories, but needs to open the way to discovering them. Perhaps questions like, "Is it a familiar smell? Can we allow the smell to bring us back in time to a place where it was first important somehow? Is it an old musty, or something-wet-drying-out musty, or . . . ?"

Helping the Client Find Meaning

When the unconscious offers a spontaneous memory to follow, there is a clinical choice between leading through being what Kurtz called a "magical stranger"—who shows up in the memory and relates to the child as a compassionate, understanding adult who was not there originally—or asking the client's larger self to relate helpfully to the younger part. Magical stranger: "Oh, you are three years old and your older brother keeps fooling you, and scaring you by inviting you to look at new things that turn out to be scary snakes, or something that looks like a rat that turns out to be a guinea pig, and then he makes fun of you." Larger or organic self: "Notice what is going on with this younger you? Or maybe have him tell you what is most painful about his situation."

Comforting and Providing Nourishment

Once the pain of the formative memory is clear, and the younger part's strategy for dealing with it becomes more obvious, the needed antidote or missing experience usually becomes clearer. The therapist can lead through introducing it, though always without attachment, with an exquisite tracking of whether the person is in accordance, and with an immediate willingness to be corrected. Magical stranger: "So, you really learned how to be cautious about being fooled in new situations, and got very careful about taking invitations from people. You were a very smart little boy who learned how to not trust everybody and let them take advantage of you. And now that you are not back there being suspicious of your brother every day, I can tell you that it is a bigger world out there. Some people will try to trick you sometimes, and it is good to know how to be cautious and protect yourself. But some people are very nice and just want to share nice things with you that will make you happier. So, we have to learn how to look twice at people to check out whether they can be trusted or not." Larger or organic self: "So what wisdom and truth can you offer this three-year-old you who needs to know the difference between mean older brothers and people who just want to share?"

Integrating the Processes That Engage the Client in the Larger World

Since everyone has a multiplicity of parts that compose a delicate, inner ecology (Schwartz, 1995), it is never clear how the parts worked with in a session will play out in the client's larger world. It is clear that in the therapy, a skill or defense is never taken away from anyone, but new possibilities previously organized out are added in to make a more complete, more organic system (Johanson, 2015). The therapist can lead in exploring a life-world integration in a number of ways. One might be to suggest, "How about picking one of the troubling examples you have mentioned—your girlfriend wanting you to explore new things in dancing or yoga, or your boss wanting you to try new things—and notice how you organize around those possibilities now. . . [?]"

In each of these endeavors, the therapist takes the lead or does something to influence the client's consciousness and experience of the process as it unfolds in the present moment. With such a long list of skills to employ, one might imagine a rather busy process, but that is not necessarily so. For example, building relationship might take place through the use of curious, compassionate tracking—which conveys a profound sense of attunement. When performed with skill, it is experienced as being listened to fully and deeply, with connection and understanding that goes beyond listening to words alone. While this is going on, the therapist, through her safe and spacious manner, influences the client in the direction of slowing down. As that slowing down occurs, there will be space for mindfulness and a deeper consciousness of the present moment.

At the same time that contact statements are encouraging mindfulness, trust, and relationship, they also draw attention to present-moment experience and lead the client deeper. With almost every well-made contact statement—for example, "sad now. . .[?]"—there is a pronounced shift in the client's process; the amiable chatter pauses, the client checks his experience, and then replies, "Well, yes, now that you mention it, I do sense a sadness here." Thus with a well-chosen word or two, the process is led deeper. This might be followed with an acknowledgment by the therapist in just the right empathetic and accepting voice: "I see your sadness now." Once again, the experience that was about to be glossed over, lost, or dismissed by the client's narrative or story line is held in awareness long enough to deepen.

We could also call this deepening a form of accessing (see Chapter 15). Contact statements and acknowledgments have accessed an unconscious feeling and brought it forth into conscious awareness. Simultaneously, the acknowledgment has reached out to assure the client that he has been heard in a deep way and that he is not alone. The therapist might also have noticed the sadness and asserted a more active form of leading. This might require that the therapist intervene in the narrative to suggest an experiment. She might help the client to become mindful and use a theoretically nourishing offering (a verbal or nonverbal probe). An example might be, "Your feelings are safe here." Such a "little experiment in mindfulness" can help the process deepen, access the barriers to such a notion, or be nourishing.

Going for meaning also does not need to be a busy activity. Sometimes we just sit and let the client find the meaning without helping or getting in the way. We might describe this as "leading by being still." While we sit, we hold a definite intention and we watch for little signs that the client is working and the process is moving. If we see it bog down and notice worried lines between our client's brows, we might contact it; for example, "hard work, eh. . . . [?]" Again, it takes merely a word or two. At other times, we might evoke the meaning by asking the client, "What does that sadness say?" or "What kind of sadness is that?" or "What does that sadness remember or imagine?" There are many evocative phrases like this that are designed to direct the client's attention toward some sort of meaning. The meaning can be found as words, an association, an image, or a memory. The meaning of a feeling is not necessarily a verbal formulation. Memories, images, and felt-sense experiences contain meanings, and within them one may find the words or the personalized, generalized belief, or the unconscious anticipatory structure (Kurtz, 2006) that determines patterns of constraint and suffering in present time.

The therapist may also lead the client toward accepting nourishment once deemed impossible. Again, simplicity and economy are the Hakomi way (Kurtz, 2006). With an experienced client, the therapist may simply extend her hand, or hand out a tissue, then let the hand linger to see if the client looks longingly or reaches out. Asking, in this instance, might force the process toward some kind of neocortical decision, for example: "What should I say?" or "If I say no, will I hurt her feelings?" By asking with the hand and leaving it open, we can speak at the limbic level, and allow the process to unfold without neocortical intervention that calls attention away from the experience.

Another approach would be to use the voice in a suggestive way. For example, "Would a hand feel good right now? . . . Just a soft hand on your shoulder to let you know that there is someone here with you . . . to tell you that you have someone in your corner." Here is a sentence that starts out sounding like a question but transforms into an evocative suggestion, and ends up as a nourishing offering. In Hakomi, life is the ultimate healer, which means we need to take in the nourishment it offers. Instead of avoiding gratifying a client as in classical psychoanalysis, gratification is offered experimentally, where it is either mindfully integrated in a nourishing manner or barriers to taking in gratification are evoked for further exploration and processing.

With words like those in the paragraph above, spoken artfully and at the right time, actual touch might not be necessary. The voice can be made to reach out and touch. But when it is appropriate and safe, touch may be offered and either accepted or explored. After giving the client some time to sense into a touch, the therapist might use the situation to move toward meaning. "What does that hand say to you?" or "If my hand were using words, what might it be saying?"

Finally, in integration the actions can be so natural and subtle that one hardly recognizes them as some kind of deliberate work or leadership skill. We have often marveled at Kurtz's genius at creating a little game to encourage a client to try out a new growth step. For example, he might set up a game in which he plays the client's father. It might go something like this: "Okay, you be yourself and I'll be your father. I'll say, 'Don't speak until you're spoken to!' just like your father did, only maybe I'll exaggerate a little. Then you give me a great big old raspberry! Shall we try that?" These invitations can be so appetizing that the client has a hard time refusing. Kurtz then typically overacted the part enormously, with just enough reality to conjure an image of the stern and disapproving father. The client would respond with a big raspberry (which, in itself, might be a new experience), and then Kurtz would fall over in a heap as if blown away by a great gust of wind (Pesso, 1973), and both would join in a conspiracy of hilarious laughter to celebrate this newfound pluck, holding their sides as they rolled around the floor.

Conclusion

Every act of knowing brings forth a world.

HUMBERTO MATURANA AND FRANCISCO VARELA,
The Tree of Knowledge, 1992

Life, at its best, is a flowing, changing process in which nothing is fixed. In my clients and in myself I find that when life is richest and most rewarding it is a flowing process. . . . I find I am at my best when I can let the flow of my experience carry me in a direction which appears to be forward toward goals of which I am but dimly aware.

CARL ROGERS, *On Becoming a Person*, 1961

While Hakomi resonates with the humanistic ethos of nondirective client-led therapies, it is not a derivative of Rogerian therapy, and it would be inaccurate to describe it as nondirective in the Rogerian sense (Raskin, 1948). It differs from Rogerian therapies in its preference for the implicit, its use of the body and nonverbal communication, and its attitude toward leadership. Unlike the so-called nondirective approaches, Hakomi does not avoid or advocate the abolition of leadership from the therapeutic alliance.

By a similar token, one might question the use of the word "nondirective" to label Rogerian therapy or the approaches of its predecessors, Jessie Taft (1933), Otto Rank (1936), and Frederick Allen (1942). While these pioneers did much to liberate therapy from the power inequities in what has been called "Freud's fundamentally authoritative orientation" (Raskin, 1948), they consistently overlook their own exercise of influence in their confinement of therapy to an explicit and verbal dialogue. They do not seem to recognize that they unwittingly assert a subtle, yet very powerful, form of leadership that channels awareness away from attention to the body, body sensations, and subtleties of felt sense experience—and the wealth of information that is accessed through nonverbal channels. The magnitude of that oversight has been underlined through the discoveries of Kurtz in the late 1960s and the subsequent development of Hakomi from 1970 to the present (Barratt, 2010).

In addition, when we view the process of Hakomi through the concepts of following and leading, the Western notions of absolute and formal opposition, within which those early "client-led" therapies developed, dissolve into a flux or flow of two distinct but complementary intentions. The Taoist notion of yin and yang is an especially useful view through which to interpret Hakomi, with its practice of "leading within following" and "following even as one leads." And it is from his grasp of this Eastern perspective that Kurtz developed the Hakomi approach.

However, in spite of the differences, in practice there are numerous points of similarity and plenty of room for cross-fertilization between Hakomi and more conventional humanistic approaches. Certainly, both eschew an overbearing use of the power differential between client and therapist; both are gentle and yielding as opposed to confrontational and challenging of the client. They also share a great respect for the cultivation of empathy, compassion, and experimentation, and mutually refrain from imposing or projecting an absolute system of values or an overarching theory of human development upon their clients.

Furthermore, the concepts of leading and following, when reframed as relative and complementary intentions, are clinically useful. Just as Hakomi therapists keep watch on their own internal state with regard to loving presence, personal agendas, getting hooked by their own countertransference, and other qualities related to personhood, it is well to keep checking on leading and following, for they provide us with valuable feedback about our use of influence and power. We can find ourselves erring on the side of too much following or too much leading. Stopping and realigning with the client's unfolding organic wisdom can help the therapist repair the breach and regain the traction of the session. Finding time to reflect on one's own disposition to lead or follow overmuch can serve as creative material for the therapist's continued personal and professional growth.

CHAPTER 13

Ethics: Right Use of Power

Cedar Barstow

RIGHT USE OF power is the use of personal and professional power to prevent and repair harm and to promote the well-being of all (Barstow, 2005). Body-centered psychotherapies, such as Hakomi, invite an experiential, integrated, and relational approach to the development and practice of ethical awareness and accountability. Right use of power and influence is understood as the heart of ethics (Knowlan & Patterson, 1993). It is my experience that using power skillfully and wisely requires more than good intentions. It requires a lifelong engagement of increasing awareness and sensitivity to our personal and professional impacts.

In the Hakomi method, ethics in the broad scope of the right use of power is embedded in the method itself. The Hakomi sensitivity cycle (Chapter 17) describes the process of increasing sensitivity as a dynamic and spiraling movement. Inspired by the usefulness of this cycle and the positive framework of this Hakomi map, I have identified a power spiral with four aspects of the right use of power. Right use of power is (1) informed, (2) conscious, (3) caring, and (4) skillful. The focus is on developing an increasing level of skill and awareness in each of these dimensions as a positive power model, as outlined more fully in Barstow (2005).

This chapter does not cover the whole range of ethical issues addressed within these four dimensions, but focuses instead on the topics particularly relevant to psychotherapeutic work using the Hakomi method. The principles, theory, and skills of the Hakomi method encourage and support a deep level of ethical awareness, sensitivity, and wisdom. Hakomi, as a method, includes a refined ability to track subtle clues about a client's internal experience and to contact them in the present moment. Hakomi therapists also work in a collaborative way, insisting that clients offer their experience and their feedback in an ongoing and present process. The Hakomi method also focuses on establishing safety (see Chapter 14). These practices significantly reduce the possibilities of unacknowledged misunderstandings and harm from power-over directiveness. They also tend to very quickly create a therapeutic atmosphere of special intimacy, vulnerability, and depth. This atmosphere of loving presence calls for an increased sensitivity and watchfulness to not become personally entangled.

Power Differential Ethics

The core of ethical sensitivity comes from acquiring a felt sense of the power differential. The power differential is the inherently greater or enhanced power and influence therapists have compared to their clients (see Table 13.1). The impacts of this enhanced power are many and varied. Written ethical codes designed to prevent harm to clients are based on the effects of the power differential (Hunter & Struve, 1998).

In the Hakomi therapeutic relationship, the power differential has great value. Used wisely and appropriately, it creates a safe, well-boundaried, professional context for growth and healing. More specifically, when used ethically, the power differential offers clients some very important assurances:

1. Confidence in the caregiver's knowledge, training, and expertise
2. Security and safety

Table 13.1 Power Differential Role Differences

Caregiver (Power-Up Role)	Client (Power-Down Role)
Is in service	Is served
Has increased and enhanced power and influence	Very often experiences a decreased felt sense of power and influence
Is paid for time and expertise	Pays for service
Sets and maintains appropriate boundaries	Accepts or challenges boundaries
Own needs and personal process are not focused on	Own needs and personal process is known and focused on—self-revelation is important
Less vulnerability	Greater vulnerability to rejection, criticism, undue influence, being taken advantage of, disrespect
Depended on for trustworthiness, earns trust	Needs to trust
Ultimately responsible for tracking and repairing relationship difficulties	Coresponsible for naming and working with difficulties
May be idealized or devalued	More susceptible to idealizing or devaluing
May need to assist client in being more empowered	May unnecessarily disempower self
Makes assessments and evaluates results	Collaborates with or responds to assessments

3. Direction and support
4. Role boundary clarification
5. Allocated responsibilities

Because the power differential is role dependent, it is easy to overidentify (that is, get inflated or addicted) with this increased or enhanced power. It is just as easy to misuse this increased power by underidentifying with it (for example, disowning or disregarding one's power or role-generated impact). Here are several misunderstandings that illustrate the multiplicity of the impact of the power differential for both helping professionals and clients:

1. Using the Hakomi method, we may find ourselves unaware of the amount of transference that the context of loving presence creates.
2. Believing in equality, we may find it difficult to accept that our role creates a power inequality, and that this inequality is actually essential to our effectiveness.
3. Out of fear of manipulative and wounding abuses of power, we may find it difficult to understand that we must own the power that we have, to be able to use it for good.

Underuse of power is also a misuse of power.

4. Motivated by a desire to be of service, we may find it difficult to comprehend that our impact may be different from our intention—that it may be experienced as confusing or harmful.

While training in the Hakomi method, students deepen their sensitivity to the dynamics of the power differential through an experiential exercise in which they sit with a partner and silently role-play being in both the power-up role and the client role. Here are some reflections from therapists when in the power-up role:

> I have always equated power with power over, force, and manipulation. I am now seeing power as a skill, as knowledge, as sensitivity and awareness. This is so different.

> I now understand that my clients and I are equals as humans, but we have different roles. These roles have significant differences.

> The new paradigm of power requires therapists to educate their clients about their use of power.

Ethics of Working in Nonordinary States

A nonordinary state of consciousness is a "mild to deep trance in which awareness is focused in a different way than in ordinary life" (Taylor, 1995, p. 50). Nonordinary states of consciousness can spontaneously arise through many experiences such as ecstasy, shame, trauma, grief, fasting, and peak experiences. Mindfulness, as used in the Hakomi method, is a nonordinary state of consciousness that facilitates profound personal awareness and healing. In teaching and inviting clients to turn their awareness inside to notice whatever their present experience is, we are deliberately encouraging our clients to enter a nonordinary state of consciousness. In a technical sense, mindfulness is not a hypnotic trance state that diverts conscious attention (Wolinsky, 1991). It actually enhances awareness and breaks the trance of everyday habits. Still, when using the Hakomi method, this nonordinary state of mindfulness engenders special concerns about the right use of power. When invited into the state of mindfulness, clients lower their defenses. This puts them in an exposed and vulnerable position, without their normal level of protection. Because of this, the impact of the power differential is heightened and expanded when clients are in such a state.

Qualities and effects of nonordinary states include the following:

1. Time distortion
2. Increased intensity of feeling and sensation
3. Greater need or capacity for faith and trust
4. Increased sensitivity and awareness through all senses
5. Consciousness expansion
6. Relaxation or diffusion of boundaries
7. Increased felt sense of the truth
8. Increased sensitivity to authenticity (Taylor, 1995, p. 54)

When working with clients in mindfulness, it is helpful to make appropriate and effective interventions, assessments, and adjustments like the following:

1. Find out how the nonordinary state of mindfulness is being experienced by the client.
2. Pay especially close attention to setting and maintaining boundaries for privacy, time, confidentiality, touch, and safety and security needs.
3. Learn how to distinguish between a healing process in a nonordinary state and a process in which the client is being retraumatized.
4. Increase sensitivity to subtle safety needs and to body, emotion, energy, and cues.
5. Stay connected to present felt experience.
6. Slow down and be spacious.

Ethics and the Therapeutic Use of Touch

Touch is necessary to both physical health and emotional well-being (Ford, 1993; Montagu, 1978; Peloquin, 1990; Rubenfeld, 2000). Johanson (personal communication) maintains that not to use the power of touch (therapeutically, nonsexually, and appropriately initiated) might be considered unethical since it withholds a powerful therapeutic tool from clients, who then must invest increased time, energy, and money in therapy to the unfair gain of therapists.

Restoring a satisfying and healthy relationship to touch may indeed be considered a worthy goal in therapy. The body is a rich source of wisdom. The use of body information and informed and conscious touch are powerful tools for healing, self-awareness, establishing good boundaries, and cultivating more satisfying connections. Years of cultural, theoretical, and ethical controversy surround the use of touch in the helping professions (Causey, 1993; McNeely, 1987; Smith, Clance, & Imes, 1998; Thomas, 1994). In many states, using touch is illegal or uninsurable—laws often based on traditional psychoanalytic strictures. The United States Association for Body Psychotherapy is an organization focusing on the therapeutic value of including the body and ethical touch in healing work, whose purpose is to increase the attention, validation, and respect afforded to the modalities of body psychotherapy.

Ethical codes for helping professions and state laws related to the use of touch vary greatly. Therapists need to take personal responsibility for researching relevant codes and laws. Controversy arises from the following factors:

1. It is never ethical for psychotherapists to use sexual touch with a client or to engage in or imply sexual intimacy or the future possibility of such. The strong healing power of touch may be undone and contaminated by the betrayal of sexual intimacy in a relationship with a power differential supposedly characterized by trust. The prohibition of even nonsexual touch in helping relationships by some organizations is intended to prevent the egregious harm caused by inappropriate touch.
2. Human beings automatically and uniquely assign meaning to touch. Thus, therapeutic touch is easily misinterpreted by clients as sexual, forceful, serving the caregiver, or controlling. Touch is deeply longed for and a source of deep vulnerability. Use of therapeutic touch is ethically and relationally complex and requires assessment, sensitivity, good tracking, and clarity of intention on the part of caregivers.

Jaffy Phillips (2003) succinctly describes the values of the use of touch, and the ways in which touch can support healing and the deepening of self-awareness: "When you touch someone, everything changes." Touch is a physical and relational experience that is generally imbued with layers of historical, cultural, and psychological meaning. The meanings evoked by touch are often unconscious or nonverbal, and they often manifest somatically or relationally before the client is able to articulate anything about them. Boundary issues, transference, and countertransference are common examples of this kind of response. If unaddressed, the unintended consequences of touch can wreak havoc in the therapeutic relationship and ultimately damage the client.

The Hakomi method has been a bodymind psychotherapy since its inception. Several techniques consciously and deliberately use touch to assist and support therapeutic change. Taking over and supporting spontaneous emotional management are two specific techniques where touch may be employed. Touch may be used in other creative little experiments in mindfulness (see Chapter 16). This exploratory, mindful context for touch builds in safety, as it invites the client to notice and report the impact of touch in the moment. Still, the therapist's sensitivity to impact and awareness of the possible risks is especially important when using touch in clinical practice.

Hakomi's ethical guidelines in the use of touch are as follows:

1. Client knows how and why touch will be used in the therapy.
2. Client understands limits and boundaries of touch (for example, nonsexual).
3. Client agrees to this and gives permission.
4. Clients know that they can stop or discontinue the use of touch at any time, and that they are always in control of when, where, how, and for how long they are touched.
5. Therapist continually tracks for indicators of how the client is experiencing the touch—whether it is as intended—and checks in with the client on the impact of the touch.

Additional factors to consider:

1. Touch should always and only be used deliberately, carefully, and consciously.
2. The use of touch should be accompanied by assessment and a clear clinical rationale that is in the service of the client's process.
3. Time should be taken to become clear about one's intentions and feelings toward the client. Lack of clarity about intentions is often a sign that shadow material or countertransference is present.
4. Become familiar with one's own touch issues and potential countertransferences.
5. Be mindful: stop touching when the intention is complete.

Avoid touch when:

1. The therapist does not want to touch.
2. The client does not want to be touched.
3. The client is likely to misinterpret the touch.

The Ethical Importance of Resolving Difficulties

Ethics and power are all about how we treat others through our attitudes and our behavior. Relationships are what make ethics necessary. Being sensitive to our impact and staying connected even in conflict is at the core of ethical relationships. Relationships are most effective and grievances are avoided when we are able to resolve problems and repair connections.

We must assume that there will be relationship issues and that our clients will experience feeling hurt. No matter how good our intentions: we make mistakes; we have a complex impact on others; we misunderstand power dynamics; we are naive; we project and are projected on; and harm is caused. We may automatically and habitually link present conflict with past trauma. When conflict triggers old trauma, we may disengage from relationships, dissociate, lose touch with our resources, feel hopeless with shame, or blame others.

When acknowledged and attended to, most mistakes can be corrected and most harm can be repaired. A number of studies have shown that what people need when they have been harmed in a helping relationship is surprisingly simple, as summarized below (Stolorow et al., 1987). Unacknowledged hurt feelings can escalate toward an ethical grievance at an alarming rate. Rather than getting defensive, feeling ashamed, or referring to clients as resistant, we can attend directly to the difficulty.

What Clients Need When They Have Been Harmed in a Helping Relationship

1. **Acknowledgment**
   They want their experience acknowledged, understood, validated, and empathized with.
2. **Understanding**
   They want to know what happened, or what our intention was.
3. **Regret**
   They want an apology, or an authentic expression of our sorrow or regret.
4. **Learning**
   They want reassurance that we've learned or understood something about ourselves or how to better care for them.
5. **Repair**
   They want to reconnect and participate in repair of the relationship or in gaining clarity and letting go.

The more immediate the attention to the problem, the more clear and complete the resolution. Skills of tracking and contact—so central to the Hakomi method—are of great help to therapists in noticing and attending to safety and relationship issues in present time. By approaching ethics and power reparationally, we can put our attention toward skillful resolution, relationship repair, and self-correction.

Case Example

The phone message said, "I want to come in for a completion session because I need to use my financial resources for something else." Steven, a body psychotherapist, wondered what else might be going on for this client, who had not yet met the goals she had set for herself. When Carrie came for her completion session, she focused on how great therapy had been and how thankful she was, and how unfortunately she just couldn't afford to come anymore. Steven sensed some tension and asked Carrie, "Is there anything at all that you are disappointed about?" Carrie answered, "No, you have been such a good listener and so patient and insightful." Steven checked again. "Thank you. As I think about the work we've done together, I wonder if you feel discouraged that the problem you came in to work on hasn't resolved even though you've gotten clearer about it."

Carrie was silent for a time and then, apparently feeling safe and encouraged, took what was a big risk for her. She spoke thoughtfully. "Yes, actually, I am disappointed. I've done a lot of therapy and once again it seems like it hasn't worked. If it was working, I'd feel like my money was being well used." Steven contacted her feelings and her courage and thanked her for being so honest. Carrie went on, "And something else—I have felt a little uncomfortable with how close to me you move your chair, and sometimes, like when we did the experiment when we were pushing hands so I could find out about anger, touching was too much. But I thought, you're the therapist and I really want to change and so I never said anything."

Steven took a breath and responded, "Thank you for telling me. Again, that must have taken courage. I am so sorry that I wasn't tracking the cues you have given me about your discomfort. Could we spend a few minutes with this? I'll start moving my chair back and you tell me when the distance feels just right." After finding and experiencing the right distance, which turned out to be about 6 feet away, Steven suggested an experiment in mindfulness in which he would move slowly closer. She would hold up her hand when she began to feel uncomfortable and they could both notice what happened. Steven described tracking a slight tensing in her cheeks, but otherwise, everything about Carrie's demeanor and posture seemed visibly unchanged to him when she was uncomfortable.

Carrie had an insight: "I feel it all inside me and I put a lot of effort into making sure that you won't notice anything that might not be agreeable." Steven responded, "So it seems that you have been working hard for me not to be able to notice. And you succeeded, but it cost you a lot of suffering. I'm imagining you might be a bit angry that I didn't notice." She said, "Well, yes. You're the therapist. You're supposed to notice. I don't want to have to tell you. Then I feel like I'm doing your job!"

From this interaction, Steven was able to self-correct by being more attuned to Carrie's discomfort cues and her fears of not being liked. Carrie had had a successful experience of revealing discomfort and not being rejected. She took a several-month break and then returned to work successfully, this time, with being more personally engaged and self-disclosing in her relationships. Had Steven not found a way to help Carrie talk about these concerns, her sense of betrayal and distrust could have escalated into a grievance and kept her away from seeking successful therapy in the future.

Ethical Proactivity

Responses to issues of power and ethics can be unconscious and history based, and littered with automatic behavior and outdated beliefs. By actively exploring our ethical edges, taking care of ourselves, and asking for and using feedback constructively, we become more sensitive. We can increase our skills, change ineffective habits, and use lessons from our history to grow. Focusing on proactive right use of power takes ethics to a deeply refined level.

Case Example

He was a well-loved music teacher. He loved his students. After several months of therapy, he told his therapist that he was ready to talk about something he hadn't had the trust to bring up before and even then wasn't sure how it would be received. He had felt for a while that something about the way he loved his students, especially the boys, wasn't right. He had noticed that when he gave one of the boys a hug, he was grasping on, wanting to father him, wanting to give him more than a teacher should. He had then had a dream that he was holding one of his students and then in the dream the student was holding him. The therapist appreciated his courage and helped him explore what was going on. His father had died when he was six and he had experienced an aching longing for father love and attention that he felt as an adult as a deep, vacant place in his chest. In paying attention to this place in his chest, it became clear that this was the emptiness he was trying to fill when he was hugging his students. Understanding this strong need from his childhood helped him find other ways to connect and be nourished—filling himself with his music, reaching out more to friends, being more playful. His love for his students then shifted dramatically to more appropriate expression. His courage in bringing this issue to therapy resulted in proactive behavior that prevented harm to his students.

Conclusion

The Hakomi method is highly tuned to the establishment and maintenance of ethical decision making and ethical therapeutic relationships. Therapeutic relationships are intended to be empowering. The power differential role can be used to support self-discovery, rely on internal wisdom, become more lovingly present, reduce unnecessary suffering, and create new possibilities. This use of personal and professional power promotes empowerment and well-being.

Right use of power is the heart of ethics. Empathy and compassion can inform often complex and challenging situations, so that both caregivers and clients will be empowered to self-correct and grow into increased sensitivity. The development of compassion, "as being an ability to imagine—to see—the connection between everyone and everything, everywhere" (Barasch, 2005, p. 304), is the salve for wounds and separation, and the inspiration and motivation for those who are in positions of power and trust. In becoming increasingly ethically sensitive and aware, we can and must link our power with heart.

Technique and Intervention

CHAPTER 14

The Skills of Tracking and Contact

Donna Martin

HAKOMI HAS BEEN described by Ron Kurtz as a method of assisted self-study. Two of the most important skills for the therapist that support this approach are called tracking and contact. Tracking is an active form of witnessing, which involves paying attention to the outward signs of the client's internal, present-moment experience and the way her experience seems to be organized by core beliefs and habits. Contact is the skill of verbally responding to the client, to demonstrate presence and understanding as well as to help bring something into the client's consciousness for the purpose of self-study.

These are the most fundamental skills in the method, and the rest of the process unfolds from how well these are practiced. Contact and tracking are a big part of creating the kind of limbic resonance on which the therapeutic relationship and process of therapy are based. In *A General Theory of Love*, limbic resonance is defined as "a symphony of mutual exchange and internal adaptation whereby two mammals become attuned to each other's inner states" (Lewis et al., 2000, p. 61). The authors go on to say that the first part of emotional healing is being limbically known—"having someone with a keen ear catch your melodic essence" (p. 168). In the Hakomi method, we consider the concept of limbic resonance to be similar to what is being described as "attunement" or "mindsight" (Siegel, 2006). The skills of contact and tracking can be honed further and further, and will eventually become the skill base for an attuned therapeutic relationship—a crucial aspect of therapy in the context of attachment theory (Cozolino, 2006; D. Siegel, 2010; Wallin, 2007) as well as in common factors research, where the therapeutic alliance is understood as a core indicator for therapeutic success (Ardito & Rabellino, 2011; Hubble, Duncan, & Miller, 1999; Wampold, 2001).

Tracking

One of the distinguishing characteristics of the Hakomi method is the use of little experiments done in mindfulness for the purpose of self-study (see Chapter 16). Helping clients to "lower the noise"—to quietly slow things down in order to notice and study what is happening in their bodies, their thoughts, and their feelings—is a fundamental aspect of this approach.

Tracking is the key to setting up experiments through the observation, by the therapist, of much more than the verbal story being told. The therapist is taking in information all the time from such things as tone of voice, pacing, gestures, posture, facial expressions, and the many ways that clients communicate their internal world and the models they hold of their reality.

Daniel Goleman (1996), in his book *Emotional Intelligence*, estimates that more than 90% of someone's emotional experience is expressed nonverbally. Research has shown that "we can learn a lot more about what people think by observing their body language and facial expressions . . . than by asking them directly" (Gladwell, 2005 p. 155). Yet most of us have not learned to pay much attention to more than the verbal content of someone's story—to listen to the narrative beliefs behind the story being told, to the storyteller behind the stories.

Tracking is about taking in information about the client on as many levels as possible. The key to this, more than anything else, is the state of mind of the therapist. So to talk about tracking, as therapists, we must first look at our own states of mind.

There is an old Chinese tale of a man who came out of his home to chop wood only to discover that his axe was missing. He looked around and noticed his neighbor's boy playing in the yard next door. As he looked, he noticed that the boy looked like a thief, sounded like a thief, moved like a thief. Suddenly the neighbor from next door came back with the axe, which he had borrowed. Now the boy, when the old man turned to see him again, looked like a child, sounded like a child, moved like a child.

It is easy to demonstrate to yourself that your perception is altered by your state of mind. Sit in a public place, for example, and take a moment to imagine this fantasy: All the adults you see are only five years old. This is a kindergarten setting. Now look around. Can you see the child in everyone? Imagine another fantasy: Everyone around you has saved someone's life. Look around again. Can you see bravery, kindness, dignity, humanity? Ordinariness and greatness all rolled up in one being?

We cannot begin to observe or track another without attending first to our own states of mind and habits of perception. Kurtz developed a practice for shifting the attitude of the therapist in a way that cultivates a state of mind most conducive to working with others in a healing way. He called it the practice of loving presence (see Chapter 9). It involves being very good, as a first step, at mindfully noticing our automatic tendencies and habits of perception and attention. We want to become more conscious of what Malcolm Gladwell (2005) calls our "blink" perceptions, or Kahnemann (2011) calls "system one," namely the way our adaptive unconscious (Wilson, 2002) reacts to people and situations.

The next step in this practice is to create a kind of spaciousness—to clear away the habitual projections and attitudes that obscure clear perception. In that new state of spacious mind, we learn to look more receptively, more intuitively, and more appreciatively (Johanson, 2008).

We then create an intention to see something in the other that inspires us. We invite and search for those qualities in the other that nourish us—qualities like courage, vulnerability, sensitivity, gentleness, determination, and intelligence. The natural result of finding this— something that inspires and nourishes us—is twofold. First, we relax. We are touched and reminded of the client's strengths and innate beauty. Our heart opens to see this person in her wholeness.

Amazingly, the person begins to realize, unconsciously at first, that she can reveal herself safely. She feels invited, accepted, and appreciated, and begins to express even more of herself. This is noticed by the therapist, who then feels even more inspired and nourished. A reinforcement cycle is underway that deepens the connection, and this creates the context for assisted self-study and discovery to occur naturally and spontaneously in ways that will serve the client and begin the healing process.

Tracking for Signs of Present Experience

In any case, tracking is best done from this calm, receptive, appreciative state, noticing any signs of the client's present-moment experience. We watch for nonverbal signs such as the client's breathing, body movements, skin tone, angle of the head, quivering, twitching, tension patterns, facial expressions, tears, sighing, tone of voice—anything at all that gives us a sense of what is happening internally for the client. We pay special attention to tracking the level of nervous system arousal in the client—how activated he is. When the person has been traumatized, we want to look for signs that he is outside the window of tolerance, either too highly aroused to be able to use mindfulness, or too numb and dissociated. We need to be able to recognize signs of hyper- or hypoarousal, dissociation, or trance. We need to notice when the person is in flight-or-fight mode, and to help him calm down. We want to be able to see, sense, and recognize even fleeting signs of the client's internal state as it changes from moment to moment. Since collaboration is so important in therapy (Duncan, 2010), we also enlist the client, when appropriate, to become sensitive to tracking himself, and naming his present felt experience while staying with it, as opposed to coming out of it to report to us about it from a distance.

A simple but important sign to track for is the client's readiness to speak, when ready to express her experiential truth, at which point the therapist needs to stop and listen. We also track for when the client is doing work inside, which also signals us to wait. We let the client follow her internal process, find congruent thoughts and ideas that arise from emotional states, and come up with her own insights and answers. We must track for the difference between the client falling into old trances, which we need to interrupt, and doing important inner work, which requires that we wait patiently for a signal that invites us to engage. We watch for signs of social engagement. We also pay attention to our own feelings and bodily experience. We learn to track and to trust the degree of limbic resonance that is happening between the client and ourselves.

Tracking Nonverbal Indicators

Once we are observing what the person's moment-to-moment experience seems to be, we begin to detect nonverbal indicators of core material. These include signs of how the person is organizing experience—things that seem significant or characteristic about the person. We want to notice something that suggests how the client sees himself, how he sees the world, what he expects from others. We remember that all we can actually do is guess about this. We don't need to be right, but we want to collect some possible ideas as hypotheses for experiments, and to check them out when the time is right. We are looking for patterns of emotional management behavior, of meaning making, and of social engagement skills.

So we learn to pay attention to the client's eyes, postural habits, gestures that repeat themselves, the expression etched in the face (the default expression), patterns of speech—anything that goes with the client's unique personal style. We want to continually see these characteristics in the light of loving presence, not to pathologize them or make them a problem in terms of the person's being. To foster this, we might take on the characteristics of a person's style the way an actor would, not to caricaturize or mimic them, but just subtly embodying them to get a more compassionate sense of what the client's world is like. We are interested in inhabiting the client's world in order to understand his fears, his needs, his experience of life, his ideas about himself and others. The result of this kind of understanding is a natural feeling of warmth toward him, of compassionate appreciation. Barasch notes, "Being able to feel our way into another's soul, to sense what is going on behind their social mask, is the passkey to kindness" (2005, p. 58).

There are many possible nonverbal indicators of how people organize their experience and model their world. Just the voice alone offers these possible indicators: tone, intonation, cadence, intensity, loudness, speed, long pauses, word order, editing, laughing, swallowing, whispering, repeating words or phrases ("you know," "because," "uh . . ."), using past tense, saying "you" instead of "I," repeated throat clearing, and so on.

We could notice, for example, that someone tends to speak quickly, in little bursts. We could imagine or guess that this habit might go back to a situation where the person as a child wasn't listened to enough, or with enough patience. We then hypothesize a generalized belief the person might have that others have limited attention available for him—that he needs to speak fast or the listener will be gone before he gets it all out. We could contact this possible dynamic by saying, "I notice that you seem to speak quickly," with an invitation to curiosity implied in our voice. We could also suggest, as an experiment (see Chapter 16), "Notice what happens if you speak slowly." Or we could just leap in with our guess about a missing experience and offer a statement like, "I'm listening to you. I'll stay while you finish saying what you want to say." Or simply, "I'm interested in you," while closely tracking the client's response for parts of him that agree and parts that might not.

Other indicators include facial expressions (as so delicately researched by Ekman & Rosenberg, 2005), such as position of the lips, licking the lips, biting the lip, chin forward, chin up or down, jaw tension, blushing, smiling or not smiling, furrowed brow, eyes wide open, looking up, direction of eyes, no eye contact, eyes seem forward or pulled back, narrowing of the eyes, dimming of the light in the eyes, movement of the eyebrows—there are perhaps hundreds of these little signs that can serve as indicators. Significant nonverbal indicators might also include body gestures, postural tendencies like curling inward, turning away, or leaning forward, raised shoulders, shrugging movements, rigidity, rocking, hand movements, position of the feet, containing (by holding arms in tight to the sides), rubbing fingers, stroking a leg, covering mouth while speaking, incongruent gestures, facial expressions, or speech—all those outward signs of internal experiences that body psychotherapy has explored for decades (Marlock & Weiss, with Young & Soth, 2015).

Tracking is one of the ways that Hakomi therapy is present centered—the skill of paying attention to the outward physical signs of the person's present experience. Nonverbal indicators are usually outside a person's conscious awareness. They are habitual, reflecting the core material that organizes a person's experience, as well as her sense of self. One of the main goals of the Hakomi method is to bring this core material to consciousness. The first step is to notice the signs of implicit beliefs in the way someone expresses her experience. Tracking allows a therapist to do this and not ask unnecessary questions or wait for the client to tell him.

Contact

Once we have an idea of what the client is experiencing, we can make explicit contact, though hopefully we have been in a nonverbal level of contact all along. Verbal contact is naming the client's present experience. We contact something we have tracked—something the other person is doing, feeling, or focusing on in the moment. It can be something the client is conscious of, or something that is outside of her awareness. We generally avoid contacting the content or story unnecessarily, beyond letting the person know we are listening and following what she is telling us.

In Hakomi, we consider it more skillful and clinically useful to contact the experience the person seems to be having while she telling us about it: "That brings up some feelings. . .[?]" "You're remembering it now, huh. . . [?]" "That makes you happy. . . [?]" A contact statement is actually a short phrase that lets the person know (1) that you are listening and really present in a heartfelt way, (2) that you're interested and in a nonjudgmental state, and (3) that you understand her feelings and internal experience. A contact statement is open ended, almost like a question: "That was intense for you . . . [?]" "Hard to talk, huh. . .[?]"—so the other person can easily accept, reject, or modify it. Contact, therefore, invites the client to slow down, explore deeper, be more specific, and find out what is really going on inside.

The Practical Skill of Contacting

While the verbal skill of contact is quite simple and is sometimes used by people intuitively in everyday life, it needs a background of the therapist "being in contact." This means that through tracking and by being in a state of mindful connection and awareness of the client's present experience, the therapist can empathically sense what is going on behind the words and other expressions of the client (Marks-Tarlow, 2012). Since many therapists are trained to focus on the story being told, the state of the client may become lost as secondary. This change of focus from story to storyteller often takes therapists long periods of relearning. With this way of being present in place, contact flows without any effort from the therapist, if no other conflicting factors are in play.

When we teach contact in the Hakomi method, we focus our behavior on the following guidelines that tend to become second nature after some practice:

- A contact statement addresses only one aspect of the client's experience—a simple, one-dimensional observation—nothing that invites complex mental work. It is meant to be easy to grasp and to lead to deeper internal observations.
- Contact statements use the present tense and rarely address the content of the verbal exchange.
- The statement is short, sometimes only one word, like, "sad. . .[?]," "nerve-wracking . . . [?]," or "confusing . . . [?]." More often it includes a small number of words, such as, "several parts here . . . [?]" or "hard to stay present . . .[?]."
- A contact statement isn't a true question, but has a questioning tone and is open-ended enough (indicated by the [?] symbol) to let the client know that the therapist is guessing and not attached to being right. The therapist's tone invites curiosity and slowing down. That gives the client the freedom to search inside himself, to confirm, reject, specify, reflect, or add, because there is nothing in the therapist to resist that takes the client's attention away from his own process. Ultimately, this supports a deepening exchange in which a client can feel well understood, and trust that he is on a collaborative, curious search together with the therapist, mining the wisdom of the client's experience.
- Full diagnostic questions are avoided because they lead the client, and create a doctor-patient system (Chapter 22) where it is implied that the doctor is going to magically or scientifically do something with the response. Questions such as, "Did you ever feel this before? Why do you think you are feeling this kind of emotion?" often trigger left-brain efforts in clients, and encourage them to come up with a theory about their experience rather than immersing themselves mindfully in it.

Questions can be used skillfully to keep clients in a mindful exploration: "Oh, some emotion comes up with that, huh. . . [?] Why don't we hang out with that longer? What does that part of you seem to need?"

- Skillful contact statements might not even be noticed by the client. The therapist is very simply demonstrating understanding to create attunement in and for the therapeutic relationship. Later on in the process, a contact statement can be used to shift attention to something the client could then study (only if he or she becomes curious). It is an invitation for the client to become aware of or go more deeply into what is arising in him with the therapist coming along as a companion. It can often bring attention to something the client has not been aware of, and opens the door to the assisted self-study which is the main characteristic of Hakomi.

Using Contact

We may contact something in order to help the person be more aware of some part of his experience, or to help him stay with an experience: "Your breathing starts to change as you think about that, huh. . . [?]" "So, that feeling is in your chest. . . [?]" "Maybe you notice some tightness in your jaw . . .[?]" "Your hands seem to be saying something. . . [?]" At some point, we want to shift the person's attention to one of the indicators of what we imagine to be core material. We want to do this with good timing, sensitivity, and grace.

Contact serves several purposes in a Hakomi session. It is part of building the relationship and, as such, it must be an expression of the therapist's state of mind—loving presence. Any hint of a critical attitude or implication of something wrong can jeopardize the relationship and compromise the therapeutic alliance. The therapist doesn't need to verbalize the experience she is having that evokes in her a spontaneous state of loving presence, such as the client's sweet nature or determination or courage, but she could at times: "I am so touched by the courage you show." But the conscious intention to be seeing the client in this way not only influences what the therapist can perceive, it also gets communicated in the tone, energy, and words the therapist uses whenever she makes verbal contact. Being in loving presence, of course, does not mean we cannot be curious about countertransference reactions that are evoked in us by the other, which can also give us clues about how the other is organized (Feinstein, 1990; Natterson, 1991).

Our attitude in working with our experience or our client's remains crucial. Just the tiny shift of saying, "That was really frightening, huh. . .?" instead of "You were frightened?" conveys a different message to the client. Therefore, the skillfulness involved with contacting the client is less about getting the words right than it is about the state of mind from which the therapist does or says anything. It comes back to working on our own presence and habits of perception. It comes down to, above all else, the practice of loving presence.

In the last part of a session, we often contact the parts that are working well, and the nourishment that is going in ("You feel a little more relaxed now. . . [?]") whereas earlier in the session we might contact what seems to be in the way ("Hard to let that in, huh. . . [?]"). Contacting the shifts in the client's experience toward nourishment and transformation helps him anchor these shifts in his conscious awareness and felt experience, so that he may find his way back to them in his daily life outside of the therapy room.

Mastering Tracking and Contact

To develop mastery in the Hakomi skills of tracking and contact, it is most helpful is to practice:

- Staying calm
- Staying present
- Staying aware
- Opening ourselves (being accessible and receptive)
- Loving presence
- Listening (to the body—our own included)
- Responding wisely and compassionately

In short, this means that the therapist needs to be practiced and experienced in being in a mindful state while being present to another person.

Listening—deep listening—means listening to emotions, to the body, to embedded attitudes and themes, to more than just the verbal story someone is telling. The philosopher Heidegger (1966) talked about "releasement" (*Gelassenheit*)—the capacity to be available to what is in a way that lets things be just as they are. In deep listening, we release ourselves to the reality we are encountering, waiting for it to come to us while letting go as best we can of our preconceptions. In Hakomi, listening to emotions skillfully means we specifically try to learn to tell the difference between emotions based on limiting ideas and beliefs, and the natural feelings that are an authentic response to the painful experiences of life. The indicators of someone's inner experience and world are mostly nonverbal. Our own body is also constantly communicating information about the mutual experience we are having as we resonate limbically with another. We may even consider that the heart might be a kind of brain with a large "energy field" that receives and sends signals to and from the immediate environment (Barasch, 2005). From this perspective, we learn to release ourselves to listen to and from the heart to get the best chance of understanding someone's experience in a way that allows us to be helpful.

Responding wisely is the act of verbally or nonverbally expressing what the other person needs from us. It may require staying quiet or speaking, moving away or closer. A wise response moves a client nearer to her own truth, strength, goodness, and freedom. There is no formula for a wise response; it comes from clarity and kindness, wisdom and compassion, courage and sensitivity. However, there is a maxim in Hakomi that says, "When in doubt, collaborate" (Duncan, Miller, Wampold, & Hubble, 2010), and a training exercise called "doing therapy the easy way." In doing therapy the easy way, the therapist collaborates with the client by putting out whatever she is wondering about and allowing the client to choose what is most alive for him in the moment. "We could deepen into this doubt we are contacting, or stay with the image of your brother you noticed. Do you have a sense of which one is best for now?"

Tracking is a kind of loving attention, offering our presence and perceptual skillfulness to another. We demonstrate that we are paying this quality of attention by our demeanor, our nonverbal expression, and by verbally contacting the experience of the talker so that she realizes we are a loving, curious witness. We are always tracking to notice the client's reactions to how we are being. If anything seems to disrupt the limbic resonance or disturb the relational field, we want to name it and shift it if possible. We could do this simply by changing our posture or facial expression, or by contacting what seems to be happening: "So, something doesn't feel quite right here . . . [?]" (see Chapter 22).

What we contact is what we draw the client's attention to, and it demonstrates where our own attention was drawn. In this way, it expresses our state of mind and influences the state of mind of the client. It has the power to direct the flow of attention and in this way to direct the unfolding process of the client and of the therapy session.

The way we do contact, as the outward demonstration of what we are tracking and understanding, as well as of our state of mind as therapists, either invites the process with the client to unfold toward pathology or allows it to move in the direction of nourishment and expanding growth. It determines the degree of nonviolence, nonforcing, and nonjudgment that is possible in the therapeutic relationship. What and how we contact has the power to move the process in the direction of what is now being called "positive psychology" (Johanson, 2010b; Seligman & Csikszentmihalyi, 2000) or to be held by the historical perspective of "damage repair." It either perpetuates clients' ideas that there is something fundamentally wrong with them, or it shifts them in the direction of remembering their wholeness (Monda, 2000), of becoming interested—in a mindful and accepting way—in what and how they do things. In Hakomi, inviting mindfulness is an affirmation that the person was at least cocreative in organizing his experience in the first place, and retains the creative potential to reorganize his life in new, more complex, satisfying ways now. Mindfulness and what Lewis and his coauthors call the love that "is the tether binding our whirling lives" (Lewis et al., 2000, p. 222) empowers clients naturally and respectfully in the direction of finding the kind of emotional nourishment they need at this point in their lives.

Since research shows that the client is the most potent variable affecting outcome of therapy (Wampold, 2001), it is essential that as therapists we remember that we are supporting someone to have a positive experience. This means that therapy

- must be a collaborative process,
- demonstrates that the client's experience guides and directs the process,
- uses experiencing and mindfulness to access the limbic system,
- sees the client as primary agent and the therapist as a support person,
- is experimental, rather than directive or mechanical,
- stays with experience to allow insights to arise,

- respects the needs and goals of the client,
- adjusts for the reactions of the client to the therapist and the process,
- places nourishing self-study, exploration, and self-discovery as a priority, and
- realizes that insight is not enough, but seeks the missing experiences that can counteract and transform previous limiting experiences.

Our ways of perceiving, receiving, and responding to the client, through what we call tracking and contact, form the basis for the therapeutic experience in Hakomi. They are how we show up for the client, and they help to create an alliance that is a powerful context for healing.

CHAPTER 15

Accessing and Deepening

Carol Ladas Gaskin, David Cole, and Jon Eisman

Consciousness: a reflexive aspect of mental process that occurs in some but not all minds, in which the knower is aware of some fraction of his knowledge or the thinker of some fraction of his thought.

GREGORY BATESON, *Angels Fear*, 1987

"ACCESSING" IS A word borrowed by Kurtz from the vocabulary of information technology. It describes a phase in a typical Hakomi session, which progresses from the opening phase of establishing an interpersonal therapeutic alliance to the intrapsychic phase of exploring in mindfulness. It is a move from ordinary consciousness to mindful exploration of emergent, unconscious experience (Kurtz, 1990a).

In the field of information technology, accessing refers to data retrieval from memory storage or from a source remote from the processor. Its metaphoric meaning within Hakomi refers to language and actions initiated by the therapist with the intention of helping a client attend to previously unattended-to experience. By "unattended-to experience," we mean thoughts, feelings, sensations, images, desires, and impulses that exist outside the client's normal purview of awareness. In psychoanalytic language, we are helping clients become aware of their "'pre-reflective unconscious'—the shaping of experience by organizing principles that operate outside a person's conscious awareness" (Stolorow et al., 1987, pp. 12–13). In the language of neuroscience, we are providing a way for clients to access core organizing beliefs (see Chapters 7 and 19) embedded in implicit memory (Schacter, 1992, 1996).

In order to understand this, we might imagine client and therapist exploring a dark landscape together with a flashlight. Prior to the accessing phase, the flashlight of the client's attention has been drifting in habitual patterns that inform a limited cognitive map of the client's internal world, a map based primarily on habituated and stereotyped patterns of attention (Bargh & Chartrand, 1999). Through the skillful use of language and the interventions described below, the Hakomi therapist invites the client's hand gently to alter this automatic scanning pattern, and bring into the light experiences that are otherwise consigned to darkness.

This redirection of attention—sometimes surprising, painful, relieving, or refreshing—gives clients access to new information about their inner ecology (Schwartz, 1995). Accessing in the context of safety and support leads into the deepening phase that helps clients come to understand and take ownership of previously unconscious interpretations, decisions, beliefs, agendas, and positions thought of by Ecker and Hulley (1996) as including emotional wounds, presuppositions, and protective actions. Kris (1982) and others have suggested that possible organizers of experience could be frustrated desires, forgotten fears, rekindled injuries, internal conflicts, memories of relationships, or enduring character traits.

In Hakomi, we are helping our clients study how they have unconsciously organized experience, usually with regard to certain areas of concern, such as unwanted behaviors, constraints, and forms of suffering or perturbation, that motivate them to seek help.

Hakomi's Constructivist Roots

What we do not make conscious emerges later as fate.

CARL JUNG

A personal past that acts silently to make someone repeat patterns at any and all scales and in any and all conditions can only feel like an intrinsic constraint reducing the degree of freedom in the present.

DANIEL STERN, *The Present Moment in Psychotherapy and Everyday Life*, 2004

Hakomi has a constructivist view of human psychology (Mahoney, 2003). Hakomi therapists operate on the premise that human beings are active agents in at least the cocreation of a world of meaning and experience. Not only do humans consciously and unconsciously interpret their experience and give it meaning, but they also organize and manage it. This organization and management places some things in the domain of conscious awareness, and consigns others to the forgetfulness of the unconscious. For example, Siegel (1999) writes that implicit memory carries emotionally loaded memories such as those experienced in disorganized or chaotic attachments (Karen, 1998). They are stored in the limbic brain and are often preverbal memories or experiences where insight is blocked. These memories when retrieved have no feeling of being a memory. In a sense, a great deal of experience is organized outside of the mind's limited scope of attention into the domain of the unconscious, where it continues autonomously to influence affect and behavior in the interest of perceived self-survival and self-fulfillment.

Given the limited capacity of the human mind to be reflexively aware of experience in a present moment, at any given time most of what we know is known unconsciously (Stern, 2004). Also, given the difficulty humans encounter when they deliberately try to change habitual patterns of behavior—dieting, getting more exercise, managing temper, learning to be less judgmental, or learning to slow down, even when that behavior results in frustration, failure, pain, and discomfort—one must assume, as does contemporary science (Lipton, 2005), that what is unconscious has a far greater capacity to motivate behavior than what we consciously know, want, or desire. It follows that by making the unconscious conscious, we render it less powerful and less likely to determine our feelings, thoughts, and behavior. As Ecker and Hulley (1996) suggest, clients normally present in an antisymptom way that desires the riddance of a symptom. However, a little experiential work, such as accessing and deepening in Hakomi, inevitably reveals a prosymptom level where the presenting problem makes perfect sense in terms of fulfilling unconscious needs with originally limited resources (Johanson & Taylor, 1988).

Or, as Watzlawick has often put it in books and lectures, consciousness is the problem (Watzlawick et al., 1974). The inherent predicament with many talk therapies that occur in ordinary consciousness is that consciousness is already organized. Both perception of and response to external and internal stimuli have already been organized by the core filters, beliefs, schemas, or maps of our unconscious imagination by the time we are perceiving and responding. While verbal discourse can provide many things such as support and analytical insight, it is basically recycling already known material at the mercy of unknown organizers (Wilber, 2006) influenced by subtle but powerful social-cultural as well as personal-familial forces (Paniagua & Yamada, 2013; Sue & Sue, 1990; Thomas & Scharazbaum, 2006). This is why Watzlawick and others opted for paradoxical and/or hypnotic methods in therapy to negotiate this conundrum of consciousness.

If these presumptions are correct, then accessing the organization of experience through mindfulness is indeed a powerful way for human beings to relate and interact (Fisher, 2002; Grayson, 2003; Siegel & Hartzell, 2003). Within the therapeutic interaction of a Hakomi session there is born a capacity for freedom that exceeds the freedom an individual can achieve through acting alone, even through meditating alone (Wilber, 2006). The attention of the individual acting alone is constantly constrained by these unconsciously determined patterns we have been naming. The therapist equipped to facilitate accessing nudges the hand that holds the beam to break the self-reinforcing patterns of attention that sustain habitual ways of thinking, interpreting, and reacting.

This is so because the basic assessing move toward mindfulness induces a shift in consciousness away from simply talking about one's experience or simply acting it out in some expressive way and toward talking from direct, present-moment experience. The mindful qualities of slowing down, letting go of agendas, becoming open, receptive, exploratory, and befriending experience as opposed to changing it allow us to be present to immediate, felt experience in a way that opens a place of mysterious not-knowing that makes possible the discovery of new material (Chapters 10 and 15). At the same time, bringing bare awareness to our present experience allows us to take it under observation or disidentify with it (Kegan, 1982). No longer being fused or blended with our experiences, we now have them instead of simply being them, thus achieving a freedom that overcomes Watzlawick's problematic. A short answer, then, to the question, "What do you do in Hakomi?" is "We manage states of consciousness," in a way that helps us access unconscious experience in a mindful state.

We suggest that this accessing movement is a coconstructivist endeavor in which client and therapist conspire in the creation of freedom to act nonreactively, thereby honoring complexity, diversity, and response flexibility. As Stolorow and colleagues (1987) point out so clearly, everyone, therapists and clients alike, creatively organizes experience. This means that therapy must indeed be intersubjective, since neither side can claim objectivity in our postmodern world. In Hakomi, this translates into working in a radically collaborative way that always honors the organic wisdom of a client's experience (Duncan, 2010).

The Unconscious Is Organic, Knowing, and Close at Hand

Living things are called organisms because of the overriding importance of organization and each part of the pattern somehow contains the information as to what it is in relation to the whole.

ROBERT O. BECKER, *The Body Electric*, 1998

The accessing metaphor connotes that the needed unconscious information is close at hand and can appear quickly once the right accessing code and context are discovered. Indeed, in Hakomi, we believe that the unconscious figuratively shines through the conscious persona like flakes of gold in the ore of the present moment. It is right there before our very eyes wanting to be discovered. There is an impulse, which manifests in multiple ways, of the organism to heal—to move toward greater wholeness (Monda, 2000). As Ilya Prigogine won the Nobel Prize for discovering (Prigogine & Stengers, 1984), there are not only entropic forces in life that tear things down, there is a negentropic force that moves parts toward increasing complexity. Gendlin (1996) thinks of this phenomenon in terms of "the life-forward direction," while Fosha (2008) refers to it as "transformance."

Gold-accessing codes are often revealed in body posture, which can be employed for efficient retrieval of normally unconscious information. For instance, a therapist reflected with curiosity to a client he was working with while standing:

THERAPIST: I notice your left foot is not parallel with the right, but pointed out a bit[?].
CLIENT: Oh, yeah.
THERAPIST: Are you curious about that?
CLIENT: Yeah, it makes me wonder.

THERAPIST: Okay, how about just bringing your awareness to it, and maybe notice if there is any movement associated with it.

CLIENT [Puts more pressure on the outward foot]: Oh! It is the beginning of a movement toward the door.

THERAPIST: The door. . . [?]

CLIENT: Yes, like that is my escape route.

THERAPIST: Oh, escape. Like some part of you needs to know that is an option. How about making space for it, and allowing it to tell you more about itself?

CLIENT: Uh . . . so . . . it is something about humiliation. If there is any form of disrespect, it wants to head for the door.

THERAPIST: That sounds reasonable. Can you stay with it and sense into what it needs around that?

CLIENT: Yeah. . . . It needs to know its opinions . . . its opinions won't be shut down because someone thinks they are smarter.

THERAPIST: All right then. So, let's tell it clearly, from me and from you, that we really want to respect its opinions or hear about it if it starts to feel humiliated.

CLIENT: Okay. Yeah, it's getting that. It's calming down.

THERAPIST: Great. And I'm thinking it would not have that sensitivity if there were not some good reason for it. Would this be a good time for us to make room for it to lead us toward any foundational memories it might have in its consciousness around this issue?

CLIENT: Yeah, this is a familiar one.

This is an example of a therapist trained to relinquish a habitual fixation on the content of the client's speech—the repetitive recital of stories, complaints, explanations, cycles of figuring out, and automatic systems of interaction. More positively, the therapist is trained to attend to the client's present-moment experience as revealed by literally everything else the client characteristically does, including the placement of his feet. Various forms of body language—tone of voice, facial gestures, breathing patterns, hand gestures, speech rhythms, tics, and key words—may all reveal (Kurtz & Prestera, 1976) core narrative organizers, all of which can be used as a royal road to the unconscious (Johanson, 2015). This is also an example of accessing by going from ordinary consciousness to a more mindful state, and then deepening by maintaining mindful curiosity about what comes up next. The deepening process moves from an example of the client's creation (placement of feet, in the example above) toward the level of the creator, the core narrative memories and beliefs organizing the feet.

Preconditions for Success With Accessing Skills

When a limbic connection has established a neural pattern, it takes a limbic connection to revise it.

THOMAS LEWIS, FARI AMINI, AND RICHARD LANNON,
A General Theory of Love, 2000

Since a living, organic system has inherent, self-protective dispositions, accessing requires that the first agenda be that client and therapist become allies and collaborators in order to create a perceived environment of emotional safety (Chapter 9). It is important to move slowly as well as with sensitivity and respect. It is essential that we adopt an anthropological attitude—one that realizes the relativity of all systems of meaning and value, and refrains from expectations and impositions of external frameworks and absolute ideals and standards (McGoldrick et al., 1996; Paniagua & Yamada, 2013; Thomas & Schwarzbaum, 2006). Toward this end, the five foundational Hakomi principles of unity, organicity, mind-body holism, mindfulness, and nonviolence must constantly underlie all methods and techniques. In addition, Kurtz (1990a) has recommended somewhat overlapping, but worth repeating, guidelines for accessing: Create safety; concentrate on present experience; go slowly—always within a therapeutic bubble of loving presence.

Essential Accessing Skills: The Accessing Four-Step

All accessing in Hakomi follows a basic four-step formula:

1. Contact experience.
2. Ensure mindfulness is present.
3. Immerse fully in the experience.
4. Study the nuances of the experience or allow the experience to summon other related experiences.

The information or summoned experience from the fourth step then becomes the subject of the next, first-step contact statement, and the sequence repeats. Each round reveals wider and deeper elements of the client's experiential system, all the way down, eventually, to the core organizing material from which the experiences arise.

While we may, for the sake of conceptual simplicity, describe the process in metaphoric terms of up and down, in fact it is essential to hold the more accurate perspective that the client's organization is actually holographic. More an interactive sphere than a ladder, our psychological-neural-somatic-emotional selves are held and therefore accessed using these four steps in a serpentine meander through an otherwise subconscious labyrinth.

Let's clarify each step.

Step 1: Contact Experience

Contact, described in Chapter 14, is used during the accessing phase for three main purposes. First, we want to demonstrate to the client that we understand his current experience. Such demonstration provides both acknowledgment and acceptance. "So you tighten your shoulders as you say that . . .[?]" lets the client know both that we grasp that this is happening, and, by virtue of our embracing tone, that we are interested in a curious way while not judging it.

Second, contacting the client's present experience spotlights the experience, and focuses awareness on this particular experiential location. By naming the tight shoulders, it supports the client tuning in more deeply to the nuances of that experience.

And third, we can use a contact statement to steer the flow of the session in some ostensibly useful direction. There may be several events occurring, with some seeming more closely aligned with the client's present or longed-for need. We may work more efficiently by directing the client toward some less aware or more charged aspect of his world. For example, the client may be talking about and focused on a complaint about his relationship, and we notice that his shoulders are tightening. By contacting the shoulders, we steer the client away from the exclusivity of his verbal focus to include a somatic element he may not otherwise have noticed.

Even more strategically, we may steer the flow of the session by contacting some element we, as clinicians, assume or guess is present. "There's probably something familiar about this tension . . . [?]," we might offer, or—guessing at the underlying meaning of his story—guide the client toward his deeper need by stating, "So what you really want is to be respected. . . [?]" Like a good tennis player placing the ball in a particular part of the court, a skilled therapist can use contact to direct the session and the client's awareness toward deeper or more inclusive aspects of his process.

Of course, as always in Hakomi, we are careful to track diligently for the impact of our attempts to suggest and steer. We are hoping our attempt at guiding his flashlight of awareness evokes a deepening curiosity in the client, but we are fully prepared to back off and reorient if we get hesitant responses to our suggested direction.

Most of the time, more than one kind of experience is present. In the above example, we are tracking both the verbal and the somatic: the complaint story and the tightening shoulders. We may also be aware of affect (client seems cranky) or breath (shallow and rapid) or facial expression (determination) or any number of other emergent features. As practitioners, any or all of this may be the best to focus on, including umbrella statements, such as the simple "So there's a lot going on. . . ." As a part of accessing, we need to develop the skill of intuiting (Marks-Tarlow, 2012) where the energy seems to be, the complexity of experience, and the need to somehow keep things simple enough so that the client can proceed without distraction.

Step 2: Ensure Mindfulness

As discussed previously, mindfulness is central to Hakomi, which has pioneered its use in psychotherapy since the early 1970s. If we are to assist clients in studying their experiences, so they are enabled to notice the internal sources of those experiences, then awareness will be absolutely essential. When we are accessing, once we have invited the client into some present experience, we need to be certain that she is in the proper state of awareness that will allow the careful investigation and revelation of all that is actually happening. Just as it would be fruitless to enter a dark cave without a flashlight, so engaging experience without awareness typically yields only superficial or rote insight into its qualities and origins, and tends to reinforce its habituated nature.

So, as our second step of accessing, we want to be sure the client is sufficiently embodied in the state and skill of mindful self-observation. We do this by tracking for signs of self-attention, verbal quality and content, and a sense of energetic settling (however simultaneously activating the presenting experience may be). If we are not satisfied that mindfulness is present, and sufficiently deep to examine experience carefully, it is our job to help the client get more fully induced into mindfulness. There is no point in proceeding toward accessing core material if the client is not able to observe, as opposed to being carried away by, the organization of her experience.

This monitoring of mindfulness is an ongoing task throughout accessing that we refer to as managing consciousness. Clients may be fully mindful one moment, and then pop out for any number of reasons: they are more comfortable reporting in conversational mode; they got distracted; they became anxious about what they are finding; and so on. Therefore, we need to stay diligent about tracking the level of mindfulness present in the client at any moment, and attend to maintaining a suitable depth of awareness as the session proceeds.

Step 3: Immerse Fully in the Experience

The third step in the accessing formula is to have the client be completely immersed in whatever experience is pursued and studied. We want him to embody fully the richness and nuance of the experience or experiences that have been contacted. If it is tight shoulders, then we want his entire world at the moment to be anchored in the sensations, movements, and details of holding tension in those shoulders. If the client is sad, we want her to feel that grief deeply, purely, attentively. We're about to study that field of experience with great care, and so we want the person fully in the field, not on the edge, not looking from above, but so fully grounded in that field that every blade of experiential grass, every breeze that shakes that grass, the size and smell and sounds in that field are all available for recognition and investigation. Imagine the difference between trying to describe the taste of chocolate right now, and how much more specific and nuanced that description would be if you put a piece of chocolate in your mouth and then articulated its specific subtleties while letting it dissolve there.

The immersion into an experience is achieved by the use of what we call accessing directives. Accessing directives are suggestions and commands that lead a person toward mindfulness of a specific activity, focus, or event: "Go ahead and turn your attention toward that sadness. Maybe let yourself really feel how that sadness lingers inside of you." "Take your time, and just let this sadness be here. Let yourself really sink into this feeling. . . . Notice how it registers in your body." These are examples of accessing directives.

Because we are directing clients toward an experience they hope to deal with or learn more about, such commands and suggestions are usually met with compliance. They tend not to be experienced as forceful control of the client's will, because we are actually supporting his own organic wish to do the work. If I hold out a glass of water to a person crawling out of the desert, and say, "Here, drink this!" he won't reply, "Don't tell me what to do!" because his need and the directive to drink are well aligned. Of course, if I tell a client to do something that is not in her interest, or that feels like a promotion of my agenda as opposed to an interface with her, then I will likely get resistance or tense compliance that needs to be contacted to get back on track: "Oh, exploring the chest sensation is not quite right. It would be better to . . ."

Immersion in experience is not a familiar construct in Western culture. Our expressions of experience are not typically met with invitations to plunge into and marinate in them. "I'm scared, Mommy," is more likely to be met with, "Come here and let me hold you" than it is with, "Oh, that must feel yucky. Go ahead and be scared and notice what your body starts to do. . . ." As a result, there is usually a learning curve for practitioners to develop the habit of immersing clients fully into their experiences before invoking the more seemingly glamorous interventions of inquiry and problem solving. "I'm sad" will likely evoke something such as, "What are you sad about?" A reasonable, though left-brain, question, but in the Hakomi framework much better asked after the client has been invited to feel his sadness mindfully. That way, the client will be responding from full access to the exactness of the sadness, and not from some possibly abstracted or less specific place, that is, from a more experiential, right-brain place. He will be reporting about his sadness from within the sadness itself, just as the actual eating of the chocolate will yield a greater source for its description.

Step 4: Study the Experience (Deepening)

After contacting, ensuring mindfulness, and immersing the client in her experience, the final step is to have her explore the experience for its connections within herself, either to relevant information or to linked experiences that are summoned by association.

Any experience that is personally or psychologically significant will be laden with details, nuances, and meanings. An obsessive thought, for example, cycling at a particular speed, may seem to be happening on the right or left side of your head, or may, upon examination, reveal itself to be in the voice of your third grade teacher. If your palm is sitting face up on your leg, studying it may clarify whether it is reaching out to give, or waiting to receive something. Focusing on your excitement about a new job may surprise you by the way it stops abruptly at your belly, below which there is a kind of dark emptiness.

One function of this accessing step is to bring such information into awareness, which is moving from accessing (inviting mindfulness) to deepening (maintaining mindfulness). Not only is it an integral, if often unconscious, aspect of your experiences, but it begins to complete the picture of the world in which you live and operate. Something from third grade is still shaping your current life. On a subtle level, you are hoping that someone will give you something important, even though you don't trust that can happen. You can't just celebrate life, for some murky void undermines your joy. Through accessing, the contact statement steered you toward this experience; the mindfulness gave you the inner frame to discern it; the immersion took you fully into the unconscious' "file" on this experience and now the study phase lets you read what time has written and stored in those archives. Again, we call this part of the process "deepening."

Details and meanings

Some of the information accessed and deepened into may be details about the nuances of how you are organized: the specific location of somatic events ("It's on my right side, just below my shoulder"); the subtle flavor of your sadness ("It's more wistful than grieving"); or the intensity of an impulse ("It's like just the tiniest pulling back from you"), to name just a few examples.

Equally necessary, some of the discovered information may be about meanings: the subjective psychological significance an experience holds or expresses, its importance or relevance, the "why" beneath the "what." You keep your right hand on top of your left hand, because you need to hold your anger back. You don't finish your sentences while speaking, because you don't believe anyone is listening. You're anxious all the time, because your family was reckless and insensitive, and you need to stay alert to avoid otherwise inevitable disaster. That shallow breathing? Perhaps protection from letting in love and losing your freedom.

It's crucial to note that Hakomi's pursuit of meaning through deepening seeks natural revelations from within the immersed study of experience, and not from analytical inquiries or theories about the experience. We don't typically ask the client, in conversational form, "Why do you think you're anxious?" or "How come you breathe so shallowly?" The aspect of self that might answer those questions is likely to be somewhat removed from or lacking access to the full psychological significance of the event. Such questions, in the abstract, often lead to guesses: "I think it's because . . ."; "Well, my astrologer says . . ."; or to partial understandings: "I don't want anyone to know" (while lurking underneath, we later discover, is, "I really need help . . .").

The meaning-experience interface

As we work with a client, we typically move back and forth across what we call the meaning-experience interface. We'll study a present or evoked experience for its details: "Notice exactly where that tension starts and stops. . . ." or "Is that voice angry, or stern, or just determined?" Then we shift over to evoking the experience's meaning: "From inside that tension, notice what it's doing for you. . . ." "As you hear that voice, how does it feel about you that makes it need to tell you this all the time?" When meanings begin to seem more distant, we deliberately return to studying the experience itself, so that the work remains a continuous exploration of the experiential rather than just the interpretive realm: "Oh, so the tension is creating a wall between you and others. So take your time, really be mindful, feel the tension and the need to have a wall, and let yourself notice if this wall is completely solid, or can you find places where something can get through?"

Accessing questions

Notice as you examine the above examples that, in terms of technique, we use three main language structures: contact statements, accessing directives, and what we call accessing questions. We have previously described contact statements ("You start to smile . . .") and accessing directives ("Stay with that smile and see what else you notice . . ."). Accessing questions are questions that can be answered only by immersing in and studying the present experience. The opposite of abstract analysis, accessing questions require the client to move more deeply into the present constellation of events to discover the embedded information. In fact, we will pose such a question only after we have established mindfulness and immersed the person in the experience. We can ask a miner on the surface where he thinks the gold will be found, but we won't know exactly where it is, or even if it is there at all, until we are down in the dirt, digging slowly and carefully, headlamp turned on bright. Accessing questions are among our most useful shovels, once we are inside the mine.

Here are some examples of accessing questions:

- Where exactly in your back does this pain start[?]
- How is your body participating in this sadness right now[?]
- Which of the two feels bigger right now: your fear or your desire to speak[?]
- What impulses show up when you talk about your brother this way[?]
- As you turn your head, are you turning toward something or turning away from something[?]

All of these questions can be answered only by examining carefully the present experiential circumstances. (The [?] symbol, once again, indicates the tone of the therapist's voice that invites the client's own mindful curiosity, as opposed to a doctor-patient interrogatory tone that implies the doctor is going to do something with the information requested.)

Unfolding

As important as gathering such information is to the understanding of ourselves and our core organization, the fourth step provides an additional essential function: to summon up or deepen into related experiences. As discussed in Chapter 8 on character, experiences happen because a specific collection of brain cells (neurons) fire in concert with each other, activating thoughts, emotions, bodily events, and so on. When they fire, a link develops among them, creating a network. Even after the firing ceases, this link—like a kind of channel dug between the cells—remains.

When we immerse in an experience, the links between that experience and others in that network slowly become activated in concert. The more we sink into an experience, the more we fire the neurons associated with that experience. As those neurons become saturated, they send messages along those established channels to other linked neurons in the network. It's like pouring water into a system of channels; gradually, the flood moves from the original location to inundate another. The original neural activation begins to flood connected neural structures. As those linked neurons begin to fire, they generate further related, but distinct, experiences. In the above example, the person complaining about work automatically began to tighten his shoulders. Remaining with a particular experience in mindfulness causes related events to erupt. Staying with the way I point my finger while talking may evoke first a sense of determination, and then gradually a memory of trying to convince my dad about something. Submerging myself in my tendency to sigh may yield a feeling of collapse in my chest, and then a great sense of hopelessness. One distinct, heavily invested experience leads to the arousal of another, linked experience and a fuller sense of the network's organization.

We call this process "unfolding." Like a long ribbon of scarves in a magician's pocket, tugging on any one experience in a neural network gradually pulls all of them out—they unfold piece by piece until the entire system is revealed. Honoring unfolding is the ultimate expression of faith in the client's organicity. We trust that keeping the client mindful and immersed in one aspect of his being will gradually reveal his entire world. Because present experiences are organized by the core images and beliefs that we hold, a seemingly banal experience on the surface of awareness—your palm, say, turned up in your lap—is actually the gateway to a path that leads down into the deepest psychological wellsprings of your being.

As a fourth step, we promote this unfolding by encouraging the client deliberately toward allowance and unforced connection. Rather than seeking details ("Where in your body do you feel this?" "Notice if the voice is coming from inside or outside of you. . . .") or meanings ("What does turning away like this do for you?" "Study what's so important about keeping your eyes open. . . ."), unfolding uses directives to encourage the whole network to wake up: "Go ahead and let whatever wants to happen next, just start to happen. . . ." "Follow that feeling and let it take you where it wants. . . ." "So as you hang out here, without trying to do anything else, notice whatever starts to come up all by itself." We are using directives to encourage the awakening of all intertwined elements of the neural network, gradually spiraling from expressed conscious events down into unconscious core material.

Actually, all four of the steps in the accessing process serve this unfolding function. Contact steers you into an experience. Mindfulness lets you dwell upon it, further activating the neurons. Immersion with its intention of summoning the full experience directly seeks neural arousal, and then fourth-step directives to unfold finalize the process by enlisting the client's cooperation to just allow the unconscious to lead us where it will.

The overall combination of (1) unfolding and (2) pursuing details and meanings allows Hakomi to be potent and comprehensive. In a typical sequence, the therapist may patiently invite unfolding (after contacting, ensuring mindfulness, and immersing), and then explicitly explore details of what has unfolded. She will likely then return to unfolding, excavating, if you will, another corner of the psychic web, followed by more detail work on the new unfolded piece. Here's an example of such accessing:

CLIENT: Every time she turns away, it drives me crazy.
THERAPIST: It's really aggravating.
CLIENT: Yeah, I just want to . . . [trails off]
THERAPIST [noticing fist forms in the left hand]: Looks like your left hand has something to say about it.

CLIENT [looking at his fist]: Huh, I didn't even realize I was doing that.

THERAPIST: Why don't we pay some attention to it, and see what comes up?

CLIENT: Okay. . . .

THERAPIST: Great. So your hand is making a fist. Go ahead and turn your attention inward. Let yourself start to move into that part of yourself that can just notice things. . . . [Seeing the client settling into mindfulness.] Yeah, that's it, just settle into noticing yourself . . . and begin to notice your fist. Just go ahead and really clamp your hand down like that, press your fingers into your palm, all that tension in your arm, really feel exactly the way you experience it. . . .

CLIENT: Hmm, it's really intense. . . .

THERAPIST: Yeah, you're really clamping down. So just stay really focused . . . paying careful attention, still holding your fist like this, just being in this place where your fist is so tight, go ahead and let yourself notice anything at all that starts to happen here by itself—a thought, a feeling, something your hand wants to do, anything at all. . . .

CLIENT [after several seconds]: Huh, it's weird. I start to get this sense something bad is happening and I have to fight. I have to fight or I'll die or something. Something like that. . . .

THERAPIST: Yeah, so it gets even more intense, life or death. Urgent.

CLIENT: Yeah, urgent. . . .

THERAPIST: So let's hang out here. Really staying aware, focusing, feeling into your hand and your arm, and this sense of needing to fight—it's urgent—and study carefully, what is the rest of your body doing[?]

CLIENT [nodding]: Yeah, my jaw is tight. I'm starting to lean forward, just a tiny bit. . . .

THERAPIST: Great! Your jaw and your body are starting to get involved. So just let all that happen, your fist and your jaw and leaning forward, and paying very careful attention, go ahead and scan around in front of you, and see or feel what's out there—is there something, or someone or anything out there with you[?]. . . .

CLIENT [breath stops, slight shudder]: Yeah . . . something. . . .

THERAPIST: Take your time, sense your body—you know something. Feel into that space in front of you, and just let anything at all that wants to show itself to you . . . begin to show itself. . . .

CLIENT [long pause]: I see my mom. She's walking away. . . . She's getting into the car. . . . [Starts to cry.]

In this example, the therapist:

1. contacts the client at each step ("You're really clamping down." "It gets even more intense"),
2. returns several times to keeping the client in a mindful state of focus and awareness ("Go ahead and turn your attention inward." "So just stay really focused. . . paying careful attention. . . "),
3. consistently encourages the client to immerse himself in his experiences ("Go ahead

and really clamp your hand down. . ." "Feeling into . . . this sense of needing to fight. . . ."), and

4. then uses a combination of accessing directives and questions both to flesh out details and meanings ("What is the rest of your body doing?"), and also to encourage the unfolding of further material ("Let anything at all that wants to show itself to you just start to show itself. . . .").

By following this basic accessing structure, the client deepens readily from presenting narrative to core revelation.

In addition to using relatively simple accessing questions and directives by themselves to elicit details, meanings, and unfolding in the fourth step, Hakomi also works experimentally to evoke core experience in more sophisticated ways. Using the first three steps precisely, the therapist can also create and offer what we call little experiments. These provide situationally appropriate, momentary explorations through which the client's innate experiential structure will further emerge (see Chapter 16).

Fourth-step interventions

To summarize, there are four kinds of fourth-step interventions Hakomi uses to evoke experiences and deepen toward core beliefs. All use the groundwork of contact, mindfulness, and immersion in direct experience. Each provides essential elements that synergize with each other, both to allow and to pursue, to make space for the client's own structure to reveal itself, and to permit the practitioner's wisdom and expertise to impact the process. The four kinds of fourth steps are:

1. We ask and direct to uncover details and nuances.
2. We search for embedded meanings.
3. We encourage innate, self-generated unfolding through patient self-association within the network.
4. We design and employ little experiments to evoke complex experiential constructs.

By embracing both allowing (that is, trust in the client's organicity and neural network self-activation) and pursuing (the willingness to take charge, pursue, and help the client stay with exploring significant elements), Hakomi accessing maintains a balance between the organicity and unity principles, and between the client's organic wisdom and the therapist's learned expertise (see Chapter 12).

Issue, Theme, and World

The basic four-step formula and its component techniques yield powerful evocation and exploration of experience. However, simply evoking experiences does not guarantee an efficient path to arriving at the core. Often, simply applying the techniques, even in a skilled way, can lead to a kind of rambling—a serial awakening of related, but not transparently connected, incidents. A bodily tension leads to an abstract thought, and the thought to an image of a field, which in turn summons a different tension. When we add a sense of strategy to the unfoldings and evocations, we minimize the randomness and optimize the capacity for focus.

Strategically, by understanding the way in which psychological networks are logically structured, we can follow that structure toward its origins. The basic structure is this: core organizational beliefs and patterns develop around specific developmental tasks or, in practical terms, around themes. These themes describe the life resources needed for a person to thrive: belonging, protection, support, autonomy, respect, inclusion, and so forth. When one of these fails to lodge fully or successfully enough within a person, we say they have an issue around that theme. Issues describe the fragmented relationship a person has to a theme—the skewed perceptual frames we hold, the distorted meanings we have constructed, and the life problems we endure around that theme. A person who didn't get enough early support will have an issue with abandonment or nourishment. If a child's reasonable requests for attention and love are met with scorn, the child may have an issue with alienation or intimacy. And so on. Formative events can also happen in later life, like going to war at age 20, and often involve issues that require trauma processing.

Issues are what clients typically present; they are feeling the pain of not being well-resourced around some (often unrecognized) theme. Because the actual, necessary resources of the developmental learning are missing or incomplete, the person has had to create various adaptations: postures, voice usages, breathing patterns, beliefs, and so forth. (This process is described in Chapter 8.) These adaptations are the experiences with which we work in our sessions.

It follows, then, that if we pursue the issue shaping the experiences, it will lead us to the theme around which the issue formed. Together, the experiences, issues, and themes create a perceptual and behavioral world in which the client lives. This world is the sum total neural network around which the client operates in distress and for which he has sought help. We can track this world back to where the theme became an issue, back to its core history, woundings, latent resources, and needs, and begin the search for evolution and transformation—the purpose of the therapy.

This process of interfacing and untangling experience, issue, theme, and world—informed by various maps like character and the sensitivity cycle (Chapter 17)—provides the basic strategy for efficient accessing and deepening. To the power of the four-step techniques, it adds the wisdom of making informed choices in how to manage the otherwise semichaotic evocation of experiences. Instead of just digging all over the place to find the gold, we use sophisticated knowledge of inner geology to focus our combined efforts.

We make these choices in four ways:

1. Being curious about, tracking, and deliberately moving toward issue, theme, and world

   Hmm, she keeps avoiding my input. . . .

   What is the pattern emerging here?

   What must it be like to have that thought all the time?

2. Recognizing them: understanding what are typical issues and themes; having a personal and clinical database about how people are and what they do

   Hmm, he said he feels vulnerable. . . . That rings a bell. . . .

   Tightening up is often defensive; he must be protecting against something. . . .

3. Fishing for them: deliberately steering toward, evoking, and naming issues, themes, and worlds

   Let yourself notice what all this tension is doing for you. . . .

   Is there something you wish you could do besides protect yourself?

   So there's a certain world you live in where all this is necessary. . . [?]

4. Using them as context as you process various evoked experiences, both to keep from rambling and to deepen into the core

   Go ahead and protect yourself, have protective thoughts, let the tension in your hands protect you as much as you need to. . . .

   So notice what kind of a world you live in, where you need love, but nobody cares about you. . . .

As we proceed toward establishing a sense of the world in which the client operates, we follow a particular sequence, deliberately shifting from level to deeper level: experience to issue to theme to world. For example, the following sequence, using contact statements and omitting all the necessary language, immersion, and study in between, demonstrates a typical progression:

You haven't been feeling well. . . .

You're noticing this is the third time in just a few months that you've been sick.

It's a real problem being sick a lot.

And yet, as you feel into it, there's something pleasurable about it.

It gets you lots of attention, huh?

You get sad when you think about the issue of attention.

You know you should be loved just for being yourself.

So you live in this world where you have to get sick to get attention, when all you really want is just to be loved.

There's probably something familiar about this. . . .

Yeah, you remember being little and your mom staying home from work when you had a fever. . . .

To make these transitions, we specifically word our contact statements (in these examples) or fourth steps in a focused direction. "It's a real problem being sick a lot" directs the client to the issue level: not just the event or particulars of the illnesses, but the way that having them impacts the client's life negatively—he has an issue with it. Similarly, "You know you should be loved just for being yourself" invites the client to consider the underlying theme of being attended to without having to do anything. A statement tying them all together evokes the larger frame of a world: "So you live in this world where . . ." By working all four steps skillfully, we create a solid, mindfully immersed platform for study, on which we can then elegantly evoke, explore, and ultimately resolve the issues and developmental themes that have corrupted the client's sense of self and world—and organized out certain currently realistic possibilities, limiting the client's decisions and resources.

Time and Space

To do all this, we need to sustain dual frameworks in both time and space as we work. In terms of time, we need to be fully located in the present moment, working carefully and lovingly with exactly what is here right now, and we also need to be scanning ahead, anticipating both where all this might be going and how to nudge the process carefully and lovingly in that direction, all the while maintaining a complete, experimental openness to whatever arises, wherever things lead, in either time zone.

Spatially, we need to be able to access both horizontally and vertically. We need to stay with a present experience, going wide to extract every bit of relevant information, keeping the client carefully and lovingly immersed and involved with what is here. And we need to anticipate and then proceed toward other related or deeper aspects of the network, sliding from thoughts to sensations, sensations to emotions, emotions to memories, or memories to core beliefs. We are working here now, and we also know there is an entire network, framed around themes and issues, creating an experiential world in which the client lives, and it is our therapeutic job to evoke, engage, and reveal all of that.

In the accessing and deepening phases of the Hakomi process, we do all this. We use contact to focus, mindfulness to recognize, and immersion to stabilize, all so that we may help clients to use their flashlights to study experience, and in that study and revelation to access their organizational core. When we arrive at the core, our accessing and deepening is complete, and we move to the next stage of the Hakomi method: processing at the core (Chapters 17–20 and 23).

CHAPTER 16

Experiments in Mindfulness

Shai Lavie

EXPERIMENTS IN MINDFULNESS are perhaps the most signature elements of the Hakomi method. They can also be the most dramatic. Experiments allow the therapist to study the organizing schemas that underlie how a client relates to the world: how the client "does" relationships, work, nourishment, family, life purpose, and community. Experiments provide windows into the inner workings of the client: the deepest self-protective mechanisms and the strategies used to meet psychological needs.

Our ordinary consciousness is always already organized when we relate normally in the world. This means our organizing beliefs for experience guide our perceptions and responses to a large extent on autopilot, repeating and reinforcing our previous ways of perceiving and responding, resulting in what Bargh and Chartrand (1999) term the unbearable automaticity of being. Or, as Piaget might voice it, regarding important things that challenge emotionally charged tenets of our core beliefs, we tend to assimilate new material into the organization we already have, instead of accommodating our organizers to make room for the novel material (Piaget & Inhelder, 1969). Hakomi experiments transcend these powerful limitations by using a mindful state of consciousness that allows us to observe the automaticity of self-organization from a distance, which also allows for its eventual modification or transformation.

It is a crucial aspect of experiments that they also allow clients to try out and integrate new possibilities. A client, for example, can get to experience what it actually feels like to receive support in a new way, or what it feels like in her own body to experience both grief and connection with others at the same time. Experiments engage an experiential learning that is simply unachievable through cognitive intervention alone. Experiments give the Hakomi method a therapeutic efficacy that is emotionally cogent and undeniably powerful. Through the experiment, the client's nervous system may discover a new experience of what is possible (Simpkins & Simpkins, 2010). The experiment can become part of the client's inner repertoire, creating more options for how the client relates to her world (see Chapter 20).

There are many kinds of experiments in mindfulness: verbal and nonverbal probes, taking over, slowing down, acknowledgments, referencing the neutral, physicalizing, and others. Before we look at these particular kinds, let us first talk about their general function, and then see a case example.

Hakomi experiments generally function in one of two main ways. First, the experiment can appeal to organic yearnings, such as the desire to be loved and accepted, the ability to rest and be nourished, or the experience of being able to feel good in one's own body in the presence of other people. By invoking these core-level yearnings, this kind of experiment usually has the paradoxical effect of engaging the defensive strategies that the client adopted for self-protection, usually in childhood, when inhabiting organic self-states proved problematic for the client. For example, a client may never have felt loved for just being himself. As a child, this client learned he had to accomplish things in order to get recognition from his parents. The therapist might offer the client a verbal experiment called a probe such as, "You deserve love just the way you are." Upon hearing this experimental probe, the client, in a deeply mindful state, might notice that he embodies a rejecting response, for example, shaking his head, sticking out his lower lip, and pulling inward, accompanied by a statement of disbelief or mistrust. This response, if studied in mindfulness, allows the accessing of the defensive strategies that have protected the client from painful feelings. Such theoretically positive probes in Hakomi are often designed specifically to address what the client has organized out as not possible, and thus immediately evoke the client's core barriers to realistic nourishment.

A second kind of experiment works in the opposite direction: the therapist actively supports the client's defensive strategies as a way of illuminating organic needs, yearnings, and potentials. The therapist might notice situations in which the client is working to provide a sense of protection or internal cohesion, and then actively support this effort. The magic of this approach is that the client gets to experience, often for the first time, what is beneath his habitual efforts. The client has the opportunity to feel the yearning for connection, for nourishment, for acceptance, the yearnings to release old pain or grief that are being held in the body, or whatever else has been just beneath his self-protective strategies.

For example, a client is grieving the end of a significant relationship. As she begins to feel more of her grief, she finds herself holding her torso with both arms. "I need to hold myself together . . . but I can't get all of myself covered," she says with a sense of desperation. "This is where I start hating myself, telling myself all the reasons I messed up, and why it's my fault my boyfriend left me." The therapist sits with her in her deep distress, staying empathic and attuned. At the right moment, the therapist offers her a blanket to wrap herself in. "Take a few moments and let the blanket support the holding you are trying to do. Allow yourself to really feel the blanket. Notice the places you feel warmth, the places you feel the blanket's thickness or texture." The client pulls the blanket around her and begins to feel her arms relax. She describes a huge sense of relief. "I feel my whole body settling, as if the blanket is telling me, 'You're okay right now.'"

In this example, the therapist has engaged in an experiment called taking over, in which the therapist offers the client support in doing something the client is already doing herself for self-protection, self-cohesion, or in service of another core-level need. When we use taking over, the client no longer has to fight by herself to maintain her protective strategies. Rather, her defenses are actively supported by the therapist. This allows the needs underlying the client's tension to emerge, with all their vulnerability, authenticity, and beauty.

Both of these types of Hakomi experiments are paradoxical in nature. One supports the organic yearnings in order to evoke the defensive structures. The other supports the defensive structures as a way of evoking the deeper yearnings. Each offers a powerful opportunity to study the organization of experience. In working with clients using the Hakomi method, we often find ourselves alternating between one type of experiment and the other; as if, like yin and yang, the illumination of one side supports the illumination of the other. Here we often see the possibility of a third category of experiments, those (like physicalizing or equivalence) that allow us to gently explore either side of the continuum, or to shift back and forth between the defensive structures and organic yearnings, creating more fluidity between them.

Let's now look to a case study to illustrate the use of experiments in the Hakomi method.

Case Study: Experiments in Mindfulness

Ariel is a 39-year-old physical therapist. She is recently divorced and just starting to date. She is telling me, in a very hurried way, about the latest developments in her dating life. She complains about how anxious she is with men, how desperate to get responses from them. It is our fifth session, and I am noting that she has talked very quickly each time we've met. I bring this up gently (being careful not to shame her), and wonder if it relates to her anxiety around men.

In earlier sessions, we have done a few simple mindfulness exercises, which Ariel has enjoyed. "I like getting to slow down and really feel myself," she told me at the end of one session. Today I ask her if she would like to use mindfulness to study the theme of trying so hard to get attention. She agrees, and I guide her into a general experience of mindfulness of sounds, body sensations, and breath. I ask her to report on her experience, and she tells me that she can hear the tree leaves rustling outside, and that she feels her lower back against the couch. Satisfied that she is fairly mindful, I ask her if I can say a statement to her as an experiment in awareness or mindfulness.

First, I tell Ariel, "Your job will be to notice whatever comes up—an emotion, a sensation, an impulse, an image or thought, a 'yes' or a 'no,' or nothing at all—in response to the statement."

When Ariel indicates she is ready, by nodding, I set up the experiment by saying, "Notice what happens, Ariel, when I say the words [pause] . . . I'm here to listen to you." At first, she takes this in deeply. "It feels very good." But then she also notices a strong impulse to push me away. I invite her to stay with this impulse, to notice all the sensations, tiny body movements, and images that go with it. She observes her hands wanting to go up, as if to block me, and she reports her belly feeling very tight. Suddenly an insight emerges: "I am pushing people away through my barrage of talking. I tell myself I want more contact with people, but I am also putting up this barrier at the same time!"

"Yes, you're having an insight that feels so valuable here," I acknowledge. "I also see that your hands have come up in an important way. . . . Why don't you let yourself really feel your hands making this barrier in front of you? Take your time, and let the movement happen slowly, with mindfulness."

Ariel looks at me with curiosity, as if ascertaining whether creating a barrier between us is actually fine with me. She lets her hands go up a little more, and they now push outward. "I hope it's okay to say this, but I feel better knowing I can push you away."

"Sometimes it's important to know that," I suggest, and we both laugh. There is now a deep sense of connection between us.

"You know, this is interesting," I say. "You've set a boundary with me and now we both feel so at ease with each other." We continue to integrate what has just happened, in a relaxed way, until the session ends.

We see two experiments in the above example. First, we see a verbal probe in mindfulness, "I'm here to listen to you." I choose this experiment because I predict it will conflict with Ariel's core-level belief that people are not really going to listen to her. The words, at first, evoke a sense of deep nourishment, but, as commonly happens, this sense of nourishment quickly becomes eclipsed by a defensive response that emerges to protect Ariel from the vulnerability associated with the nourishment. In the Hakomi method, we see defenses as organic attempts to manage experience according to felt safely needs, and so I invite Ariel to study the experience by bringing her awareness to it.

When Ariel studies her experience in mindfulness, she deepens into an insight about herself: that despite what she likes to tell herself, she is often pushing people away in relationship. This insight is not an analytical speculation, but something that emerges from the experience itself (Johanson, 1996). We do experiments precisely because we want meaning to emerge from experience. Here Ariel has discovered something about how she organizes herself in relationship to others.

Notice that while I honor Ariel's insight, I also invite her to return to what her hands are doing. An intelligent process is revealed through her body (Kurtz & Prestera, 1976), in this very moment, which I don't want to lose by going too far into the cognitive realm. Here I am experimenting with slowing down, an essential aspect of mindfulness; directing Ariel's awareness to a movement that her body knows it wants to do, and seeing what happens as she slows it down, feels it, and gives it space to unfold. When Ariel allows herself to really feel her hands pushing me away, she notices how good it feels to create this barrier in a conscious way. She also gets to experience something new: that she can consciously set a boundary while still feeling connected to others, paradoxically even more so.

In this case example, the experimental probe appeals to the organic yearning to be listened to while paradoxically eliciting the defensive structure of pushing people away. Experimenting with mindfully slowing down supports the same self-protective impulse, which paradoxically evokes the underlying longing to feel more connected to others while embracing a need for boundaries.

The Structure of Hakomi Experiments in Awareness

There is a general structure for the many kinds Hakomi experiments.

1. The experiment begins with collaboration (Duncan, 2010), with asking the client for permission to do an experiment while carefully tracking to make sure the client is willing and not simply being compliant. "Is this a good time to explore the anger more deeply through doing an experiment in mindfulness?"

2. The next step is some form of induction or invitation into mindfulness. This induction is often longer for newer clients than for more experienced ones. "Notice what happens when . . ." "Study, be curious about what is evoked in you spontaneously when . . ." "Without effort or doing anything, just be aware of what comes up when . . ." Here the inductions are designed, following the wisdom of neurolinguistic programming (Bandler & Grinder, 1975), to open the client to a broad range of experience. Asking clients to notice what they feel or see narrows the field to feelings or visual material, which should only be done if there is some clinical warrant. Especially with new clients, it is sometimes helpful to orient them to the possibilities of a broad range of responses. "Notice what goes off or bubbles up within you . . . any sensations, tensions, feelings, memories, thoughts, images, or not much of anything . . . when . . ."

   Next we describe the nature of the "when," that is, the experiment to come. For example: "When I say these words . . ." "When I reach out and touch you on the shoulder . . ." "When I start walking and begin to close the distance between us . . ." "When you reach toward me with your arms . . ." "When I block your arms from going forward . . ." "When you imagine asking your boss for a raise . . ." "When you put this rope on the ground to symbolize the boundary between us . . ." "When I take over the tension in your shoulders . . ."

3. We then insert a pause between the invitation and the actual experiment to encourage deeper mindfulness. The instructions themselves cause ripples in the pond of consciousness and need to settle so that the client can study the specific ripples evoked by the experiment. "Notice what happens when you hear the words [pause]. . . . It is okay to take up space."

4. If the client does not offer it himself, we ask for a report of what the result of the experiment was. A report is what the client witnessed about how he organized around the input. "I noticed a sensation in my stomach that had a quality of nausea." A report is distinguishable from a reaction that is not mindful (for example, "That's yucky!"). If the client simply reacts, the therapist can invite further mindfulness. Therapist: "So what signaled you that it was yucky? Was that a thought or feeling or sensation or . . . ?" Client: "Oh, yeah. It started like a sensation in my stomach that had a quality of nausea that flipped into a yuck." There are many other possibilities for what can happen while working with experiments.

Types of Hakomi Experiments in Mindfulness

Having looked at one case example, let's now get a general sense of the range of experiments we might use in the Hakomi method.

Verbal Probes

These are verbal statements, designed to be potentially nourishing and offered to the client in mindfulness, like the ones discussed above. There are countless formulations of such statements. Here are some general examples. In clinical practice, the specific words would organically arise from the client's process—from the themes evoked or the nourishment being defended against.

- You're safe here.
- You can ask for what you want.
- You don't have to do it yourself/alone.
- I'll listen to you.
- You're important.
- You can show me who you are.
- Your life belongs to you.
- You can do what you want (and still be loved).
- You don't have to prove anything.
- You're lovable the way you are.
- It's okay to rest/slow down.
- You can be your full self.

Nonverbal Probes

Instead of words, gestures, movements, or any number of nonverbal experiments can be offered to the client in mindfulness. Examples include extending a hand toward the client, offering an object to the client, smiling lovingly at the client, or opening one's hands to the client. Often the best ones are those that emerge from the present-moment process. Classically in Hakomi, Kurtz (1990a) would build experiments around indicators (see Chapter 3) of missing experiences the client learned how to organize out of her experience (Johanson, 2015) because they were perceived as threatening.

Nonverbal probes, like verbal ones, are generally positive or neutral offerings. If they are designed around the opposite of a client's core beliefs, they will usually evoke the barriers or the client's defensive systems, thus giving the client an opportunity to study how he organizes around relevant themes such as being cared about, supported, opened to, respected, and so forth.

Taking Over

To best understand taking over, we can start with the very first time that Kurtz discovered its possibility. This encounter was, in fact, a beginning point of the Hakomi method itself, as Kurtz began to modify his approach from his previous training in Gestalt, bioenergetics, and other modalities (see Appendix 3). It showed Kurtz two essential things: the power of conducting experiments in mindfulness, and the power of supporting defenses rather than trying to break them down.

> The first time I took something over was at a workshop in New Mexico. I was working with a woman who was getting close to something important and charged with feeling. She was lying on her back on the carpet and, as we focused in on her experience, her back began little by little to arch. After a few minutes, her body was a bridge with only her head and her heels on the floor. I was still into Bioenergetics then. My approach to defenses was to force them to yield. Since I saw the arching as a defense, I was prepared to put a lot of weight on the woman's abdomen until the bridge came tumbling down. In my mind, that would have been the logical, defeat-the-defenses approach. . . . [But] I knew how terrible it would feel if I tried to make the client collapse. I couldn't bring myself to do it, even in the name of therapy. *Instead, a light bulb went off, and I put my hands under her back*—and I told her that if she wanted to, she could relax her back and I would hold her up. Well, she tested my hands a little, giving them some of the weight at first and then, little by little, all of it. This took a minute or less. As she let herself give the weight of her body to me, she also let herself feel and experience the things that she had been fighting against—a painful memory and the feelings and insights that went with it. She eased into that and we worked with it. . . . She let herself relax, slowly, at her own pace, into the experience she'd been running from. (Kurtz, 1990a, pp. 102–103)

Taking over is an intervention in which the therapist, assuming that there is organic wisdom in the defense, supports the client in doing what she is already doing to protect or manage herself. In doing so, the client gets to experience what is beneath the protections:

yearnings, needs, or painful feelings that have been shunned from consciousness. People invest tremendous energy keeping underlying material from entering consciousness. Reich's (1949) central teaching about body armor is that tension masks sensitivity. Taking over allows clients to temporarily give the therapist their protective strategies, thus providing the safety of the defense while freeing up energy and attention to study the underlying needs, feelings, and yearnings.

Some examples of taking over:

- The client is leaning her head to one side; the therapist offers to take over the support of the head so that the client can study more clearly what the head is doing or needing.
- The client is putting his hands in front of himself, as if to strike something; the therapist offers the client some large cushions to put in front of him that take over the worry about hurting anyone. When the client still cannot assert, the therapist takes over what is holding back the assertion by restraining the client's arms, thus allowing the client to safely explore the impulse to strike out.
- The client reports a voice in her head saying, "You've got to do this right"; the therapist takes over the words, coached by the client to say them in the same tone, volume, and intensity that the client was hearing.
- The client feels an impulse to scream, but blocks the impulse; the therapist (working in collaboration with the client) finds just the right place to put her hands over the client's mouth to take over blocking the impulse and sound, paradoxically freeing the client to follow through with the now-muffled scream.

As we have discussed, taking over typically has the effect of opening the client to what is yearned for at the deepest levels. A carefully chosen experiment in taking over, implemented with sensitivity, respect, and full collaboration with the client, can be one of the single most powerful therapeutic experiences. It honors and supports the defense the client obviously thinks he needs while trusting it to the therapist to maintain, thus providing the safety for the client's awareness to explore deeper levels of his organization.

The above examples demonstrate both passive and active taking-over techniques. In Hakomi, the therapist is always active, doing something. "Passive" and "active" refer to the client. In the above example of the therapist supporting the weight of the head, the client passively allows the support while mindfully studying what is evoked. In the example of the therapist taking over the client's holding back his arms from striking out, the safety is provided for the client to then actively explore his impulse to hit (Kurtz, 1990a).

In terms of signal-to-noise issues, taking over is an example of how Kurtz tended to lower the noise in a system in order for a signal to come through more clearly; this as opposed to trying to exaggerate the signal to come above the noise. This is also an example of the Taoist wisdom that Kurtz (Johanson & Kurtz, 1991) brought into psychotherapy, which serves as an Eastern example of nondoing and nonviolence that balances the more current Western impulse to do or to overcome. While Kurtz integrated a number of existing techniques into Hakomi in line with Hakomi principles (see Chapter 5), taking over represents a potent original contribution to the field of therapeutic intervention.

Referencing the Neutral: Peace With Gravity

Here the therapist observes how the client is using body posture, referencing an alignment that would be most at peace with gravity if no physical or emotional issues were present. The therapist then suggests an experiment that will work with a displacement toward that alignment, such as uncurling the shoulders, tilting the chin, shifting the pelvis slightly, and so forth. The therapist must make sure that the client only displaces in tiny increments, and with solid mindfulness, so that the internal changes can be tracked and explored. Large movements or displacements tend to produce too much noise in the system. Often if deep, core-level beliefs have been powerful enough to affect the voluntary muscles shaping posture, they will emerge in response to postural displacements. The therapist must be especially careful about anything that could feel shaming or judgmental toward the client. In addition, the therapist must keep in mind that any experiments that invite a shifting away from defensive structures or compensatory postures will tend to draw out those very structures and compensations.

Referencing the Neutral: Exaggeration

This experiment is basically the opposite of peace with gravity. Here the therapist invites the client to exaggerate habituated postures, movements, or sounds, more in line with classic Gestalt work. Again, the therapist must make sure that the client is enacting only in small increments, and with a keen and spacious mindfulness. Exaggeration can be used in combination with peace with gravity to take the client back and forth between defensive structures and organic yearnings—termed "rocking" in Hakomi. Especially in the integration phase of a Hakomi session, rocking consciously between old defensive structures and new, more open organizations can create more fluidity and control for the client to navigate between these polarities.

Physicalizing

In this experiment, the therapist invites the client to turn an internal experience into an external physical experience. For example, a client says, "I just want to push everything away from me." The physicalizing experiment might be to have the client push against something, and to study that experience in mindfulness. Or the client might say, "The whole thing is such a burden." The experiment could then be to let the client hold up a weight while studying the experience. Likewise, if the client feels pulled in two directions, this can be physicalized. Sometimes physicalizing calls for strenuous exertion, but normally with the aim of coming back to subtle movements that can be mindfully explored for their wisdom.

Verbal Equivalence in the Mind-Body Interface

In these experiments with deepening, the therapist invites the client to turn a physical experience into a verbal meaning. Equivalence is somewhat opposite to physicalizing, as the therapist will ask the client to express in words the meaning of what his body is doing. For example, a client feels his throat tighten, and the therapist has him find the words that express the tightening. "I have to hold my feelings back," the client reports. Or a client averts her gaze repeatedly, and when asked to find the words that go with it, she discovers from a mindful place, "I need to avoid contact."

Equivalence is typically used when a client is immersed in her kinesthetic experience and the therapist senses that by using words, the client may more fully own her experience. It is similar to focusing (Gendlin, 1982), where a client is first immersed in a felt sense of an issue physically, and then allows words to come up that have a felt sense of congruence. Equivalence functions to engage the client's cognitive capacity to get the meaning of an event. As Johanson (1996) notes, words can bear the birth or death of meaning. Hakomi therapists have an ear out for when words are alive and expressive, and when the words are becoming abstract and distancing, signaling that clients should immerse again in the physicality of their experience.

Slowing Down

This experiment is used informally in most Hakomi sessions since slowing down is a general characteristic of mindfulness as a state of consciousness. Hakomi therapy is sometimes called "slowing down therapy" informally, and a therapist will often ask the client to slow down and notice her experience more carefully, more receptively. As a formal experiment, slowing down is used to study a movement, gesture, or voice tone that is happening automatically in the fast pace of ordinary consciousness. As in the earlier case example, the therapist will get the client's permission to study the experience, guide her into mindfulness, and then invite her to be aware of what she observes. Slowing down allows clients to access the experience more deeply, whether it is something edgy they typically avoid or a new internal resource that their body is waiting to show them.

Acknowledgments

Acknowledgments are similar to experiments with verbal probes. While probes are normally addressed to intuited core beliefs, Kurtz (1990a) used acknowledgments to slow things down and address the emotional import of what the person was saying. Most people habitually name and gloss over some aspect of their story as they continue in ordinary consciousness to another part. They are talking about their experience, as opposed to being with it and reporting from it. And they rarely expect anyone to really get, acknowledge, and honor the emotional meaning of what they are saying (Schore, 2003). So Kurtz would politely interrupt someone, ask permission to experiment with an acknowledgment, set it up formally as above, and use words that summarized the poignant significance of what the person was saying. The effect of such an experiment was often to make a profound level of contact (see Chapter 14) and to deepen into (Chapter 15) the person's core issues. Some examples:

- I know you tried hard.
- You really had to be strong.
- It is really a great grief.
- It meant a lot to you.
- You were really scared.
- You really struggled.
- It was really confusing.
- You couldn't find anyone to help.
- You were left having to figure it out by yourself.

Creativity

The previous nine possible experiments are standard Hakomi possibilities, but only suggestive of the infinite opportunities that can come from creative collaboration with clients. In Hakomi training, it is often said that what define Hakomi are the principles. Techniques are secondary and are often invented within a session. For instance, there is the famous Rainer Scheunemann probe, invented in the south of France: "Notice what happens when [pause] . . . I eat your cookie for you."

When We Do Experiments

We do experiments only after we have established three foundational elements. First and foremost, we need a solid and trusting relationship between therapist and client (see Chapter 9). Everything we do in Hakomi requires this. At the neuroscience level, we cannot access the emotional patterns held in the limbic brain and its linkages with the right prefrontal cortex until we have first established a right hemisphere–to–right hemisphere connection with the client (Badenoch, 2008; Cozolino, 2006; Fosha, Siegel, & Solomon, 2009; Schore, 2003; D. Siegel, 2010). At the colloquial level, "People ain't going deep if they don't trust you."

Second, we need to establish and monitor the client's capacity for mindfulness. Hakomi experiments rely on mindfulness to elicit data from the experiment. We might tell the client, as a verbal probe, "You don't have to work so hard." This experiment will register completely differently depending on whether the client is mindful or not. If the client is not mindful, the statement will most likely be heard and responded to by the left hemisphere's abstract thought and semantic centers (McGilchrist, 2009). "Oh sure, I know that," might be the mental experience of the client. If the client is mindful, the statement will more likely impact the right hemisphere, with its linkages to the limbic brain, where the emotional "operating systems" are running. The client may experience a dropping of the shoulders, a leaning forward of the head, followed by a tightening up in the body accompanied by anger. For experiments to be effective in this way, we must be able to use mindfulness to immerse clients deeply into their experience. A collaborative culture around immersing into experience in this way can take time to develop, depending on the strength of the therapeutic relationship and the client's comfort with turning inward. But once we have this shared intention, the therapy can go significantly deeper.

Third, and most important in determining when to do an experiment, is the therapist's attunement to the client (Marks-Tarlow, 2012; Siegel, 2007). Experiments work when congruent with the client's rhythm, energy level, and in-the-moment needs. The therapist may have a great idea for an experiment, but it will fall flat if the experiment is out of sync with the client, for example, if the client feels a strong need to talk about other things in that particular moment.

How We Choose an Experiment

The linchpin of doing a Hakomi experiment is choosing what experiment to use and when. The big question is this: Of the countless aspects of our client's presentation (voice tone, hand movements, posture, story content, facial expressions, and so on), how do we know what to make the launching point for the experiment? And how do we choose among all the kinds of experiments listed above?

Ron Kurtz (see Chapter 3) used the term "indicator" to denote an aspect of the client's presentation that warrants special attention. An indicator can be almost anything: voice tone, hand movements, posture, facial expressions, foot movements, changes in breath, eye movements, a pattern in the client's relationship with the therapist, or a way the client talks about a particular person, just to name a few. An indicator catches our attention because it seems to stand out energetically. The client brightens, dims, opens up, closes down, gets more intense, relaxes, or appears stronger or weaker. The indicator also appears to be a manifestation of a person's core organization; as such, it can be used to help access the core level of psychic process that generated it.

In the earlier case example, a particular indicator preceded each experiment. The first indicator was Ariel's pattern of talking quickly, as if pulling for my continued attention. Using that indicator, I offered the verbal experiment, "I'm here to listen to you." The second indicator was when Ariel moved her hand in front of her body, in a way that somehow felt important. That was when I invited Ariel to slow down the movement and to explore what emerged next. This brought her deeper into an authentic experience of herself and her own boundaries.

The therapist's own subjective sense, coming from a place of emotional attunement with the client (Fogel, 2009; Siegel, 2007), is the most critical factor in deciding what may be an indicator and thus worthy of more attention. For one client, tapping her feet may seem minor, but for another client the same kind of tapping can be very important. The therapist is working from his own intuition. If the therapist senses something important is going on, he can say without attachment, "Something important seems to happen as you tap like that. . . . Can we stay with this tapping a little while?" Bringing attention to an experience is itself an informal experiment, and oftentimes, just this attention alone takes the session in a new and important direction. In this way, a Hakomi therapist learns to trust his own subjective sense of what may be an indicator, trusting that by paying attention to the indicator, the right experiment will begin to emerge organically. There are a few key types of indicators that therapists can look for as sources of potentially fruitful experiments.

Indicators of Physical Effort

Physical effort can take any number of forms. A client might be holding his head in his hands, or leaning on his forearm, or pushing against the couch, or pushing out his feet, or embracing himself tightly, or extending his head toward the therapist. It can be helpful to think of these efforts as ways of holding the self together, protecting the self, or reaching for support.

Our task as therapists is to bring a new level of consciousness to the activity of making effort, and Hakomi experiments help us do this. In situations of physical effort, we will often choose taking over as our experiment: after invoking a mindful state, we provide the support, holding, or reaching that the client is trying to do on her own. As discussed earlier, these experiments often open the client to the organic needs that had been previously been invisible, but lingering just beneath the effort.

Indicators of Closed Systems

A closed system is defined as a network of information and relationships that relies on rigid patterns and excludes new inputs. Each of us does things in highly patterned ways—from mundane tasks to how we conduct relationships—that from the outside appear fixed and limiting. Closed systems (see Chapter 22) restrict fluidity in expression, communication, and internal experience.

Indicators of closed systems are usually the hardest to detect within ourselves. Most of us have learned to meet our needs in very indirect ways. We have learned to fish for compliments instead of acknowledging that we feel insecure, to act tough instead of asking for support, or to achieve great success at work to compensate for an underlying sense of unworthiness. Hakomi character theory (Chapters 8 and 23) helps us understand some of these common patterns. One thing that is common to all of the typical character strategies, as well as other closed systems, is a sense of disconnection—that something is split off from the whole. As Wilber (1979) suggests, some part of the mind is split from another part, the mind is split from aspects of the body, the mind-body is split from the fullness of the environment, or the autonomous self is split from the larger unity of all life. The therapist will perceive a disconnect within the client, or between herself and the client. In essence, the sense of disconnection reveals the indicator that can be employed for healing.

Hakomi therapists will think about and, more importantly, feel into what is missing for clients. What have they organized out of their experience or split off from as not possible? What are they not able to do that is realistically possible at this point in their lives? When we get a sense of what is missing, we can offer clients the potential nourishment they have not yet integrated, evoking in the process the underlying defensive pattern that pushes the nourishment away. This is where various experiments can be so effective. They allow us to move directly toward the client's underlying protective needs. As we get to this level of the work, we experience the client's authentic being: Now the client is engaging the truth of his fear, sadness, or confusion, rather than the typical pattern that manages his experience to avoid underlying pain. Here we also begin to feel more connected to the client, as both therapist and client usually feel that something very important is happening.

In the earlier case example, Ariel's pattern of talking quickly made me feel more distant from her. This countertransference (Cooper, 1999; Feinstein, 1990; Field, 1989; Natterson, 1991) clued me in that a closed system was at work. I offered potential nourishment through a verbal probe: "I'm here to listen to you." This evoked her underlying protective need: to be able to push people away, to set a boundary when appropriate. When we got to this level, we both began to feel more connected and more relaxed. Moving from the closed system to the underlying protective need, we were now able to access the frustrated, organic yearnings immediately beneath the self-protection.

Indicators of Resources

Resources can be seen as experiences of relative cohesiveness, clarity, fluidity, aliveness, and integrity. What is a resource for a given person is relative: for an anxious person, a resource might be an experience of calm; for a depressed person, an experience of aliveness; for an overly rigid person, an experience of being more flexible.

In the Hakomi method, we pay special attention to any gestures, movements, or postures that seem to indicate nascent resources. We might do this early in a session or early in the course of therapy as a way of building resilience for deeper work. When working with trauma, it is normally essential to begin with resourcing (see Chapter 24; Ogden et al., 2006). And we often do this later in the session, or later in the course of therapy, as a way of consolidating gains made in the work. With Ariel, for example, later in my work with her I suggested, as an experiment, that she try to imagine a challenging person in her life while holding up her hand to set a boundary.

Some of the other indicators of nascent resources include the following:

- A client who tends to be very timid, sticking out his chest with pride
- A client who tends to run from topic to topic, taking a pause
- A client who diminishes her value with men, shaking her head with "attitude" as she talks about not being taken in by a man's lies
- A client who struggles with addictive tendencies, reaching out to a friend for emotional support, instead of the bottle

Notice that all these examples contain action verbs. Slowing down in Hakomi can be very effective in helping clients mindfully immerse in the actions that resource them, study how these actions ripple through the body and mind, and become more centered and grounded in larger self-states of awareness, compassion, and wisdom. In this way, these new action possibilities can firmly take root in our clients' nervous systems, reinforcing new neural networks (Cozolino, 2010; Craig, 2003; Perry et al., 1995; Siegel, 2003, 2006).

What Happens After the Experiment

Because experiments can be so evocative, it is essential that the Hakomi therapist hold a strong container for the emerging experience. Most important are the therapist's intention and skills related to attunement, compassion, curiosity, and connectedness. When these elements are in place, the therapist is usually on solid footing. Often after doing an experiment, the therapist will want plenty of time to process the experience at all levels. The client may need time to just sit longer with his own bodily experience, to deepen into core material, to process the experience verbally, to integrate through associating it with other situations in his life, or to engage the therapist relationally. Kurtz (2006) often extolled the virtue of doing something and then waiting for the client to process internally, allowing the next step to emerge. Sometimes an experiment touches so deeply that the client finds himself riding the rapids of spontaneous emotional release (see Chapter 18). If so, the therapist must gauge the amount of time left in the session, making sure there is plenty of time to process what is emerging from the experiment. Some experiments might be relevant, but not indicated when close to a time boundary.

In addition, the therapist must make room for any dissonance that may have occurred as a result of the experiment. Once a client told me he felt "freaked out" after an experiment, in which I had offered the verbal probe, "It's okay to trust yourself." After the experiment, he had felt a notable aliveness throughout his body and, unusually for him, in his legs. I commented, "Your legs seem to know something important." I had meant this to suggest that his legs knew what they wanted to do (to move, to run, and so forth), but he interpreted my comment as implying repressed abuse memories. We needed plenty of time to process his concerns, reassure him about my intentions, and collaborate on where the therapy was focused.

These kinds of misunderstandings can happen at any time. What is key is having a collaborative relationship in which misunderstandings can be cleared up and repaired (Barstow, 2005; Goldfried & Wolfe, 1996), and also being in tune enough with our clients so that we sense when something has gone wrong. As has been said in previous chapters, the most important thing is our relationship with the client. This is especially true when we are engaging such profoundly deep material. It is also true that Hakomi processes are self-correcting. If something comes up that was unintended or not taken as intended, this can be contacted, and once again the process gets on track as the two-party dance continues.

Following an experiment, we continue to engage the basic repertoire of Hakomi skills: tracking, contact, accessing, deepening, and processing in mindfulness (see Chapter 21).

We use these skills to integrate what has emerged from the experiment: insights, questions, newly discovered capacities, and the reowning of formerly split-off parts of the self. We also work to reaffirm and maintain our role as caring witnesses, midwives for our clients in their extraordinary process of self-discovery.

Conclusion

A client is deeply immersed in mindfulness. The therapist softly says, "I'm going to say a phrase to you, and your job is to notice whatever you experience when you hear the phrase. It could be a 'yes' or a 'no.' It could be a sensation in your body, an impulse, or a movement. It could be an image or thought in the mind, or a shift in mood or emotion. Or you might not notice anything at all. So give me a little nod when you feel ready. . . . All right, notice what happens when you hear the words, 'It's okay to rest.'"

Hakomi experiments in essence engage the two basic dimensions of core-level psychological organization: What the client's deepest yearnings are (for example, personal wholeness, connectedness, authenticity) and how the client organizes protections against the vulnerability that accompanies these deepest yearnings.

Experiments in mindfulness provide Hakomi therapy a richness that is palpable to both therapist and client. Clients learn to explore their deepest organizing patterns with curiosity, acceptance, and fluidity. Core material is evoked through experiments in awareness, which is why Kurtz (2008) sometimes referred to Hakomi as the method of evoked experience. As this journey continues, clients will report much greater degrees of choice in their day-to-day lives, in relation to when they want to engage familiar defensive strategies, and when they discern they no longer need to in a given situation. For a Hakomi client and therapist, this is a profoundly rewarding experience leading to in-depth transformation.

CHAPTER 17

Exploring the Barriers: Hakomi Perspectives on Working With Resistance and Defense

Jaci Hull

SINCE THE LATE 1930s the field of psychology has evolved in its understanding of how the body relates to psychological process. The concepts of defense and resistance have been important factors in the study of human behavior, becoming key elements in virtually all strands of psychodynamic therapy.

"Body armoring" (Reich, 1949) was the term used in body-oriented psychotherapy for how a person uses muscle tension or physiological numbing to protect himself from experiencing or expressing challenging emotions and impulses evoked by external stimuli. Over the past five decades, this concept has been refined by numerous leaders in the field of somatic psychology. Alexander Lowen (1958) and John Pierrakos (1990) further elaborated on the idea of body defense by including more than just the musculature of the body. They saw that the whole of the personality could be found in musculature and energetic flow. Early painful events that caused armoring affected not only body stance and freedom of movement but the entire organization of a person's experience—behaviors, life choices, reactions, and so on. Lowen (1958) went on to develop a character theory based on common patterns of behavior, emotion, and body stance.

Ron Kurtz incorporated these theories but emphasized a particular perspective that set the focus of his work apart from that of his antecedents. He showed that in the therapeutic process, clients seem to defend against the very thing they long for, such as safety, help, good news, or the possibility that they deserve something beneficial to happen to them. Clients came to therapy often describing a stuck place around a lifelong yearning. When Kurtz would experimentally offer the freedom to move beyond the stuck place, the client would often dismiss the offer, respond with adverse emotions, tighten up, shut down, turn away, or freeze.

Realizing the significance of such automatic reactions, Kurtz proceeded to study the dynamics of avoidance and rejection. By having his clients report to him from their mindful, present experience, he was able to hear descriptions of what was happening beyond the automatic response. He heard beliefs, memories, voices, images, and other aspects of what was mostly unconscious yet self-organizing material. There seemed to be a number of behavioral ways in which clients would attempt to avoid the anticipated negative impact of the very experience they longed for. Nourishment had become toxic. Kurtz learned that when a person is missing a certain essential nourishment in their lives it is because it either doesn't exist in their environment or they are keeping it out (defensively, for instance, in order to avoid the pain of losing it again). Thus, Kurtz generally interpreted defensive patterns as intelligent measures of the client's adaptive unconscious (Wilson, 2002) to protect him from further harm.

It became clear that in order for it to be safe enough to explore these defenses, the therapist had to be open and curious about anything that emerged spontaneously in the client. Guided by the principles of mindfulness, nonviolence, and organicity, Kurtz emphasized the importance of using an experimental attitude when working with defense systems in the client. Rather than attempting to fit the client into a previously established category of defense and personality theory that would suggest a certain set of treatment goals, he stayed open and curious toward what the client presented. Not only did this attitude assure clients of a safe and unencumbered exploration of painful material, it also had the effect of encouraging them to approach the investigation with the same kindness and openness given by the therapist. Together, therapist and client could cocreate an environment where defenses could be appreciated, respected, understood, and reevaluated.

From this perspective, a defense is an intelligent way in which a person keeps out a potentially nourishing experience because it has become associated with painful memories, such as neglectful or abusive parenting or a tragedy. The adaptive unconscious has learned to expect more traumatization and pain and makes sure it will not happen again. This is very different from a defense against internal drives, as in Freud's (1900, 1938) concept of the struggle around a "primitive wish."

Working With a Barrier

A pragmatist, Kurtz renamed these habitual defense patterns barriers. The Hakomi therapist sees a defense as an indicator that a psychosocial, developmental task was interrupted, causing an inability in the individual to easily move toward needed nourishment, freedom, or growth.

Barriers are made up of several physiological and psychoemotional components. In the Hakomi session, both therapist and client work together to identify and define the barrier and its components, and in so doing they accomplish three tasks:

1. make conscious the unconscious manifestations of internal wounding,
2. create a sense of choice around future responses to life events, and
3. explore new options in the experience of painful material within the safety of the therapeutic relationship.

The Hakomi therapeutic stance involves, again, a sense of openness about the barrier. In order to fully understand a barrier, its meaning and function, there has to be enough safety in the therapeutic relationship for a barrier to emerge and to be observed, explored, named, and validated without fear of judgment or of having the same offense occur that created the barrier in the first place. The particular principle the Hakomi therapist invokes that helps her create this environment—the principle of organicity (Chapter 5)—allows for three things:

1. The therapist anticipates that the defense will arise and so is not thrown off when it does. In fact, the therapist recognizes that the client's mindful study of the barrier is one of the important steps to transformation.
2. The therapist's expectation is held within a window of compassion and curiosity, meaning that compassion and curiosity already exist as part of the attitude of the therapist before a particular defense has even appeared or been named.
3. The therapist knows to meet this defense with a kind of acknowledgment that will evoke little or no added defense in the client.

The therapist then slows down the process, interrupts the sharing of content, and gently directs the client's attention toward the verbal or nonverbal indicator of the defense to study and explore it in mindfulness.

Case Example

Jim, a 34-year-old accountant, came into my office saying that the new job he'd gotten required that he do some public speaking. He noticed that when he thought about it, his anxiety became overwhelming. He was terrified of his first public speaking event, and it was beginning to affect other aspects of his work and his personal life. To begin exploring this issue, I asked him to imagine himself at a public speaking event in order to evoke the mental, physiological, and emotional components of his anxiety. After some time spent in mindful exploration of the sensations and feelings involved—the tightened shoulders and jaw and a sense of feeling younger—he had a memory of being humiliated by an elementary school teacher during a reading lesson when he was having trouble pronouncing

*a particular word in the text. Long-forgotten feelings emerged as well as the impli-
cation of the teacher's actions, which he interpreted to mean, "You're ruining this
for all the other students because you're not keeping up. We can't wait for you." We
explored this further, acknowledging the pain he felt and the unconscious belief he
had established about himself: he was not good at speaking in front of others. He
would fail, annoy everyone, and be left behind.*

*I then created an experiment by offering an experience that was clearly missing
at that time: patience and support for him to learn. I offered a probe (see Chapter
16), saying, "Notice what happens inside your body and your being when you hear
the words . . . 'You can take all the time you need.'" Jim tightened his shoulders,
stopped breathing, and frowned, indicating a defense or barrier against this kind of
relieving, but seemingly impossible, perspective. Having designed the probe to elicit
such a barrier, I then said to Jim in a very gentle way, "Hard to believe, huh?" and
told him of the body changes I had witnessed. "What does your body seem to be
saying with that response?" I asked. Jim studied this response and heard an internal voice that said, "Don't cry—it'll get worse. You'll be humiliated. Don't be stupid." Again, I gently contacted his feelings and watched his shoulders loosen up as
he took in the compassion in my voice and words. Small tears appeared in his eyes
and, with quiet sobs, he released the internal pressure he'd been holding onto,
including the frustration he'd been directing toward himself all these years. His
breathing became more full and regular and he began to relax.*

*We continued to deeply explore the experience and the memory that had been
buried in his unconscious but was now uncovered by staying with the initial tension, still somewhat alive. He became very aware of how this barrier was made up
of body tensions, movement, memories, and thoughts—that when he needed to
muster up the courage to speak in public, this was what interrupted that process.
As we talked, Jim began to feel two things: (1) anger toward the ignorance of the
teacher who shamed him in a learning environment, and (2) a disengagement from
the identification with the old negative introjections he'd been holding about himself. The habitual self-organization that reflected those beliefs started to relax, and
a new perspective of possibilities became alive inside. He began to feel that he now
could succeed at public speaking.*

Once safety has been established and is refined with each continuing session, the client
and therapist can explore the nature of a given barrier. This may happen quickly or over
the course of several sessions depending on the nature of the wounding. There are three
main lines of inquiry for the therapist:

1. When and how does the barrier arise?
2. What is it composed of? (For example, movements, thoughts, memories, body
   stance, tensions.)
3. What does the client need to experience? More precisely, what developmental needs
   does the barrier indicate have been missed?

In answering the first question—when and how does the barrier arise?—the Hakomi therapist uses the techniques of tracking and contact. She is trained to notice any kind of change in the client's nonverbal behavior and demeanor and to verbally contact present experience, techniques designed by Kurtz to encourage self-study (Chapter 14).

To answer the questions "What is it composed of?" and "What's the missing experience?," the therapist most likely uses little experiments in mindfulness (Chapter 16) to complete the understanding of the barrier. As the client reports from inside his experience, and his barrier is being received with kindness and precise understanding by the therapist, he may begin to yield physically and psychologically to the nourishment being offered or go on to explore deeper levels of defense that reflect formative experiences that may need more time to be worked through (Chapters 15, 18, and 19).

Referring to a defense as a barrier directs a more specific approach to character work, allowing the therapist to help the client see the ways in which he rejects potential nourishing experiences—not just conceptually but with his body, emotions, and behaviors. Having a direct, affective experience of one's barrier draws it into the conscious realm, making it more recognizable and available for change. The less conscious the barrier, the less change can happen.

Relating to the Defense

Understanding a defense as a barrier and meeting it with compassionate curiosity also changes the therapeutic relationship. No longer does either party become frustrated by the client's inability to change. No longer does the client have to go into the shame of resistance and the therapist into the dangerous role of pushing the client. Now the therapist can simply help the client explore her barrier, allow her to become aware of it, deepen her understanding of its meaning and function, and then see if this understanding opens up opportunities for new experiences that would create change.

Case Example

Mary, a 30-year-old wife and mother of two young children realized, at one point in a session, that she rarely allowed herself to feel really happy. After inviting her to go into a mindful state, I offered her the probe, "It's okay to be happy." Her arms and shoulders started to tighten up and she heard a voice say, "Yes, but what about the others?"

"You are worrying about somebody, huh[?]" I inquired. She described a picture of her parents—her very unhappy parents. As we slowly proceeded to experience that relationship, we got clearer that if she were to feel happy, she would be seen by others and would feel herself to be selfish.

At this point, as with any client, I encouraged us both to become curious about the barrier rather than get lost in a debate about its validity. Instead, I said, "Impossible to believe, huh[?] . . . You feel guilt when you imagine being happy[?]." Suddenly, we were into something deeper than whether or not Mary accepted my invitation to be happy. We were into the story of how happiness came to be experienced as toxic to her.

Mary recounted instances of hearing her mother complain about her life, her unhappy marriage, and the life she'd given up by marrying Mary's father. She remembered her mother's sad face and drooping body, which made Mary tighten more and feel the hopelessness of a child who couldn't help her mother to feel better.

Further exploration, which included the experiment of taking over Mary's shoulder tension (Chapter 16), showed her that tightening her shoulders yielded more distance from the oppressive unconscious beliefs. Mary realized that the burden of her mother's sadness was too much for a little child to carry alone. As she learned to take in support for herself, she was also more able to let go of her sense of responsibility for other people's happiness.

The more a client understands the origins of her limitation and is able to remove self-blame for defending herself, the easier it will be for her to embrace experiences that create the safety and support for risking new possibilities in therapy and eventually in the world (Chapters 19 and 20).

The Sensitivity Cycle

In order to map out certain types of metalevel barriers that appear to interfere with the growth process of the different character styles, Kurtz conceptualized the sensitivity cycle—a theoretical map of optimal life functioning emphasizing the need for sensitivity to one's internal experience in relation to four essential stages (Figure 17.1). In this theory, it is the experience of freedom and ability available at each step of the cycle that the individual defends against or misses.

The emergence of a defense is related to existential needs, which were left poorly met, often very early in life. These core life issues, referred to in the chapters about character (Chapters 8 and 23), show up as typical barriers within a character process.

In general terms, the sensitivity cycle suggests that for a satisfying life an individual needs to:

1. be aware of or sensitive to his own essential situation and needs,
2. take appropriate action based on this clarity,
3. experience satisfaction as a result of successful action, and
4. be able to rest and regenerate in order to become aware and clear about what is needed next (a return to Step 1).

Once the cycle is completed in a satisfying manner, it makes the next loop back to Step 1 easier. When sensitivity is impeded via a barrier, the loop is either stalled or becomes a shallow or unsatisfying journey (Kurtz, 1990, p. 177).

A wounded person may learn to avoid contact with a painful world as well as with his

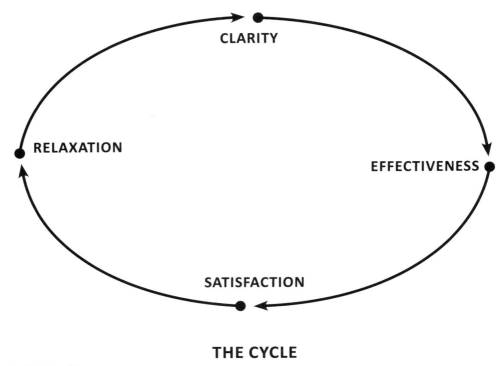

THE CYCLE

© 1981 Ron Kurtz

Figure 17.1. The Sensitivity Cycle. With permission from LifeRhythm Publications, *Body-Centered Psychotherapy: The Hakomi Method* by Ron Kurtz, Copyright 1990, Mendocino, California, USA.

own needs. Or he denies himself the freedom of taking action to get a need met for fear of possible consequences. One may reject the sensory pleasure of satisfaction for fear of a hurtful experience, whereas another may turn against the idea of relaxation or completion for fear of not having done enough to be "good enough."

Each of the indicated barriers has a name specific to the stage in the cycle (Figure 17.2): The barrier to clarity is defined as the insight barrier. The barrier to action is called the response barrier. The barrier to satisfaction is referred to as the nourishment barrier, and the barrier to relaxation, the completion barrier.

The sensitivity cycle serves as a diagnostic tool for determining where a person may be stuck in her life as well as a procedural guide for therapy. For example, if the client struggles with clarity, the therapist will know to work with the insight barrier. In this case, and in terms of Hakomi character theory, the therapist may be dealing with aspects of a sensitive/withdrawn or an expressive/clinging process.

Hakomi therapists are taught to recognize a barrier and employ certain techniques for working though them (Chapters 8, 22, and 23). The barriers relate directly to character

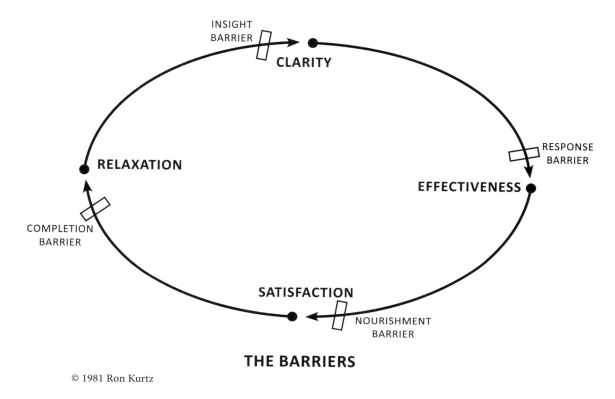

© 1981 Ron Kurtz

Figure 17.2. The Barriers. With permission from LifeRhythm Publications, *Body-Centered Psychotherapy: The Hakomi Method* by Ron Kurtz, Copyright 1990, Mendocino, California, USA.

theory, in that each barrier can be found to play a typical role within the self-organization of the different character strategies (Figure 17.3).

The ability to understand and recognize a barrier is essential to therapeutic intervention in the Hakomi method. It requires the skills of tracking and managing consciousness while helping the client discover the nature of his obstacles to maneuvering through the challenges of life successfully. This process for the client involves understanding, freedom, receiving nourishment from the world, and resting to reorient himself to his new core beliefs and to how he now relates to his experience in the world.

Summary

Recognizing a barrier greatly improves the efficiency with which psychotherapy can progress. When the therapist can understand the meaning behind a somatic, emotional, or mental response, she can immediately get a ballpark idea of which nourishment or

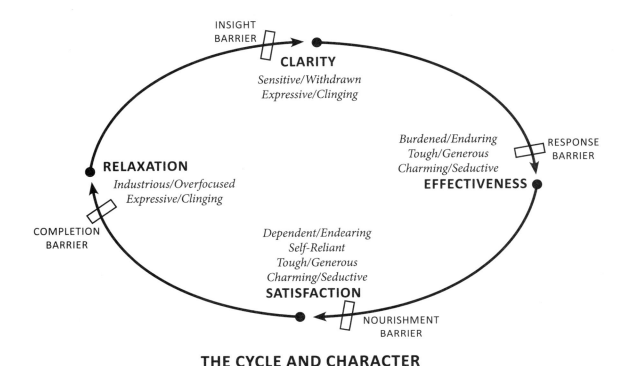

Figure 17.3. The Cycle and Character

developmental task has been compromised. The specific kinds of nourishment the client is rejecting, and the reasons for rejecting them, direct the therapist to the formative wounding events that are causing the client's current suffering, thus opening the door toward working through core material and core beliefs (Chapter 19).

The general strategy to linger at and explore the barrier in mindfulness also helps avoid subtle interactions of pressure and resistance between therapist and client. Instead, the client feels deeply accepted and often relieved to understand himself better. There is less sense of something being wrong with him. Both therapist and client can remain relaxed and curious even when the client shows characteristics within himself that appear to be problematic.

CHAPTER 18

Child States and Therapeutic Regression

Marilyn Morgan

"Mommy, Mommy," YoungerOne wails, "Mommy hold me!"
LOUISE WISECHILD, *The Obsidian Mirror*, 1988

IN PSYCHOTHERAPY, IN art and literature, and also in pop psychology and personal accounts, there are descriptions of "the inner child" (Anderson, 2000; Hall, 1993; Miller, 1986, 1988; Parks, 1994; Weinhold, 1988; Whitfield, 1987; Wisechild, 1988). The concept makes sense clinically and resonates with many clients. Working with the "child" is an important part of Hakomi therapy.

What is this inner child? Whitfield equates "the child within" with the true self. He says that when we are being our true self, we are alive and "we tend to feel current, complete, finished, appropriate, real, whole, and sane" (Whitfield, 1987, p. 11). The child is written of in spiritual traditions, as in the *Tao Te Ching*: "To find the origin, trace back the manifestations. When you recognize the children and find the mother, you will be free" (in Johanson & Kurtz, 1991, p. 79). Jung wrote about the child within: "In every adult there lurks a child—an eternal child, something that is always becoming, is never completed, and calls for unceasing care, attention, and education. This is the part of the human personality which wants to develop and become whole" (1947/1958, p. 286). The creator of psychosynthesis, Assagioli, spoke of subpersonalities (Ferruci, 1982). Eric Berne's (1964) transactional analysis detailed child, adult, and parent parts. Richard Schwartz (1995) includes exiled child parts in his internal family systems model. John Bradshaw (1990) writes of reclaiming and championing the inner child. Some more conservative Christian sects are embracing the concept: "When we access and heal our deepest wounds, we also access the deepest spaces within us where God dwells" (Linn, Emerson, Linn, & Linn, 1999, p. 9).

The Child State Intruding Into the Present—for Good or Bad

The ways in which we were not loved during childhood can be directly read from our adult relationships.

PAUL SCHELLENBAUM, *The Wound of the Unloved*, 1988

Child consciousness may feel like part of an integrated life, or it can appear to limit and sabotage a satisfying adult life.

> *Suzie, age 32, was brought up in a loving, stable family. Attachment theorists would say she has a secure base. She is a fun-loving, caring mother and enjoys her relationship with her husband. Suzie has an expressive face; her eyes are sparkling with life. When she is making mud pies with her children you can see how much her child self is there; when she is taking care of the family finances, she is very much a grown-up.*
>
> *Peter was not wanted by his parents and grew up in a number of foster families. Recently his wife, Ann, gave birth to their first child, a son. When Peter saw Ann responding to the baby's cries by picking him up, cuddling him, then feeding him, he became inexplicably furious. He yelled at his wife to stop spoiling the baby, as his son needed to toughen up. When Ann told him to lower his voice, Peter retreated in a sulk. He soothed himself with beer until he fell asleep. When Ann saw her inebriated husband on the couch she muttered, "You are more of a baby than your son!"*

Hakomi trainer Jon Eisman (1989) gives us a useful map regarding child and adult states. He describes how a child who has supportive experiences will grow into a "whole adult" in an embodied way. This was Suzie's experience. She can have, as an adult, states of childlike wonder; she can feel vulnerable and needy; and she can be spontaneous and playful. The inner child is an integrated part of who Suzie is in the world. In fact, the concept of an inner child is almost irrelevant for Suzie.

However, if the child is neglected, or suffers trauma, then a fundamental splitting occurs, such as happened for Peter. The pain, too overwhelming for the child to manage, is defended against by survival strategies. The vulnerability and natural child energy go underground, as the "hurt child," the "spirit in exile," and the "strategic child" go on to become an "assumed adult." At the same time, a "survivor part" may fight for intuitively sensed rights. Lurking behind the adult persona are child states that may inconveniently erupt. For Peter, these emerge when he least wants them—for example, when he is trying to be a good father. Peter can be taken over by his child self and he does not recognize that he is not behaving in an adult matter—furiously railing against any confrontation.

Frozen in Time: Developmental Arrest

The child will spontaneously contaminate the adult's behavior.

JOHN BRADSHAW, *Homecoming*, 1990

Eisman asserts that the natural child has core knowledge of her rights. Kohut would agree. He said that the child's "nascent self 'expects' an empathic environment to be in tune with its need-wishes, with the same unquestioning certitude as its lungs 'expect' oxygen" (Kohut, 1977, p. 85). When the conditions are not there to support normal development, then parts of the child or adolescent remain undeveloped—frozen in a time warp. "Emotional energy has the urge to complete itself" (Hall, 1993, p. 21). Physically, the person grows into an adult, but parts are left behind. Schwartz (1995) describes how child parts are often exiled and dissociated from, or disliked and disowned, as other managing parts develop to cope in the world. Some people have their child parts so hidden that they seem too adult.

> *This was so for Stephanie, who was puzzled and critical when her coworkers stopped work to joke and fool around in a lighthearted way. She told herself that they were silly and irresponsible and withdrew from them. Stephanie's colleagues teased her for being stuffy and urged her to play a little. She didn't know how.*

Child parts can emerge during the shattering pain of adult relationship breakdown (Anderson, 2000). Other people have child parts frequently dominating the adult self in present time. It seems like they are childish, or too emotional, or overly dependent on others.

> *Michael was like this. His big, soulful eyes always seemed to be pleading for something. When his wife, Marlene, was busy he hung around and complained. Marlene would get impatient, and then Michael would retreat to his bed. He wanted Marlene to look after him and was angry when she didn't.*

When a new client walks through the door for the first time, it may strike you how much she appears like a child. Sometimes the body structure itself carries something of the developmental arrest. Other clients may move in childlike ways, speak with small voices, or dress like children. Others are grown up in most spheres of their lives, but in therapy, or in intimate relationships, child parts appear spontaneously and may dominate.

Outdated Perceptions and Decisions From the Past Inhibit the Now

From the first days of life, the infant's brain is capable of creating a multimodal model of the world.

DANIEL SIEGEL, *The Developing Mind*, 1999

The child is born with most neural connections yet to be wired up. His brain development is experience dependent and is shaped by his particular environment to function in that environment. Later in life, the world the person inhabits may have changed considerably, and the abilities, emotions, automatic behavior patterns, and beliefs that were formed very early in life may no longer be functional.

Sandra was brought up in a violent home. She had to be in a constant state of vigilance. Later, in her marriage to Tony, Sandra would go very quiet and shut down when Tony was irritated. When he wanted to discuss things with her, she wouldn't be able to speak. This annoyed Tony and, as his voice got louder, Sandra became like a robot and would agree to anything.

Sandra did not know why she didn't stand up for herself. Her fear dated back to a time in her life that predated conscious memory. It can be hard to change patterns like this by willpower alone, as they are so deeply rooted in implicit memory systems.

Regressive States

Becoming so identified with my child and all her sensitivities also made me want to isolate myself in my room because it was such a safe place. So instead of my world expanding it became more and more limited.

TANHA LUVAAS, *Notes from My Inner Child*, 1992

Regression literally means returning to an earlier state of functioning. Michael Balint, a psychoanalyst, writing in 1968, describes the benign or therapeutic form of regression as involving a trusting relationship and facilitation of inner awareness, and with only moderately intense display of demands and expectations. This type of regression, he believed, could lead "to a true, new beginning," with a real, new discovery (Balint, 1992). In contrast, a person can revert to functioning in a childlike way, which is distressing and even dangerous. The client can be taken over by a trancelike state, losing access to previous resources and awareness. Sometimes this regression can last over time and can be very difficult for both the person concerned and those around him. Being stuck in such a regressed state is not therapeutic, and therapists need to do all they can to prevent such unhelpful states from occurring. Balint (1992) describes this malignant form of regression as involving a desperate clinging by the client, with frequent relationship breakdowns, high intensity of demands for external gratification, development of addiction-like states, and unsuccessful attempts at a new beginning.

> *Sally was being treated in an in-patient clinic. The methods of group therapy used were unusual and confrontational. Sally had been raised to do as she was told. She was compliant with those she saw as experts. One of the exercises given to the group was for the participants to be three years old. The facilitators starting treating them like little children, encouraging them to seek nurturing when upset. Sally had had a traumatic separation from her mother when she was three. She regressed during the exercise and began to cling to the facilitators. After a while, they became annoyed. The more they tried to get Sally to grow up again, the more she persisted in being little. Even after Sally left the clinic, she was still regressed, and she went from one professional to another in an unsatisfying search for care, validation, and love. Some mental health workers tried to give Sally what she wanted, and that seemed to reinforce her childlike, helpless state. She became furious when people refused her demands.*

The Inner Child's Dark Side

> *To worship a precious inner child is to ignore its dark side.*
>
> STEPHEN WOLINSKY, *Quantum Consciousness*, 1993

Not all child parts are sweetly vulnerable, or full of innocent wonder. Some are demanding, dependent, full of rage, obsessional, suspicious, manipulative, clinging, terrorized, stubborn, dissociated, cruel, hysterical, seductive, complaining, or even overly devoted, good, or compliant. Stephen Wolinsky describes how protective "child trances" were created in childhood to handle situations that the person could not understand or bear at the time. The child trance is a state of consciousness that the adult can later identify with. The dark side occurs when the child part acts autonomously, causing problems in the person's life. John Bradshaw, writing the foreword in Wolinsky's book, says, "The inner child is *not all precious and wonderful.* By grasping the ways we continue to use the frozen and outdated trances of survival, we deprive ourselves of some essential areas of human experience . . . like curiosity, questioning, resiliency, exuberance, and spontaneity" (1993, p. x).

Some people may inappropriately reify and glorify the inner child, and others have great loathing for their child parts. Even though child states can be problematic and limiting, it is possible to celebrate their positive origins and protective intent. In psychosynthesis, according to Ferruci (1982), they are seen as degraded expressions of higher qualities. Ferruci says, "Compassion can become self-pity, joy can become mania, peace can become inertia, humor can become sarcasm, intelligence can become cunning, and so on" (1982, p. 55). Jungian writers believe that we begin life whole, already containing archetypes within the psyche (Kaplan-Williams, 1988). Guntrip's writings affirm Eisman's assertion that the natural or organic child has an intuitive knowledge of her rights and wholeness:

> If the primary natural self, containing the individual's true potentialities, can be reached, supported, and freed from the internal persecutor, it is capable of rapid development and integration with all that is valuable and realistic. . . . The total psyche, having regained its proper wholeness, will be restored to full emotional capacity, spontaneity, and creativity. (1968, p. 195)

Regressing in the Service of Growth: Child Consciousness in Psychotherapy

Infantile, unrealistic hope is transformed into mature, realistic hope.

MARTHA STARK, *Working With Resistance*, 1994

A therapist who is overly nurturing or who promises more than is realistic can encourage an unhealthy regression. This can be a pitfall for a Hakomi therapist, who may in fact be drawn to the work because of resonance with the Hakomi values of compassion and loving presence. This can make the therapist vulnerable to establishing systems of unhelpful dependence.

To enable the child aspects of the client to grow and become embodied and integrated with the functioning adult self, the therapist needs to ensure that the client is resourced. This means that the adult witness needs to be there, alongside the child state. Wolinsky (2003) emphasizes the need for an "observer" adult self to disidentify from the child, expanding awareness and choice in the present. Ferruci, describing the psychosynthesis approach, says, "When we recognize a subpersonality, we are able to step outside it and observe it" (1982, p. 49). Schwartz talks of the Self as both observer and leader of the system: "[Individuals] can be actively engaged in their lives while in this mind set—a state the Buddhists call mindfulness. The Self then is not only a passive witness to one's life; it can also be an active leader, both internally and externally" (1995, p. 37). Self-capacity may have to be developed before it is possible to work directly with the child consciousness. The client needs to be ready (Parks, 1994). The therapist will need to set boundaries and not entice powerful, regressed longings by seeming to offer boundless mother love. Grief for what has been missed out on needs to happen along with experiences of the love and acceptance that can be offered and accepted in the present (Stark, 1994).

The path of mindfulness cultivated in Hakomi training, and with the client in therapy, assists with growth of the witness and disidentification from desperate child parts. With the witness present, a therapist and client can be with intense longings, evaluate potential nourishment, and notice when the nourishment is accepted at a deep level. In fact, the practice of mindfulness can insure against becoming trapped in life-draining systems of malignant regression.

Recognizing the Child State

As I looked at Picasso's paintings I often felt I was seeing with the eyes of the confused, uncomprehending, disorientated, but interested and curious child.

ALICE MILLER, *The Untouched Key*, 1988

As stated above, the inner child can be reified. It is rather a metaphor for a state of consciousness, which holds unintegrated, implicit memory. The metaphor of the child can be useful, but it is important to remember that the inner child is not a concrete entity. There are many child parts, and they change, move, and disappear as the overall growth process occurs (Ferruci, 1982; Schwartz, 1995; Wolinsky, 1991, 2003).

As a result of the way in which Hakomi therapists work, using mindfulness and deepening into experiences, including the bodily felt sense, the child often emerges naturally and by itself. Both client and therapist can sense this experientially. We can then use that opportunity therapeutically. The metaphor of the child can then be most useful. In fact, Kurtz developed the theory of the child and the magical stranger in response to his experience of childlike states pushing their way spontaneously into therapy sessions. Sometimes the child emerges as a first-person experience: "I am hiding under the table," accompanied by a childlike voice, words, and mannerisms. At other times the child is sensed by the adult self and spoken of in the third person: "I see her under the table, all by herself." The child may also emerge in artwork or writing.

Earning a Secure Attachment

You can live and die still a child, or move fully into adult life. You have that choice.

STREPHON KAPLAN-WILLIAMS, *Transforming Childhood*, 1988

Daniel Siegel and others talk of a person with an insecure attachment history being able to earn a secure attachment: "Although emotional relationships of all sorts can be healing and promote healthy maturation, facilitating a movement towards an 'earned' secure/ autonomous adult attachment status, at times the unique configuration of psychotherapy is needed to catalyze this growth" (Siegel, 1999, p. 287).

Working with the preverbal child-state can occur when creating new attachment "templates." This may need to be part of long-term therapy where limbic resonance processes work directly on implicit memory (Lewis et al., 2000; Schore, 2003). Loving presence, kind eye contact, reliability, and nurturing touch over a period of time may be needed. Too many words may bring the person out of present experience. Nonverbal child states of fragmentation, such as occur in disorganized attachment, can occur as a result of shock and trauma. When working with such states, the therapist needs to be safe and gentle, and go slowly. Completion of trauma sequences may be required in a safe therapeutic window of awareness (van der Kolk, 2014).

Working With the Child: Regressive States in Therapy

Holding the image of the abandoned child in our minds helps to reclaim the needy, helpless, frightened part of us.

SUSAN ANDERSON, *The Journey From Abandonment to Healing*, 2000

The core beliefs of the child are held in state-specific consciousness and are usually not available in ordinary awareness. They are available in the state in which they were first learned. For transformation to occur, the client needs to be present with his or her child consciousness, so that these early beliefs can be fully accessed and processed. An opportunity to make new decisions, due to seeing the self and world differently, can then occur. It is possible to do useful work with the child and core beliefs from the place of ordinary consciousness, but it will not have the same impact as working directly with the child state.

Other states of consciousness may be present alongside the child state, such as the adult or mindfulness. As previously discussed, it is a good idea to have the adult self, or some compassionate aspect of the adult, present as a resource (Anderson, 2000). It is not advisable to pursue the child state or do regressive work unless the client has a strong adult or sense of self as a ground and resource. Clients who generally operate out of the child state in their lives may need to develop the adult part more strongly.

During the session, the therapist can talk to the client's adult self, who internally relays the message to the child, notices any reactions, and reports back. This is especially useful for those clients who easily regress and get taken over by child trances. When the child state is present, the therapist can talk directly to that child, using simple, direct, and age-appropriate language.

Communicating With the Child

The therapeutic experience is not just that of expressing the hurt or angry or terrified feelings. . . . The real healing comes also from being listened to and understood and recognized as a person.

JOSEPHINE KLEIN, *Our Need for Others*, 1987

The therapist begins by establishing the presence of the child as a state of consciousness (see Chapters 15 and 19). The therapist addresses the fact that child consciousness is active, on a metalevel, and then can ask whether it would be okay to talk to the child directly in the present tense. It can be a very helpful, therapeutic intervention to enter into a relationship with that child part.

The child is often accessible when a memory arises in the client. The therapist can expand the memory a little by asking for the age and setting while tracking emotional and bodily expression and accessing felt sense. He may say, "You feel little now," or "You are at home now," or "Your sister is with you." The therapist can also further explore the child state with contact statements directed to the witness, such as, "This is the little boy feeling sad. . . [?]" or "A memory is emerging. . . [?]"

The Magical Stranger and the Missing Experience

The vulnerable child is tuned in energetically—it is aware of everything that is happening. Words will not fool it for a moment.
HAL STONE AND SIDRA WINKLEMAN, *The Vulnerable Inner Child,* 1990

Ron Kurtz made an invaluable contribution to psychotherapy with his ability to become a magical stranger to the inner child (Kurtz, 1990a). It was, indeed, truly magical to experience Kurtz's ability to sensitively relate to the vulnerable child in an age-appropriate way and to compassionately nourish that child with just the right input for his needs. Hakomi therapists have found working with the child in this way to be very effective in facilitating deep and lasting transformation. Moving into a magical stranger mode and providing a missing experience can be very powerful. The therapist becomes like an unknown, kindly person who has traveled back through time and who can interact with the "frozen" child, providing new experiences that were missing back then. When the client is in child consciousness, we assume that the relevant neural circuitry is active and is therefore plastic and open to revision. We must also be aware that there will be parts that tend to counter the acceptance of new, nourishing experience. These need to be worked with simultaneously.

As the magical stranger, the therapist relates to the child like a wise, loving adult—an uncle or aunt perhaps, or a friend—someone who was not actually present in the person's childhood but whose presence could have helped the child manage and understand the situation. The therapist is not acting so much as a therapist per se, but is taking on a role to provide a missing relationship experience. Even though the client's adult consciousness knows the therapist, the child does not. The therapist is a stranger to that child and has special powers. She comes from the future and appears in that magical moment when the child is back in a place that he once had to endure without solution and with no help. Now there is a magical other who understands, is patient and kind, and creates new options and perspectives. As well, the magical stranger knows unheard-of things, can answer unanswered questions, and brings nourishment that was, to the child, previously only dreamed of.

The therapist may say, "That's right. I agree you need to be out of there. Maybe I can help you do it." The therapist, of course—still working within a therapeutic frame—is conscious of session process and client state, has her own witness present, and does not promise or offer anything that is not realistic. It is important to be guided whenever possible by the adult witness self of the client, who usually knows very exactly what his child self needs in that moment.

First, the therapist should acknowledge and validate the child's experience. This is often a missing experience in itself. Take time to find out about the child's hurt, being continually empathetic, tracking and contacting experience as it unfolds. Allow spaces and silences, without abandoning the child. Usually the child, in the first instance, was alone without anyone understanding her experience. Sometimes all that is needed is for the therapist to be there, contacting and acknowledging her in an attuned way. The therapist's experience and knowledge of character styles can provide guiding maps (Chapters 8 and 23). Getting the details of the sense the child made of the situation at the time is important. Some narrative type questions can be useful here: "What did she tell herself about herself when her daddy left?" The client could reply, "It was her fault," or "It was because I was bad," or "She is too scared to cry." The therapist can then explore the core belief or decision that was made at the time. "I am no good," or "I'm not very bright," or "There is something wrong with me," or "I won't show how I feel," or "It is too dangerous out there," or explore the ways the child protected himself from the hurt. For example, he might have become extra good or rebellious, or retreated to books.

The therapist then continues to acknowledge and validate the child's experience: "You were too little to cope with that. Of course you would feel angry." It is important to accept all feelings of the child and support expression of these feelings as indicated. ("It's okay to cry now.")

In some of his later writings, Kurtz says, "Where core beliefs are limiting, destructive, unbalanced, or painful they can be challenged. New beliefs can be tried and new experiences evoked. I call these missing experiences" (2004, p. 79). He goes on to describe how the missing experience can nourish and transform outdated patterns:

> One woman, in her process, touched terror. It was set off by the statement, "You are perfectly welcome here." Her terror and fear were based on her model that she was not welcome anywhere. In fact, at the deepest level, she felt that her life was in danger. People didn't want her to be alive. These were the messages she took in as a child, and which created these terrifying core beliefs. She screamed with the terror while several of us held her very tightly (with her permission of course). She reported feeling good screaming; it was a relief to let it out. After a while the terror subsided and her body relaxed. She could finally take in that she was welcome. . . . She had this wonderful, thirty-minute experience of feeling welcome, held, cuddled, and loved. I saw her two weeks later. She told me she was . . . walking to a friend's house and she started to feel uncomfortable. . . . In the middle of an [old] internal dialogue she suddenly heard a voice saying, "You're perfectly welcome here." . . . In an easy, light-hearted way she continued to her friend's house. . . . That's how people change. They have a new model. They use it, and if it works, it becomes a habit. (pp. 80–81)

Acceptance of Nourishment

Richard is aware of a childhood memory in which he was desperate to help his depressed mother. As a four-year-old boy, he would sit with his mother, stroking her arm and offering to get her cups of tea. Richard's father would sometimes yell at him for not tidying his room or playing outside, and would pull the reluctant boy away from his mother. When Richard's mother cried, he felt that it was his fault for not being able to make her happy.

There may be parts that fight nourishment and form what Hakomi therapists call a nourishment barrier (see Chapter 17). These parts have often been created to protect the vulnerable, hurt child from disappointment, further pain, or exploitation. For example, the therapist may offer some words to Richard's child self as nourishment: "You are a thoughtful little boy." These words have been suggested by Richard's compassionate adult self who, as a father himself, can clearly see the dilemma of the little boy he once was. As these words are spoken, Richard hears a sad inner voice saying, "No, I am not. I am a failure," and a strident voice saying, "Grow up and get on with life!" The vulnerable child self does not believe the kind words. They do not nourish.

Harry Guntrip describes the complexity of offering nourishment in his book *Schizoid Phenomena, Object Relations and the Self*:

> The regressed schizoid patient wants to be treated as a baby, with the implications he should not be indulged in this. This gravely oversimplifies the case. . . . There is an infant in the patient . . . who needs to be accepted for what he is . . . but there is an anti-libidinal ego in the patient who hates this. The patient with the deepest schizoid problems of all is the patient most dependent for a successful result on the degree of maturity in the therapist. . . . One patient said simply, "If I could feel loved, I'm sure I would grow." (1968, p. 287)

The therapist cannot force nourishment against resistance, and denying nourishment tends to evoke manipulative demands and clinging. Instead, he needs to linger at the nourishment barrier, exploring responses and different parts of the client that hold defensive attitudes. A person may have experienced nourishment as insincere or toxic, so will automatically become suspicious and reject it. Another child was given nurturing, but it was always taken away prematurely. Now as an adult, she is fearful to enjoy being accepted and loved because she "knows" it won't last, and she will suffer bitter disappointment. When support is offered, she pushes it away, saying she can look after herself.

Working With the Child

General guidelines for working with the child include the following:

1. Learn to recognize the child as he appears in sessions by changes in voice, expression, posture, and so forth.
2. Be interested in that child; hold the experience in present time.
3. Acknowledge and validate the child's experience directly.
4. Talk directly to the child in simple, age-appropriate language. Attune carefully, maintaining tracking and contact.

5. Ask the adult self for comments on how the child is responding in the moment and to nourishment.

6. Check out feelings of the adult toward the child. If they are negative, there is a critical, defensive part present who is not able to show understanding and compassion toward the child. This part can be brought to the client's consciousness.

7. Encourage the child to name and express feelings and perceptions.

8. In the case of overwhelming emotions, allow for some distance to the child part (e.g., imagining placing it far away or behind a window).

9. Find out the meaning the child placed on the early situation.

10. Let the child articulate her needs.

11. Ask the compassionate adult self what the child needs to hear or know.

12. Support emotional expression as indicated.

13. Be real, realistic, and genuine toward the child.

14. Remember child-type thinking processes—magical, egocentric.

15. Remember that the child is the mapmaker, forming the core models of self and the world used throughout life.

16. Be attentive, validating, playful, compassionate, and creative, just as one would with a real child in the room. Draw on experiences with actual children. Adapt language and tone of voice according to what is age appropriate.

Progression Processes

As I've healed, Younger Ones have grown.

Louise Wisechild, *The Obsidian Mirror,* 1988

As previously discussed, it is often not helpful to explore child parts, renegotiate early trauma, or disable defensive strategies, if there is not sufficient self-capacity. Trauma therapists emphasize the need for safety and the development of ability to manage and tolerate feelings. There is the place of raw, vulnerable childhood hurt, confusion, and trauma, with the potential to overwhelm. Then there are adaptive, defensive parts, which have allowed coping. Within the majority of people who come to consult us, there will also be aspects that are strong and resourced already. The person may have had experiences that have led her to develop some of the characteristics of a secure attachment. This allows for self-reflection and self-regulation of emotion. (Certain neurological wiring has to be in place to allow this, and it grows through positive relationship experience.) When accessing these resources, the person can be visibly embodied, alive, and has a sense of wholeness. You may need to access, and even develop, these stronger parts before working with childhood hurts (Emmons, 2007).

Often the client presents in survival mode. It is important to assess self-capacity before dipping into the childhood hurts, and to honor the survival strategies that have enabled coping. Otherwise, clients can regress, becoming overly dependent, and the therapist then has to manage this for them outside usual session times, as an external regulator. Therapy should proceed in a backward-and-forward manner. The therapist may need to first spend considerable time building relationship and safety for clients with few inner or outer resources. The therapist's presence may be the main containing function, which can directly influence growth of limbic pathways and inner capacity. Psychodynamically, this process is described as internalization. When there is sufficient safety, child parts can be transformed and integrated, bringing implicit memory into consciousness and freeing energy for more functional patterns in the present. The person then no longer needs to function from survival strategies. An increasing sense of wholeness develops as the person integrates more of the split-off parts and thus gains more awareness, control, and choice in her present life.

Integrating the Natural Child With the Embodied Adult

To bring back his soul from the pit, to be enlightened with the light of the living.

JOB 33:30

Maybe we don't always need a concept of the inner child to integrate outdated, frozen memories, to bring implicit, core material into the present, and to change neural pathways to support more satisfying responses to life. Some woundings from childhood are changed implicitly, without conscious intervention from the client, but rather by direct influence on the physiology. As commented on above, this can occur when the therapist brings loving presence to the therapeutic relationship, and his limbic states of attention, attunement, and compassion directly impact the client, increasing aliveness and self-capacity (Lewis et al., 2000; Schore, 2003). It can also occur through the creation of calm, mindful states, in relationship, or through the use of selected music—enhancing the ability to engage socially (Porges, 2006). The creation of a safe environment and then sequencing through body sensations and micromovements can change frozen trauma states (Levine with Frederick, 1997; Rothschild, 2000).

Growing the Child Within

The rebirth and regrowth of the lost living heart of the personality is the ultimate problem psychotherapy now seeks to solve.

HARRY GUNTRIP, *Schizoid Phenomena, Object Relations and the Self,* 1968

Michael Balint describes the "new beginning" in therapy as happening within relationship, involving satisfaction of something that was missing, and leading to character changes: "going back to something primitive . . . which could be described as regression . . . and at the same time discovering a new, better suited way which amounts to a progression. . . . Regression for the sake of progression" (1992, p. 132).

> *Jill had therapy over a period of two years. She was an adopted child, growing up with well-meaning but emotionally unresponsive parents. She generally held herself back from people and was easily influenced by other people's moods, often feeling wounded by them. In therapy, Jill appeared collapsed; her eyes were wide and often full of tears. Her heart area was painful. A young, infant self was frequently present, needing calm words and gentle touch. The therapist gave this part attention and acceptance, reminding her that she was now safe and welcome. Jill, as adult, mindfully learned to recognize this baby part and cared for her. Eventually, Jill noticed how much stronger her body felt, how she was sitting straight, and how her heart felt warm. She said, "I feel like I belong now, and I want to be here."*

Exiled parts can be reintegrated in the present time, bringing empowerment and choice to the client. We must, however, hold the child imagery lightly, allowing these young parts to grow, change, and ultimately disappear into the complexity of the embodied adult, where they become parts of the whole, grown person. Kurtz (1978) described how the child is the mapmaker, constantly forming the core models of reality about the world and himself. Future experience is largely created through these maps. In therapy, we can return to the "map room" and show the child, who is frozen in time, a different reality that is congruent with growth. The new experience can now be integrated and laid down in the neural architecture of the brain. The maps have been redrawn. Working at this powerful, vulnerable place in therapy has a very special, sacred feel to it. Such opportunities should not be missed, for it is here that life-changing, therapeutic work can be accomplished, and the reclaiming of lost potential and wholeness can occur.

CHAPTER 19

Working Through Core Beliefs

Manuela Mischke Reeds

IN TRADITIONAL PSYCHOANALYTIC work, "working through" refers to "the process of having the client face the same conflicts over and over again, under the analyst's supervision, until he can independently face and master the conflicts in ordinary life" (English & English, 1958, p. 591). In Hakomi therapy, working through is a specific stage in the therapeutic process, called the processing phase, in which the client experiences and processes core material. "Core material" refers to the beliefs that the client's soma-psyche organizes around (Johanson, 2015). Core beliefs are often unconscious or in implicit memory (Schacter, 1992) and have a powerful impact on how a person perceives and automatically reacts to the world and relationships, giving rise to the conflicts suggested in the definition above (Chapter 7). For instance, a belief that support cannot be trusted can lead to interpersonal clashes when genuine support is offered by a friend or partner but then refused. Core organizing beliefs are often unearthed through the techniques and interventions previously outlined in this section.

Many psychotherapeutic approaches acknowledge the significance of core beliefs, but how they are worked through differs. The Hakomi orientation approaches core organizers through inviting a shift to a mindful state of consciousness, so that clients can notice and study how their core beliefs automatically affect their perception and expression (Weiss, 2008). The state-specific learning that occurred when these habits and beliefs first formed needs to be accessed through mindfulness (Baer, 2003; Brown et al., 2007) or we risk remaining at the mercy of an already-organized ordinary consciousness. This slowed-down, contemplative, or self-reflective state enables clients to experience themselves in a deeper, more truthful way (Chapter 10). At this stage in the process, the therapist trusts that if clients can experience these beliefs safely and directly, then resources or gifts from the unconscious can surface and offer expanded choices in contrast to the choicelessness or automaticity (Bargh & Chartrand, 1999) of the limiting belief systems.

In the working-through phase, clients encounter the limitations of their core beliefs both emotionally and sensorially, as well as the formative experiences that lie behind them. This experiential process brings up their grief and pain, as well as offering them insight into why these core beliefs are operating. In this phase, clients somatically experience that these limitations have produced important survival-level strategies, appropriate at the time of their conception (Chapters 8 and 23), but at the price of narrowing their options in the present. When these beliefs are experienced and transformed, clarity of mind and somatic understanding can arise, along with negotiating barriers (Chapter 17) to fuller possibilities in life.

Inner and Outer Indicators

Central to Hakomi processing in general, and working through in particular, is sensitivity to the inner and outer indicators of the core organizing beliefs manifesting in the body-mind (Chapter 3). For instance, if during early relationships the mother projects a negative or dismissive body and facial expression, the child internalizes this and reads these cues in order to navigate responses toward the mother. The child learns how to avoid the gaze of the dismissive parent, or perhaps to respond by withdrawing attention in order not to draw notice. These responses turn into internal indicators—which later in life become markers of coded experiences with a strong emotional charge. These physical expressions can be tracked from without and are often linked to core beliefs about the world (Chapter 14). Even as an adult, the client learns to track for and avoid negative responses and uses her developed strategies of not provoking, diverting attention, and so forth in response to anticipated stressful moments.

In the case of Jade outlined below, she had learned how to track for signs of dismissal and disparagement and, consequently, in our initial sessions she had a hard time taking me in. It was as if she had no inner template for experiencing kindness from another human being. These became her limitations—leading to conflicts—since she experienced intimate relationships as hostile, unreliable, and ultimately unsustainable. She was sensitive to physical cues or eye movements that would signal anger or disapproval. She could also interpret cues in that manner, illustrating Siegel's (1999, 2007) point that the brain functions as an anticipatory machine. Or, in Piaget's terms, our anticipations can lead us to assimilate the world we encounter into our previous structures of meaning, as opposed to accommodating our structures to new information (Horner, 1974, pp. 9–10).

As therapists, part of working through is learning about these somatic indicators of belief and meaning in order to track, contact (Chapter 14), and ultimately understand and unpack their message. This understanding needs to come not only in the form of intellectual understanding but also as a physical knowing in the client (Fogel, 2009). Fleeting moments of eye exchanges have a powerful impact on clients who are used to feeling dismissed. These clients can feel bad or depressed within seconds, not even knowing what has happened to them. The disposition to assimilate into or confirm inner meanings is strong, even though there are always multiple attractor states in play (Chapter 5). Clients find it generally easier to live with what they already know how to navigate than to enter into unfamiliar, possibly hurtful territory. In this regard, the work on interpersonal neurobiology and emotions as well as neuroscience is a rich field to explore (Cozolino, 2006; Damasio, 1999; LeDoux, 1996; Schore, 1994; Siegel, 1999).

Working at the Core: Jade and the "Ugly Baby" Story

Case Study

Jade was a 55-year-old consultant. She worked for a prestigious firm and felt successful and proud of what she did. A few months earlier in therapy, we had discussed her desire to broaden her horizons and add some more tools to her trade. Consequently, she found a consultant training program that seemed fitting. The training institute had a promising curriculum and stringent requirements, ending in a certification to add to her resumé. Jade was excited about this potential credential and threw herself into the learning process. Now, the test for the certification was two weeks away, and she was a nervous wreck.

As we explored why this test had so much weight for her, a theme emerged. She recalled a lifelong struggle in which her mother felt ashamed of Jade's lack of accomplishments. Jade had flunked out of college, and her mother was embarrassed. She pretended to her friends and family that Jade had actually graduated. Sworn to secrecy by her mother, Jade hid how much she was filled with anger, resentment, and shame. Now, as she approached the test situation, she felt intense pressure to perform and was riddled with insecurity and fear. She felt destined to fail, and then have to cover up the failure once again.

As Jade related her story, her body exhibited a collapsed chest. Tears streamed down her cheeks, and she would wipe them as soon as they emerged. Her tone of voice sounded as if she carried a hundred years of burden. Her body was revealing the story of a secret that had been held for a very long time (Kurtz & Prestera, 1976). I asked her to slow down her storytelling and notice what she was experiencing in the moment. As she slowed down, taking in short, heavy bursts of air, she exclaimed, "You know, this goes way back. My mom called me an ugly baby."

I was struck by the way she smiled as she said this, at the same time that she dropped deeper into her sunken chest. Her eyes were droopy and sad, and her gaze fixed on the floor in an empty stare. Her right arm dangled down beside her body, as if unattached. I was curious about the arm but sensed that this was not the right moment to invite it into awareness. Then Jade made a comment of her own: "That was the going story in the house," she said. "My mom liked to tell everyone at gatherings what an ugly baby I really was, how I came out blue and red, and how kind of disfigured I looked. She considered that entertainment."

As she finally let her secret out, she was no longer able to contain her deep sadness. Tears rolled down her cheeks, but she stopped wiping them. Her voice and cries softened, giving her a younger appearance. I contacted her by saying, "That sounds really painful, Jade," which functioned to keep her deepening into her experience.

As the rest of the story came out, Jade revealed that her mother had rejected her at birth due to how she looked. Further, her mother had birth complications and had hated her pregnancy, as well as the birth, and had refused to breast-feed the baby. Jade would cry all night long.

All this revealed that Jade was rejected at the most basic level: She was not welcomed into the loving arms of her mother. Life started out rough and harsh. She began her first relationship with a lie. This pattern became an identifying rhythm between mother and daughter. In adult life, Jade would repeat this pattern in her intimate relationships, forever lamenting that her relationships were doomed.

Jade cried as she remembered more details of the story and its impact. The meaning of the story continued to extend from an intellectual understanding into a bodily expression of it—into a visceral level of experience. She rocked gently forward and back, her tears covering the softness of her face. Her gaze was again fixed on the floor in a blank stare. Reaching out to her, I suggested, "There is so much sadness here. Just let this be here, Jade. I am right here with you, and I am sorry your mother felt this way about you."

Jade continued to rock, my gentle words entering into her, her head nodding in agreement. She was taking in my words, experiencing me as a kind adult or a gentle aunt who was validating her view. This magical stranger (Chapter 18) was siding with the child, who knew in her heart that this was no way to be treated by her mother. It was an opportunity to work through an old, formative memory and concomitant belief while yielding to the integration of new possibilities of welcome.

Encouraged by her nonverbal listening cues, the stillness in her body, and her attentive gaze, I continued as the magical stranger, offering a wider perspective than the young child could ever have had at the time: "Sometimes mothers are overwhelmed and don't know what to do with their babies. They are kind of shocked and overwhelmed by the experience. I am sorry your mom felt this way. I am sorry she could not see what a beautiful baby you were and what a lovable person you are." I was addressing the need of the child to make sense of her experience, and the inevitable choice children make in painful situations—assuming it was their fault. This is generally the child's safest choice, because it assumes the possibility of some measure of control, through finding out and correcting what the fault might have been.

Jade kept rocking, her eyes intermittently closing, as if she was soaking up the confirmation of her being, right in the moment. I was silent, waiting for what would unfold next, trusting in the organicity principle (Chapter 5) that something would. Her breath eased; I noticed that she and I had been holding our breath throughout this passage. I relaxed my breath and exhaled softly, and she began to breathe a little more deeply into her chest.

Spontaneously, her left arm moved across her chest, resting on her body as if in a cradle. She didn't even realize that she was doing this. "You just moved your arm," I whispered, and then asked her, "What is your arm wanting to do right now?" Her head turned toward the cradle; she gazed at its crook, and the rocking motion increased. She lifted her right arm, delicately cupping the left (the one she had earlier abandoned), and gazed at this arm lovingly, as a mother would do with her beloved child (the "left-side cradle"). "I love you. I love you," she whispered. She kept whispering gentle words of love and nourishment as she rocked back and forth, tears streaming down her face continuously. Her face opened up in a loving gaze.

This moment seemed to go on for a long time. I sat back, witnessing the dance between herself, her actual mother, and the beloved mother who could not be there at her birth but had now shown up as a part of herself to provide a missing experience—what Alexander and colleagues (1946) termed a "corrective emotional experience," what Daniel Siegel (2010) considers being a friend to oneself.

In that moment, I recognized with increased clarity the way in which this "ugly baby" came into the world, leaving an imprint of not being welcomed in her body, thus setting up the beliefs that had shaped her life so profoundly. Jade began to act out of a lifelong trance (Wolinsky, 1991) of not being fully acceptable, beautiful, or welcomed for who she was. She learned that only an alternate persona could be loved. The trance of her life was the belief that she was not lovable for who she was, but only for who she should have been, like her brother and other successful, beautiful people.

Jade had spoken in earlier sessions of how her brother was favored and how she had always felt less than him. She had taken these interactions between herself, mother, and brother for granted, never recognizing the dynamic of her assumed ugliness being reinforced each time her mother favored her brother. This is an example of the parallel levels of internal and external family systems in play (Schwartz, 1995) that would be ideal to address in working through in a multilevel manner.

After a long while she looked up at me. Our eyes met, and she smiled directly at me. It was a warm exchange between us. In that moment, I felt a genuine love for this client. She could see it. For the first time she knew how to recognize it and allow herself to feel it. No words were needed. The nonverbal exchange through the eyes conveyed it all. She could see in my eyes that she was welcomed and seen for who she was.

Then Jade pointed to her heart (on the right side) and said, "I can't feel my heart." I smiled and replied, "Actually, your heart is on the left side." She bolted up, sat straight, and said, "What? I didn't even know that that's where the heart was in the body. No wonder that no relationships have worked out. I have been looking for love in all the wrong places!" A huge laugh erupted from her and we laughed for the longest time, delighting in the metaphorical as well as the literal level of her discovery. After a few liberating moments of deep laughter, she settled back into the chair, filled with the experience she had traversed. Then she softly cast her eyes away from contact with mine and smiled to herself with an expression of utmost kindness. In that moment, I knew she had updated a very old belief. She had taken a significant step toward working through her sense of being unlovable by the reconsolidation of early memories.

The Missing Experience

In her body, Jade knew that the lack of physical affection and holding by her mother was painful. She had not known any other way for most of her life. The bodily experience of not having this warmth and holding had created in her a disposition to withdraw from human contact. She was unable to give this quality of warmth to herself or to others. She also had difficulty recognizing warmth when she received it. Instead, beliefs would form that human contact was cold and uncaring; that the world was harsh and limited in warmth and kindness; and that love was conditional and had to be earned. Many of these beliefs became reality in her life, confirmed with every failed relationship.

In the therapeutic moment when Jade and I had a genuine exchange of love and care, when she actually experienced being received, she became at once painfully aware of the lack of this kind of intimacy with her mother, and at the same time of the experience of having it. She was able to wake up to the intimacy in the present moment. She could experience in her body what that felt like.

The therapeutic experience between Jade and me as the loving therapist figure provided a missing experience from without that then enabled her to welcome her baby self into the world with love, admiration, and care. She was empowered to provide comfort and a cradle for herself from within, as she was not able to do before. The presence of these missing experiences was a landmark on the road toward understanding, completion, and working through.

Jade's intuitive realization of the left cradle provided her with a perfect missing experience of what should have happened in her original mothering. Alan Schore (2005) has studied this phenomenon, finding that during left-side cradling, the right-to-right hemisphere connection is significant. The left cradle encourages emotional bonding between mother and infant (Manning et al., 1997). The right hemispheres connect and enhance the attachment transaction: "The social experience-dependent maturation of the right brain in human infancy is equated with the early development of self" (Schore, 2005, p. 205). And, as Siegel (2007) has noted, when Jade can become a friend to herself and mindfully bring the essential compassion of the witness state to bear on her internal parts, the same primary attachment neural networks are stimulated.

Laughter

Laughter is common in Hakomi therapy. We initially organize our experience in life when we have few and limited experiences to go on. However, the same capacity to make or remake meaning remains with us throughout our lives. While it would not be appropriate to laugh in the presence of one who was truly a victim or at the complete mercy of his circumstances, laughter is an affirmation that life is a creative, nonlinear act, and that we all retain the capacities to be at least cocreative in the meaning process. Laughter likewise affirms that both therapist and client have a compassionate witness to bring to bear on the process of working through (Pattison, 1990), making collaboration appropriate. In fact, the long-range goal of Hakomi therapy is to empower clients to make intentional continued use of the compassionate witness state so that it becomes a lifelong resource for them beyond the parameters of therapy (Eisman, 2006).

Nourishment

Typically, clients like Jade need to have multiple experiences like what happened for deeply ingrained beliefs to change and new neural networks to be reinforced (Cozolino, 2002). The paradox of experiencing the pain of loss, coupled with the joy of receiving what has been missing, has a bittersweet quality to it. Helping clients realize this threshold experientially by having them recognize it and find the newness in it while still acknowledging the pain is a delicate balance. The therapist's fine attunement to the moment is needed. It is essential not to rush into wanting to make clients feel better, or give them explanations, or rationalize the situation. This would be a disservice in this vulnerable moment of recognition and deeply felt experience. Working through is never rushing through. Therapy happens nonviolently at the barriers (Chapter 17). When clients can relate as a larger self to their inner child through a core, mindful place of awareness and compassion in between sessions, the healing accelerates and dependence on the presence of the therapist lessens (Almaas, 1990; Eisman, 2006; Fosha, 2005).

Waiting, holding clients in the therapeutic emotional exchange, and allowing them to recognize the self-authenticating goodness of the moment is crucial when in session. Offering nourishment in the form of physical contact can be an important agent of the missing experience (Kurtz, 2004). This needs to be done with sensitivity to the potential emotional activation that physical contact can have for the client. The issue of touch in the therapeutic exchange can be highly beneficial, but it also can be a confusing terrain for both therapist and client, if the deeper core issues are about boundary violations or relational trauma of any kind. This issue requires deeper exploration than can be done here (see Chapter 13; Causey, 1993; Hunter & Struve, 1998; McNeely, 1987; Peloquin, 1990; Smith et al., 1998; Thomas, 1994; Zur, 2007).

In Jade's case, however, the nourishment of touch and emotional closeness provided part of the missing experience. "This did not happen then, but it is happening now" became the new experience. Jade's mindful discovery that she could be loved had much greater impact than if I had simply told her so in ordinary consciousness. Here, she discovered it for herself and made it her own experience, not simply an intellectual insight. How much clients can actually be present to such intimacy is a good indicator of whether particular experiments with nourishment are the right ones. The issue with nourishment or gratification in Hakomi therapy is how clients are unable to take it in—and which barriers need to be negotiated to safely allow in missing experiences previously organized out (Chapter 17). Freud indicated that working through our compulsion to repeat old patterns (Johanson, 1999a) yields to an ability to experience new situations as new. Working through old beliefs results in being able to differentiate past from present.

Affect Synchrony, Loving Presence, and Somatic Resonance

The therapist's loving presence (Chapter 9) is essential when clients are working through these moments of painful memories. Loving presence provides the container in which clients can safely and deeply experience whatever they need to go through (Lewis et al., 2000). It allows for a synchrony between therapist and client, deepening the therapist's attunement so he can track and contact the client accurately, like a parent intimately aware of and sensitive to a child (Stolorow et al., 1987). The German word *Einfühlung* describes the phenomenon of being able to resonate with another and feel what he is feeling. It literally means "feeling into someone" and explains the sensorial aspect of being with another. Sensory empathy (Zanocco, 2006) describes this phenomenon between therapist and client (Fosha, 2000). The studies of mirror neurons highlight a possible explanation for such empathic occurrences (Rizzolatti & Craighero, 2004). The minute physical exchanges of positive facial expressions, (Ekman & Rosenberg, 2005), as well as positive whole-body responses, provide a new way of being received (LeDoux, 1996).

When such processes encourage Jade to deepen, mindfully regressing (Chapter 18) into the formative experiences that gave rise to the core beliefs, she is in a dual state of consciousness, both sensing herself as the younger child and knowing she is an adult in a therapy session. The interpersonal therapist-client synchrony and affect regulation (Schore, 2005) calms the child part (Chapter 18), which in turn facilitates the empowerment of the client's adult or essential self-state to intrapsychically witness and respond compassionately to its inner child (Marlock & Weiss, 2001). An experience of working through in Jade's case came from this inner witness state embodying compassion while the same state was present in the therapist (Allen & Knight, 2005). Thus, working through often reflects a parallel intrapsychic and interpersonal process, affirming from within and confirming from without (Brown & Ryan, 2004).

Jade found access to her core through her initial grief over the loss of her mother's love. This opened her to the transformational experience of taking love in rather than defending against it.

Working Into the Core and Through

When clients are working through the core experience, a paradox arises: They are averse to going into the intensity of the experience; since there is a strong association of pain and sadness, avoidance of feelings is high. There are good reasons for clients to have such avoidance or resistance. Hakomi therapists assume that these defenses are highly astute ways of managing the client's experience (see Chapter 17; Kurtz, 1990b). Such a view depathologizes clients' defense systems, celebrates the wisdom of the often young self that devised ways to survive, and affirms an active participation on their part that creatively designed ways to protect and remain safe (Hayes, Strosahl, & Wilson, 1999).

During the working-though stage, clients face a crossroads: whether to go further into the experience or to listen to the parts of their unconscious that are trying to manage the experience. In this situation, the Hakomi method of yielding to the resistance and listening for what the unconscious is revealing through these parts is a powerful tool (Chapter 17).

Asking clients to deepen their experience is an act of faith on the part of the therapist that an organically wise unfolding is taking place. Since clarity does not come to clients all at once, instead of rejecting moments of lack of clarity as failures, they can be recognized as stepping-stones along the way to lucidity. When we proceed with an experimental attitude (Chapter 11), every result becomes new information. Hakomi therapists welcome the intelligence of clients' feelings in the moment in a gentle and noninvasive way that is able to tolerate mystery (Johanson & Kurtz, 1991).

The crucial moment in Jade's story took place when she deepened into her grief and had a sensory experience of it (Craig, 2003), tuning into what Damasio (1999) terms somatic markers. She experienced the loss of her mother's love as a felt sense (Gendlin, 1996) in the moment, as if it were occurring right now. New clarity came when she was able to stay with this experience while being fully conscious that it was happening in a new context— that of a safe and caring therapeutic relationship.

At this point, clients have a choice whether to continue to identify further with the old belief set or to disidentify (Chapter 20) with the painful experience and move toward new options. The therapist needs to help clients with this process of disidentification, since they can easily construe feeling the old pain as confirming their reality one more time (Martin, 1997; Teasdale et al., 1995). Mindfulness that results in the client having the psychic distance to differentiate between *having* reactions as opposed to *being* those reactions (Kegan, 1982) is not ordinarily taught in Western culture, and must be tracked and encouraged by the therapist (Chapter 10).

Working through, in terms of the client being able to "independently face and master the conflicts in ordinary life" (English & English, 1958, p. 591), is a process affected by many variables. When clients are able to regard their new experience as real and helpful, they see that they can impact the experience they are having in the moment. This awareness lifts their previous sense of powerlessness toward the past, replacing it with a sense of understanding and compassion for what occurred in the past. Once perception shifts, the internalized past makes sense, and clients are able to see themselves and their important relationships in a new way. The narrative of their life takes on a new order, and this coherence is one of the best predictors of future healthy attachment relationships (Siegel, 2003). When deep-seated belief systems shift, they lead to the emergence of a new, more updated story, one that includes more detail and complexity. This opens up the horizon of the future, offering clarity about what one now wants to bring into one's life that is nourishing and energizing, increasing hope, and bringing to light new and viable choices (Johanson, 2010b; LeShan, 1994).

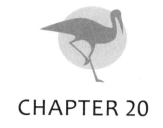

CHAPTER 20

Transformation

Halko Weiss

MANY FACTORS CONTRIBUTE to change and learning in psychotherapy (Goldfried, 1980). The factors cited in the psychodynamic literature are the therapeutic relationship, "actualization" of the problem (Grawe, 2001)—where it comes alive as an in-the-moment experience—personal conviction and experience of the therapist, expectancy of the client (placebo effects), respectful collaboration between client and therapist (Duncan, 2010), and so forth. Generally, little credit is given to method or technique, with many metastudies showing that the personality of the therapist is more important than his or her therapeutic modality (Grawe, 2001; Hubble et al., 1999; Wampold, 2001).

Consequently, there are good reasons why Hakomi therapists put a lot of emphasis on the therapeutic relationship (Chapters 9 and 14), although it is hard to find conclusive research on what exactly that relationship should look like. Attachment theory researchers suggest a number of qualities, such as presence, safety, and so forth (Cozolino, 2006; D. Siegel, 2010; Wallin, 2007), and, in recent years, a number of psychoanalysts have discovered that the characteristics of mindfulness can also powerfully shape the therapist's attitude in a positive way (Germer, 2005; Hick & Bien, 2008). According to these theorists, the state of being of the therapist is a strong component of how the relationship unfolds—a powerful support for Ron Kurtz's emphasis on loving presence.

The Hakomi tradition has approached the question of transformation heuristically, taking the path of applicable argument and convincing explanation. The models we use contain well-grounded elaborations of previously established schools of thought regarding change. Among these are acceptance (Kohut, 1984; Rogers, 1951; Segal et al., 2002), creating meanings (Freud, 1999b), sharing with another person (Catholic confession, for instance), switching logical levels (Watzlawick et al., 1974), and external regulation of internal processes, such as attention (Schore, 1994).

In particular, though, and on the level of practical intervention, Hakomi employs three strong and consistent strategies to bring about lasting change for our clients: (1) disidentification, (2) integration, and (3) experiential learning. These are discussed below in detail.

Disidentification

With the use of mindfulness, Hakomi therapists introduce a tool dedicated to establishing an internal observer. They pay constant attention to tracking who is involved in the therapeutic process as the "I" of the client: Is she yelling, "I am furious," or is she reporting, "I notice this surge of fury coming up. . . . It needs to yell"? In the latter, the observer is present and can report on her state, while in the former, the client is identified with a limiting state of being (in this instance, fury) and is "hijacked" (Goleman, 1996, 2004) by powerful emotional experience. As Schwartz (1995) would note, the furious part is blended or fused with her state of consciousness.

Hakomi therapy supports the emergence of states that are difficult for the client, but also prepares for and supports an observer to be present, especially throughout those more regressive moments (Chapter 18).

Through the concept and practice of an internal observer, Hakomi connects to ancient traditions of spirituality, those of Buddhism in particular (Johanson, 2006; Nyanaponika, 1976). Modern science shows that we can train and develop the ability to observe internal processes (Davidson & Begley, 2012; Hayes et al., 2004) through mindfulness practice. Among other benefits (Davidson et al., 2003; Kabat-Zinn, 1990; Langer, 1989), a regular mindfulness practice supports a capacity to distance persons from their own experiences without dissociating from them. In other words, the internal observer unties a person from the strong pull of identification with the different states he habitually moves through (Schwartz, 1995; Watkins & Watkins, 1997; Wolinsky, 1991).

With the cultivation of an internal witness, self-identification slowly moves into the observing position, with its traditional characteristics: calm, slow, compassionate, and interested in internal parts, with a feeling of well-being. With practice, this core state starts appearing more often. Suffering states seem more remote, and compassionate involvement with internal processes becomes possible (Eisman, 2006; Schwartz, 1995). Persons begin to move in a progressive direction where they are less likely to be overwhelmed by negative emotions. They collect the personal power to develop and find centered and integrated states of being.

This process seems to involve training effects (Hayes et al., 2004; Johanson, 2015) that create changes in the neural architecture (Brefczynski-Lewis, Lutz, Schaefer, Levinson, & Davidson, 2007; Hanson with Mendius, 2009). It has similarities with older concepts in psychotherapy like the "reflexive ego" in psychoanalysis, or with the externalization techniques of the here-and-now therapies that bring about a more outside position of observation as well.

Today, a strong movement has developed supporting the use of mindfulness in both the psychodynamic (Germer et al., 2005; Safran, 2003) and the cognitive-behavioral traditions (Hayes et al., 2004; Linehan, 1993). Humanistic psychology has used closely related approaches for several decades (Gendlin, 1996; Perls, 1973; Pesso, 1973). This general approach actually takes center stage in the so-called third wave in cognitive-behavioral therapy, where processes similar to the ones described in this book are sometimes called "decentering" (Segal et al., 2004) or "reperceiving" (Shapiro, Carlson, Astin, & Freedman, 2006).

Typically, clients who work in a mindfulness-centered way for a while report experiences similar to those of Bob, a 42-year-old engineer who started therapy in a fairly depressed state he called a "midlife crisis": "With reasons I still don't fully understand, I can see the gray fog come up. I know it has the power to pull me in, but that rarely happens now. I sit down, focus on my state, and usually connect to 'ne'er do well Bob' [a name he gave to a childlike part in himself]. I soften, warm up, and light comes in. I become aware of that hole in my chest, but I just see it clearly. It is pain and hurt. I understand it so well, but it does not have the power to dominate me."

Integration: Accommodating the New

Psychotherapy has a long history of looking at personal healing as a process of integration. In 1921, Freud pointed out that "the progressing development of the child towards a mature adult generally brings about an ever-expanding integration of the personality, a condensation of the individual drives and purposes that have grown in it independently" (1999a, p. 85, translation by author). Assagioli (in Ferruci, 1982), Jung, and other psychodynamic theorists have kept that understanding alive. Humanistic psychology (Perls, 1973) and systems psychotherapy (Berne, 1972; Schwartz, 1995; Stone & Stone, 1989; and others) are among the great variety of approaches that emphasize the importance of integrating dissociated, alienated, or polarized parts of the psyche.

Hakomi assumes both a psychodynamic and systems view of psychological processes. Internal dynamics are looked upon as parts that self-organize into a whole (see the unity principle in Chapter 5)—a whole that can have different grades of integration (Johanson, 2011c)—the quality of which is determined by the quality of communication among the parts of the whole (Bateson, 1979).

Throughout the psychotherapeutic process, a Hakomi therapist contacts those parts of a person that get activated, but are just outside awareness, or deemed unacceptable by another part of the person. By employing mindfulness and exhibiting an accepting and empathic attitude toward all parts, the therapist models and helps strengthen the client's capacity and willingness to explore, understand, and befriend internal parts that are not yet well integrated. She assists the client in finding a deeper and more complex flow of information among many elements of the overall organization—in line with Hakomi's organicity principle (Chapter 5).

Siegel and Solomon express these aspects of healing and transformation:

> [T]he mind is a self-organizing, emergent process that is both embodied and relational and that regulates as well as arises from, the flow of energy and information within us and between us. From an IPNB [interpersonal neurobiology] perspective, *healing* is the process of integration in which energy and information flow is cultivated, such that separate elements of a system are differentiated and then can become linked. *Integration* is the linkage of differentiated elements and allows the coordination and balance of a system to achieve harmony. (2013, p. 2)

The idea is that communication among parts, and especially an awareness of each part's important contribution to the whole, is essential to improve the quality of self-organization, or—according to Schwartz (1995), Siegel (2007), and others—support a well-integrated whole. Accordingly, a variety of Hakomi interventions are designed to depolarize and integrate parts and, in so doing, help end a history of dissociation. Good examples of this are sessions that unfold around the process of rapprochement between adult parts and child-type states, as the following example illustrates.

> *Caroline, a 67-year-old former school teacher, comes to see her therapist because she has had a number of strange, self-induced accidents that she feels were caused by being in a constant state of irritation and confusion, and by having torn feelings. Her main complaint centers on a "hateful and envious" part that she absolutely detests and is embarrassed about (notice her identification with that antagonistic part of herself). She is in therapy for almost half a year before she finds the strength to deal with this central part of herself that she calls the Witch. At a crucial moment, the following occurs.*
>
> *In a mindful state, Caroline is aware of a compact and burning feeling around her diaphragm that she associates with the Witch. She has identified this part as a young state (in terms of age) that threatens to overpower her. The therapist invites her to try to find a way to speak to that young being from the internal observer. (Caroline understands that this is an impartial, interested, and accepting state, which she has already learned to find in herself.)*
>
> CLIENT: *I can't stand that feeling, I want it to go away. [Client is identified.]*
> THERAPIST: *Can you find a place from where you could talk to it with compassion?*
> CLIENT: *Let's see [almost half a minute goes by]. . . . I think . . . no, I just cannot find that place. . . . I am swamped by my resentment. . . . I just want it to go away . . . to die.*
>
> *The therapist continues to explore the part of the client that so despises the client's witch-like child state. They find out that the rejecting part (she calls it her*

School Master) is worried that the Witch will dominate her existence and make her completely unlovable. Her therapist then asks the School Master whether it would be good for the therapist to talk to the child and try to make her feel better. After some hesitation, but with a glimmer of hope, the School Master gives way.

Before the therapist starts talking directly to the Witch, she asks the School Master to observe closely and step in if the therapist does something that is not okay. She also invites the Observer to be present. The School Master is appeased. Now the therapist begins an intervention with the Witch by entering into a dialogue in which the Observer keeps reporting how the internal Witch-child [for a while the terms "Witch" and "Witch-child" are used interchangeably] is responding. After contacting and exploring the Witch-child's experience for a while, the following exchange develops:

THERAPIST: [to the child] *I can see how furious you are. Can I come and sit with you? [To the observer] How does she respond?*

CLIENT: *She looks up . . . somehow surprised. But also softening . . . kind of opening a little bit. . . . She nods.*

THERAPIST: *Okay, so I will sit next to you on that log. How close should I sit? [To the observer] How does she respond?*

CLIENT: *She wants you to sit right next to her . . . actually touching. . . . She feels you. There is a cautious smile. . . .*

As they go on, the therapist explores the world of the child more deeply and shows a lot of compassion and understanding. In their shared fantasy, they sit on a log in a hidden place in the child's old backyard, as the visiting therapist has her imaginary arm around the child. It becomes clear that the Witch only protects an extremely rejected and marginalized even smaller child within Caroline whom she calls Beebee. The Observer is sometimes asked to share its observations and speak to the furious and aggressive Witch-child as well, which finally happens with ease and in a loving spirit. For example, at some point, from the Observer position, the client speaks to the Witch:

CLIENT: *Of course you hurt. . . . That is really bad. . . . I understand how they all hate you . . . and all your love . . . is stuffed down your throat. . . . Thank you for helping and protecting Beebee.*

THERAPIST: *How does she react?*

CLIENT: *She relaxes. . . . She looks at me. . . . There is warmth . . .*

THERAPIST: *What does the warmth do?*

CLIENT: *I can feel it fill my belly. . . . It spreads. . . . It is not hot anymore—it is pleasantly warm. . . . I am so glad she protected Beebee. . . .*

During the ongoing internal dialogue between the Observer and the Witch, the School Master does not intervene at all. Then, when the therapist wraps up this session's visit with the Witch, she explores with the Observer how the Witch is doing and what she needs.

CLIENT: *She wants me to not leave her again. She wants me to not push her away . . . to stay connected.*

THERAPIST: *Is that something you can do?*

CLIENT: *Yes. I want to.*

A little later the therapist contacts the School Master:

THERAPIST: *Was this okay? Did we do the right thing?*

CLIENT: *[from the Observer] She has become so soft as well. She sat down. She is nodding.*

THERAPIST: *Can I talk to the School Master directly? [Client nods.] How is that for you?*

CLIENT: *[talking from the position of the School Master] I am relieved. She is not alone anymore. I can breathe. . . . We need to make sure we stay connected.*

While such therapeutic processes can be quite complex, with different parts being triggered and needing attention, this example shows how the relationship between parts can depolarize by opening and deepening channels of information between parts, encouraged by the compassion of the observer self-state. Processes like this are well described by Richard Schwartz (1995, 2001).

When parts are no longer adversaries but instead learn how to understand each other, and know what kind of support is needed, transformation occurs naturally. In the example of Caroline above, both the Observer and the School Master find ways of integrating the Witch and learn to deal with her compassionately. This part of the client no longer holds an exiled—or rejected—position, but is more deeply integrated into the overall self-organizing system. In later sessions, some deep work with Beebee opened the way for even bigger changes in Caroline.

Experiential Learning

For Ron Kurtz, providing missing formative experiences in a psychotherapeutic process is the core mechanism of personal transformation of the client. As he saw it, unconscious beliefs (Chapter 7) are revised through powerful emotional learning when old formative memories are evoked. Insight is never enough. The tenet is: It takes experiences to counteract learnings from previous experiences.

This approach also has important predecessors: Franz Alexander, in particular, put forward his idea of "corrective emotional experiences" in the early days of psychoanalysis (Alexander et al., 1946). More recently, similar concepts have flourished. Neurobiologists Nadel (1994), Roth (2003), and many others have shown how important strong emotional experiences are for learning—and that psychotherapeutic transformative learning may be state dependent.

A regressive state, like an internal child, needs to be activated to be accessible for rewiring of the neural architecture (memory reconsolidation; Nader, 2003) by offering a healing experience, as kind of an antidote (Ecker, Ticic, & Hulley, 2012; Pesso, 1973). For many psychodynamic schools—such as Kohutian self-psychology (Kohut, 1984) or the intersubjective approach (Stolorow et al., 1987), and humanistic psychology schools, such as Rogerian client-centered therapy (Rogers, 1951) or dialogical Gestalt therapy (Hycner, 1991)—the therapeutic relationship in itself may already be a corrective emotional experience when it counteracts habitual core organizing expectations. Hakomi would add that it is best when the client is intrapsychically mindful of the corrective interpersonal experience, and how it challenges previous beliefs.

The Hakomi method emphasizes that by activating problematic formative experiences in a mindful process of deepening and differentiation (Chapter 19), particularly powerful core situations may arise in therapy. The client may regress back into such formative experiences that express some lack of specific and badly needed input: a positive relationship of some sort, a sense of safety, important knowledge, and other key experiences a growing child must have in order to complete essential developmental phases to establish a good place in the world (Chapter 8). Because these potentially nourishing experiences did not occur when they were needed, the person was forced to put appropriate protective mechanisms in place that later limited his range of experience, behavior, and satisfaction.

When such damaging formative situations arise in a live manner in a session and are explored in detail, client and therapist may experiment with what was missing in the past. When mindfulness is in place and the nature of the situation is clear, they can jointly create a new situation in the present moment that allows the client to experience the unknown, unexpected, and deeply missed experience. The assumption is that this novel experience becomes encoded in the neural architecture, especially when it is emotionally charged, and can be repeated and deepened (Cozolino, 2006). The learning arising from such an approach would then expand the client's unconscious beliefs about the world and himself. The example above, of Caroline and her Witch part, can serve to elucidate this kind of therapeutic process.

A session with Walter demonstrates a less complex way of working, where parts are not as directly expressed, but where it is obvious that transformative experiences have to be designed very carefully.

> *Walter was a 32-year-old "perpetual student" who had explored a lack of support in his life during the course of many therapy sessions. He had repeatedly been in depressive and collapsed states that were connected with the memory of losing his mother in a car accident when he was six years old. These memories had merged with even older memories that were similarly characterized by feelings of loneliness and abandonment.*
>
> *The therapist spent a great deal of time exploring the corresponding somatic-affective states and supporting the development of the connected narrative. It eventually became clear why Walter had never succeeded in becoming involved in a warm, supportive relationship. At one session, Walter repeatedly alluded to how he would like to get to know such a supportive "world" (as he called it) at least once in his life.*

At this point the therapist offered to sit next to Walter on the floor and to allow Walter to lean against him. The therapist had never touched him, so this intervention was talked over and prepared in great detail. When they tried it out, with much awareness and a slow pace, Walter couldn't feel anything other than tension and fear. These experiences were explored and processed.

After more sessions on the floor, Walter—without anything unusual happening directly beforehand, but in a state that was characterized by deepening mindfulness—suddenly yielded and was able to lean easily and without resistance into the therapist. Then an avalanche of intense emotions erupted from within: sadness, relief, joy, and pain. During later sessions, the ability to receive "backing" (as Walter called it) finally became increasingly easy and natural. Mindful observation helped to create a sense of understanding and meaning. Mindfulness also made sure that Walter did not stay identified with this internal child, and that opening into the experience did not turn into "malign regression"—a state that many psychoanalysts warn about as characterized by intense identification.

Transformation occurs when clients are able to accommodate into their structure those kinds of experiences that they had previously not been able to take in (Johanson, 2015). Here the client was able to experience something new and—certainly, for his unconscious mind—unexpected, as his body took in the information of how it feels to receive support. The underlying assumption is that only something that has been experienced as real by the emotional and implicit memory system will find its abiding representation in the neural architecture.

From the point of view of a Hakomi therapist, the form of experiential learning illustrated in Walter's case is possibly the most powerful way to reshape specific habitual, protective, and limiting patterns, which once were a healthy response to the absence of required existential experiences for the young, growing organism. As new experiences and meanings are encoded, they shift the beliefs derived from the original formative material. While these experiences are uniquely connected to the specifics of a person's life, they also address basic existential needs that every human has, and can therefore be empathically detected and pursued by the therapist.

Furthermore, it is necessary to direct the client's attentional processes to the corrective experience for transformational learning to fully take root. If the client is not mindful, or if attention is directed elsewhere, the corrective experience will not be integrated (Begley, 2007). Directing awareness to the felt sense of having a long-awaited need finally met creates the requisite conditions for moderation of the original emotional learning (Ecker et al., 2012). This, in turn, changes all the experiences that are being shaped and colored by that particular memory system.

Integration Revisited: Solidifying the New

In terms of current models of transformation (Castonguay & Hill, 2012), Hakomi's approach of transforming core beliefs based on early formative experiences—which in turn influence the person's worldview or filters that affect perception and response—is closest to Constantino and Westra's (2012) expectancy-based approach. Since there is a revision of the client's working model of the world, the way the client expects things to be or organizes her experience is altered in a manner that affects virtually everything: cognition, emotions, interpersonal relationships, posture, breathing, movement, gestures, and more. Since the old expectancies or core organizing beliefs are deeply embedded in established neural networks, there is a necessary integration phase for the new way of being to take root.

One metaphor for understanding the integration process of solidifying the new growth is to think of new corrective experiences and memories as being like a real but fragile flower beginning to grow in the garden of one's bodymind. There is still the firmly established old growth in the garden along with the new bloom. But if attention, water, protection, sun, and fertilizer are given to the new growth, it will continue to grow bigger and stronger. Some of the old growth will wither from lack of attention, except for the growth that is affirmed to have a valuable, though not exclusive, place in the garden. Some of the integrative growth and strengthening can happen within the therapy sessions or in agreed-upon homework. As with Walter, verbal or nonverbal corrective experiences can be repeated and reinforced. The new experience should be mindfully savored. The person can also voluntarily and with awareness "rock" back and forth from the bodily manifestations of the old belief system to those of the new. He can take time to reimagine going through his life developmentally while embodying the new expectations. Anticipated stressful situations at home, work, school, or wherever can be rehearsed, slowed down, and resourced through embodying the new working model of the world. The therapist can have clients check in and notice what other parts of their inner ecology support or might be nervous about the new developments. If the therapy context is a group, the corrective experience can be offered by a number of people in a mindful progression. The client can experiment in the group setting with new ways of sharing, reaching out, reacting to certain situations, or whatever is needed, again in a way that the therapist ensures is mindful as opposed to rote movements.

In Caroline's case above, she could agree to check in with her vulnerable part, Beebee, at certain times or before and after stressful situations, also checking for any dissident parts that might attempt to sabotage the progress. Every time clients check in and observe an internal part from a mindful place of awareness and compassion, they are also deepening the neural net that helps them reside in their more expansive self-state beyond the drama of ego states. Perhaps journaling about the new experience or debriefing how it played out in situations throughout the week could be helpful. Sometimes the therapist might volunteer a story that metaphorically incorporates the therapeutic journey (Weiss, 1987). For some people, developing movements, composing music, or creating art that corresponds with the new worldview can be integrative. There are endless possibilities that can be collaboratively agreed upon and supported. Stosny (2014) outlines many ways of strengthening new habit patterns.

In line with the unity principle and Wilber's holonic four-quadrant model (Chapter 5), the more integral the transformation process, the better the chances of experientially reinforcing the new beliefs. In fact, one of the largest weaknesses of individual therapy is sending someone back into a context that does not support the growth and development at stake—though the transformed person does have increased abilities to influence the surroundings as well (Deci & Ryan, 1985; Feldman et al., 2001). As part of the integration process, it might be a good time for the therapist and client to assess any helpful changes that could be made in the context of the person's daily life. For instance, should partners (Fisher, 2002; Napier, 1988), family members (Benz, 1989; Van Mistri, 2008), or friends be brought in for an integration session? Might the client benefit from group therapy (Schulmeister, 1988) for opportunities to take in experiences of being supported by peers? What cultural issues (Brown & Kasser, 2005; Foster, Moskowitz, & Javier, 1996; Johanson, 1992; Jordan, Kaplan, Miller, Stiver, & Surrey, 1991; Pinderhughes, 1989) and social structures (Daly & Cobb, 1989; Edwards, 2000; Korten, 2009) related to the multiple communities that influence the client need attention? Is it possible to modify any of the communities the client is a part of, with their various cultural values, to be more supportive, or to exit some that might interfere with progress? If the person has a spiritual community, could some sort of supportive ritual be done that symbolizes growth or transition? Is it now more possible to implement helpful changes in diet or exercise, or to benefit from bodywork, or incorporate yoga, tai chi or qigong? Is there a way to modify the client's relationship to social structures through changes in work, housing, school, transportation, and so on? Is the person now more ready to benefit from a job counselor? In general, Walsh states that these "therapeutic lifestyle changes (TLCs) are underutilized despite considerable evidence of their effectiveness in both clinical and normal populations" (2011, p. 579). Sometimes TLCs can be helpful in themselves, and sometimes intrapsychic transformation has to happen before a client is willing or able to take advantage of them.

Conclusion

Hakomi therapists work with all three approaches to transformation outlined above in an ongoing manner: They continuously track for the mindful observer; they contact, uncover, and help integrate disconnected or rejected parts; and they look for the indicators of formative beliefs that limit a person's range of experience and behavior. All of this is held by the therapists' state of loving presence, which helps repair attachment ruptures and supports a state of earned secure attachment in the client (Siegel, 2012). The Hakomi therapist then helps the client integrate these changes into the context of daily life.

Thus, the three kinds of transformational approaches are strongly interrelated: The observing mind learns to disidentify from extreme states and becomes better able to befriend, explore, and integrate different parts. The receipt of understanding and care from an empathic therapist can be drawn upon and generalized to interactions with important others. Finally, the provision and integration of experiences that counteract implicit learning processes all mix together to transform the client's internal model of reality in ways that potentially enhance resiliency, allow for a fuller range of experiences, and promote a more positive view of self and others.

CHAPTER 21

The Flow of the Process

Maya Shaw Gale

The map is not the territory.

Alfred Korzybski, *Science and Sanity*, 1933

WHILE THE FLOW of client-therapist interactions in a Hakomi session has the felt sense of a spontaneous, nonlinear, and multidimensional process, there is an underlying structure that guides its unfolding. This structure involves a basic sequence of steps that aids the therapist in carrying out the essential tasks of the Hakomi method—the intentional evoking, and then processing, of experiences in a mindful state of consciousness. It provides a pathway toward the desired destination of uncovering and transforming the client's limiting core beliefs and moves the process through clearly identifiable phases. It is linear in the sense that it has an ideal beginning, middle, and end. The structure of the Hakomi process offers a general itinerary, suggested action steps along the way, and a possible outcome—though another principle of the work is to always be ready to key off the spontaneous.

Thus, as students of Hakomi soon discover, this sequence describes an idealized trajectory that, in practice, has a thousand variations. Steps are sometimes reversed or omitted. At any given point in the process, everything might backtrack to the beginning stages. The Hakomi therapist must become comfortable with a continual dance between left and right brain functions: loosely holding an awareness of the basic sequence of the flow but surrendering moment by moment to the essentially nonlinear nature of a complex system unfolding.

Charts, graphs, and diagrams are not particularly suited to conveying the nuances of nonlinear processes, but they can offer a way to orient and to navigate the complexities of this difficult territory. Figure 21.1 was developed as just such a navigational tool. It is meant to function as a map, helping Hakomi therapists recognize where they are at any given time during a Hakomi session, what might happen at that point, where they might get stuck, and what options they have.

As when using a road map, the therapist must be prepared for surprising twists and turns or roadblocks not predicted by the map, and be willing to improvise or backtrack.

While realizing that the map is not the territory, let's take a look at the Map of the Process

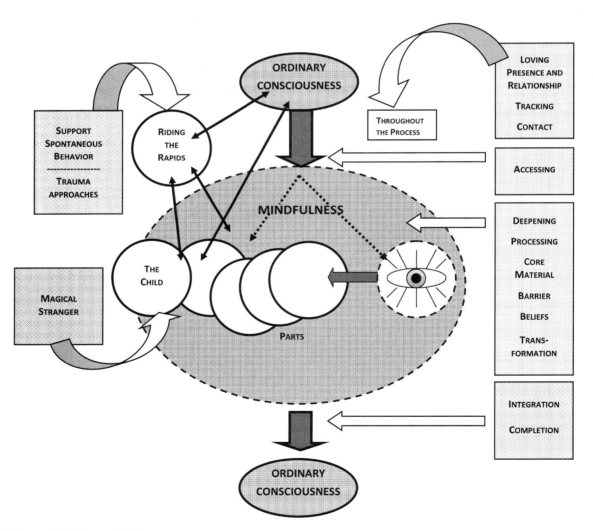

Figure 21.1. Map of the Process

(Figure 21.1). The shaded ovals in the center represent the two main states of consciousness (ordinary consciousness and mindfulness) that the client could be experiencing at different phases of the process. The smaller circles symbolize additional states of consciousness that may arise spontaneously or be evoked. The shaded rectangles identify the actions or responses of the therapist at appropriate points in the process. Large arrows indicate the overall direction in which the process moves, whereas the smaller arrows show movement between different states that may occur during the process.

A typical session begins with the client in ordinary consciousness, often focused on a problem or issue she wants to address. The therapist's initial task is to establish the healing relationship as a container and framework within which the rest of the process can unfold (Chapter 9). Imagine a larger oval surrounding the entire flowchart; this denotes the special "bubble" of safety, loving presence, and partnership that must be cultivated and tended throughout the session. The healing relationship is, in turn, informed and framed by the Hakomi principles, the largest context that supports the flow of the process (Chapter 5).

Tracking and contact are the skills that help the therapist initially connect to the client's present-moment experience and then to reflect what is observed back to the client, thus demonstrating the understanding that gains the trust of the client's unconscious (Chapter 14). A certain level of trust and safety, and an attitude of cooperation are necessary prerequisites for accessing mindfulness, the next step in the process. These qualities of the relationship are also important to maintain throughout the process, and so tracking and contacting become the therapist's bread and butter. Tracking and contacting are skills used in every phase.

Accessing (Chapter 15) happens when we help the client shift into mindfulness, a special state of consciousness where deeper layers of information and meaning become available. Mindfulness (Chapters 6, 10, and 16) involves a dual aspect of consciousness: being fully immersed or embodied in one's present-moment experience and simultaneously having the slightly detached perspective of an impartial and compassionate observer. The eye embedded in the mindfulness oval represents the self-witnessing dimension of this state.

As shown in Figure 21.1, once a state of mindfulness has been accessed in the client, the therapist can proceed to make use of the next sequence of steps that lead to transformation (Chapter 20). Deepening techniques (Chapter 15) help the client to increase the felt sense of his present experience and to experientially discover the connections to habitual patterns and themes of core material. As core material is processed, the therapist guides the client in exploring limiting beliefs (Chapter 7) and the barriers to new forms of nourishment and expanded experiences that have kept them in place (Chapter 17). Transformation happens when the client has a felt sense experience of taking in a new option, and reorganizes around including that option previously organized out (Chapter 20).

However, there are some states in which the observing consciousness temporarily dissolves or is only partially available. What we call riding the rapids is designated by a circle entirely outside the mindfulness oval, because it is a state of spontaneous emotional release during which the client's ability to mindfully observe her experience is usually not accessible (at least not verbally). As the several small arrows indicate, this state can be evoked when the client is working in mindfulness or from ordinary consciousness.

The gray rectangle to the left of this circle indicates specific strategies the therapist can follow when the client, often quite suddenly, shifts into riding the rapids. In cases where the client's experience of strong emotion seems to be embodied and following a natural arc of release and relaxation, the therapist supports the spontaneous behavior that emerges. In cases where the client dissociates, panics, or becomes stuck in a repeating loop without resolution, various trauma approaches can be used to stabilize the client and bring her back to mindfulness (Chapter 24).

The child state of consciousness (Chapter 18) is pictured in the diagram as partly inside and partly outside of the mindfulness oval. Although a client who shifts into this unique state—a kind of fully embodied memory of childhood—is often able to maintain the parallel consciousness of the adult observer, sometimes he is not. However, as soon as possible, the therapist's intention is to guide the client to reconnect with the compassionate witness.

The child state of consciousness may be seen as one of many possible parts or subselves that can emerge during the process. These are indicated by the multiple overlapping circles.

Although not every session proceeds neatly through deep mindfulness and processing to significant transformation, the natural and required course for clients is to return to ordinary consciousness in the last portion of the session. It is here that clients are supported to integrate whatever they have learned and, ideally, to complete the session in a way that allows them to translate this learning in a meaningful way into their lives outside of therapy (Chapter 20).

Overall, the flow of the process will have different rhythms and sequential patterns with each client and even in individual sessions with the same client. A client whose character style takes refuge in lots of thinking and theorizing may, at first, make little forays into mindfulness, and then continually return to the familiar intellectual territory of ordinary consciousness. Gradually, over time and a number of sessions, he may begin to experience enough safety to stay in mindfulness for longer periods. Another client may drop into deep processing in mindfulness at the very beginning of a session, but need more time to integrate in ordinary consciousness in the second half of the session. A third client may shuttle back and forth between being immersed in overwhelming emotions (riding the rapids) and moments of reviewing what happened before learning that she can be mindfully present in her experience without getting lost in it or coming out to talk about it.

Figure 21.1 can also be a map over time for the trajectory of long-term therapy. The same general structure can apply to the phases that the client and therapist will move through together over a period of weeks, months, or years. Even though all stages of the process may be visited in the beginning of therapy, at the metalevel, the early emphasis is on establishing the relationship with increasing levels of trust. As that happens over time, deeper layers of core material can be processed, with more sustained mindfulness. Then, in the termination phase of therapy, the emphasis is on integration and completion, with more time being spent preparing for closure in ordinary consciousness.

When the Hakomi principles are held as the largest frame for the flow of the process, there is no conflict between linear and nonlinear aspects. With the principles of nonviolence and organicity, there is a balance of following and leading (Chapter 12) and neither rigidly adhering to a plan nor losing a sense of direction. With unity and mindfulness, staying connected in relationship and in the present moment with one's own mindful observer keeps the process alive, fresh, and relevant. No need to consult the map at every turn.

To paraphrase Bob Marley, the process

> is one big road with lots of signs,
> So when you're riding through the ruts,
> Don't complicate your mind.

Just keep the map in your back pocket and trust the process!

CHAPTER 22

Jumping Out of the System

Rob Fisher

IT WAS ALREADY 40 minutes into the session and I was feeling intensely uncomfortable. Specifically, in my countertransference to this obviously talented and active woman, I felt useless and ineffective as a therapist. Although I have suffered bouts of low self-esteem in my life, I do not always feel this way, so the event was noteworthy. Helen, my client, kept talking, coming up with insights and feelings, which, at least outwardly, made the session look like real psychotherapy. I knew, however, that I had done very little except to squirm occasionally, as she had undertaken the session very much on her own. She was now talking about how other people never really helped her out or supported her and how, in contrast, she supported them a great deal. I realized that this was happening between us even as she spoke. Helen, a master of self-reliance, was being both client and therapist. Her expectation of help was very low, so she engaged in the session basically on her own, in the same way in which she engaged in her life outside of my office. Our relationship was a microcosm of the dynamics that occurred between her, her family, and her friends. By preempting me from helping her, she confirmed her belief that she was alone in the world and had to do everything herself. My countertransference provided the first key to exploring and working through this difficult and painful reenactment of the limiting core beliefs that plagued her in many aspects of her life.

This kind of self-reinforcing relational dynamic that includes cognition, affect, and behavior occurs frequently in psychotherapy between client and therapist. The deconstruction and exploration of this occurrence provides important clues to clients' core issues and the symptomatic problems that they present.

Systems in Human Relationships

It is inevitable that people in relationships enter into repetitive systems. These systems involve patterns of perceiving, feeling, behaving, and interacting that reinforce each other in circular ways. Systems occur in families, in intimate couple relationships, and, notably, in the process of psychotherapy. Being able to notice the system that a therapist unconsciously enters into with the client—being able to name it in a nonjudgmental fashion, connect it to the client's presenting problem, and find a way to explore it with respect, curiosity, and warmth—is one of the hallmarks of a master psychotherapist.

Actually, master therapists have been confounded by systems for a long time. Freud's vexation with being at the mercy of such systems fed into his concept of the repetition compulsion and supported in part his theory of a death instinct. He reasoned that since people resisted what he was offering to attain a more fulfilling life, they must have a fundamental wish for its opposite (Johanson, 1999a).

Likewise, Watzlawick and his colleagues at the MRI (Mental Research Institute) group (Watzlawick, Beavin, & Jackson, 1967; Watzlawick et al., 1974) noted that systems are invariant or stuck on the level of what they term first-order change. This means things change within the system without the system itself being affected. Thus, the more things change, the more they stay the same—a horror story of therapy—as when the identified patient in a family is cured of symptoms only to have some other family member become dysfunctional. Everyone is caught up in a game without end. Any changes are illusory.

Second-order change, according to Watzlawick and the MRI group (which also included Gregory Bateson, Milton Erikson, Don Jackson, and Virginia Satir), represents a change to a different logical type of system, with a different body of rules governing the structure or internal order of the system's members. It is as if the program that governs the action of the computer has been changed. The system itself has changed. Examples are changes from dream states to waking states, from position to motion, from manipulating an accelerator to shifting gears, or from scapegoating relationships to accepting, empathic relationships. The metaphor Watzlawick and his colleagues liked to use is this: being part of a system is like participating in a game that has no possible positive outcome. As long as these rules are unconsciously understood as facts, it will go on forever. Only on the higher level—the metalevel—where the rules themselves can be questioned and changed will solutions come into view. This is the kind of change Hakomi therapy is oriented toward when it attempts to help someone reevaluate their core organizing beliefs.

The problem in bringing about second-order change, according to Watzlawick, following Russell's theory of logical types, is that a system cannot generate from within itself the conditions for its own change. It cannot produce the rules for changing its own rules. Second-order change must be introduced into the system from something outside the system that does not participate in it, in the sense of being caught up in the same operating rules.

Since one's ordinary consciousness is considered a member of one's intrapsychic system, Watzlawick concludes that one's awareness is best circumvented if the goal is to bring about quick, substantial change. He recommends the use of paradoxes and the various subconscious, hypnotic techniques of Milton Erikson (Johanson, 1984).

In Hakomi, Kurtz learned that second-order change could be brought about efficiently and effectively with a person's consciousness intact the whole way. Nothing happens that the person is not aware of and does not approve of when he or she is invited to mindfully, curiously become aware of a repeating system through a technique he called "jumping out of the system" or "JOOTS." This technique allows the person to get some distance on the system, but to stay with it and appreciate it, studying it for a while to understand how it has functioned and what it is good for. When it becomes clear how it also limits one's options and how new possibilities previously organized out of the system can be mindfully explored, continuing in it unconsciously becomes difficult, and hope arises for the meaningful possibility of change.

Family therapists, of course, have also explored couples and family systems for decades (Nichols & Schwartz, 1998). They have noticed that couples reinforce each other's pathogenic beliefs and core injuries in very compelling ways. For instance, John may pull away from Mary, who then feels abandoned. She consequently pursues John more intensely, thereby provoking him to distance more intensely because he feels suffocated by her. He may have a history of interpersonal suffocation and intrusion dating back to his early years and primary relationships, whereas Mary may have a history of abandonment and neglect. Each of these wounds becomes revivified in the face of the partner's unintended, unconscious, but nevertheless wounding actions (Fisher, 2002).

Psychoanalysts have discussed these relational systems in terms of projective identification. In projective identification, the client enlists the therapist in enacting internal models of a relationship. For instance, my client Helen may have had an internal representation of others as undependable and unsupportive. Unconsciously believing that this is true about people, she will act toward me as if I were undependable and unsupportive. She will discount any information that calls into question her belief, and actively pursue and focus on evidence that supports it. Since she cannot rely on me, she has to do everything herself, including her own psychotherapy. As a direct result of her preempting me from saying anything or offering her any help, her prophecy about the relationship becomes true, and leaves me with a countertransferential experience of being a mere appendage to her monologue. Unconscious of what is happening here, I hopelessly settle back into my seat, convinced of my own ineptitude. I let her do the session entirely on her own and fail her basic test of me as a person and as a psychotherapist. Although the therapy in this example might be considered to be at a therapeutic impasse, it is actually a golden opportunity to explore and work through fundamental issues underlying the client's presenting problem. We are at the core of her therapeutic work.

Every person has a predisposition for entering into certain kind of systems. We do this by perceiving others through the filters of our own histories, treating people as if these perceptions are true and neglecting any evidence to the contrary, assimilating as opposed to accommodating in Piaget's terms (Horner, 1974). Try as we might, none of us is immune to unconsciously entering into a system that is compelling to our clients. This inevitably wounds them in ways that evoke their own history. At first glance, this seems unfortunate. However, being able to notice, name, and intervene on this level brings to consciousness the client's internal models of the world in an undeniable and visceral fashion (Aron & Anderson, 1998).

Transference and Countertransference From a Systemic Perspective

The Therapist's Contribution to the Interpsychic Field

Every therapist comes to the process of psychotherapy with her own characterological inclinations (Natterson, 1991). For instance, one therapist may be reluctant to become too intimate with his clients. It may be difficult for another to embody her own authority and set limits. Still another may need to dominate his client and give advice. Other therapists may worry about their own sense of neediness and may become dedicated to helping their clients eliminate their dependence on others. A therapist's need for attention and understanding may interfere with the ability to focus on and enter into the client's world. These examples represent just of few of the possibilities of how therapists may be internally organized as they work. Table 22.1 names the character strategies addressed in the Hakomi method (see Chapters 8 and 23) that many psychotherapists may unconsciously employ, and the type of limitation and strength each brings to the psychotherapeutic container.

Psychotherapists tend to perpetuate their own systems by enlisting the psyche of their clients. For instance, a therapist may have a tendency toward moving quickly, performing and producing in a goal-oriented fashion. She will therefore tend to create a container in psychotherapy that silently and covertly pushes clients toward results and away from connection to their internal world. The therapist might have developed this disposition because she learned in her own family of origin that she would be loved and attended to only if she succeeded in performing at high levels. Being adaptable and creative, as human beings tend to be, she learned how to perform, produce, and achieve her goals. When she grows up and becomes a competent therapist, she will be likely to conduct therapy in the same goal-oriented fashion. If a client of hers happens to have a character strategy from which he resists others in order to maintain his sense of autonomy, he will begin to resist the therapist. At the end of the day, the therapist will go home and complain to her partner or colleague about the resistant client she saw during the day. The client will go home and complain about his pushy psychotherapist, if he is capable of noticing this. Still, the client's characterological predispositions are interlocked with the therapist's. Systems between two people are determined by the meeting place of their characterological strategies and the wounds that underlie them.

The Client's Contribution

Clients also enter the therapeutic relationship with a compelling predisposition to enact the relationship according to a blueprint determined by their own history. If a therapist attends not only to the content but also to the way in which the client engages in psychotherapy, he will discover important clues to how the client most likely engages in all intimate relationships.

Table 22.1 Therapist Characterological Limitations and Strengths

	Sensitive/ Withdrawn	Dependent/ Endearing	Self-Reliant	Tough/ Generous	Charming/ Seductive	Burdened/ Enduring	Industrious/ Overfocused	Expressive/ Clinging
Limitations	Reluctant to make intimate contact with client	Difficulty taking the lead or being an authority	Discourages dependence	Must lead the client and be more powerful	Must be the therapist the client wants	Discourages expression of strong emotions; may be disapproving	Focuses on goals, not on depth or connection	Difficulty keeping attention on client; difficulty with subtleties
Strengths	Can be safe and gentle	Friendly, makes room for the other	Encourages self-reliance	Models power and strength	Attentive and empathic	Dedicated and persistent	Problem-solving orientation	Open to emotions, creative

One way to begin attending to the therapeutic system is to notice one's own counter-transference. This will provide information not only about the therapist's own psyche, but about the models of relationship, self, and other that the client brings to the therapeutic container. Once the therapist begins to sense the feelings, attitudes, and images that are rising internally, he can begin to assess what the client is doing to engender these specific experiences. For instance, one client with whom I worked in couples therapy would barely let a sentence go by without needing to reword what I said. I would say, "So, you're feeling sad, huh?" He would respond, "It's not exactly sad. It's more like feeling depressed." I'd say, "You have your right hand over your heart, huh?" He'd respond, "Well, it's really on the center of my chest." After a while I began to feel frustrated and started to doubt my ability to track what was going on with him. At that point in the session, his girlfriend was appealing to him to get married. He responded to her by saying, "Marriage is a form of slavery." I realized that he was fighting for his freedom. He did not want to be categorized or penned in any way. This battle for autonomy with her was also occurring in the present between him and me.

At this point, having understood the underlying wound, instead of feeling frustrated, I felt sympathetic toward his quest for independence. This was a just and noble cause that I could support. From this recalibrated internal place I said to him, "So this is about free-dom, huh?" He looked up at me and said simply, "Yes." I waited a moment and then, noticing that he was in a mindful state, offered a probe (Chapter 16). I slowly said, "What happens inside when you hear me say . . . 'I will fight for your right to be free'?" During the rest of the session we worked with his core beliefs around his sense of being controlled by others.

At the next couples therapy session he was grinning. He said, "Guess what happened between sessions? I asked her to marry me!" After several more sessions, we completed therapy. As we debriefed our series of sessions together, he remarked that the turning point for him was feeling like someone supported him in his quest for autonomy. This was an example of both noticing the system in place, intuiting what was driving it (Marks-Tarlow, 2012), and doing an intervention that jumped out of it.

Transference and Countertransference as a System

Each type of character strategy has its own set of transference and countertransference reactions. Table 22.2 is a very simplified chart that tries to convey some generalities about how two personal styles may become entangled. It names the character strategies com-monly presented by clients and the typical countertransference reactions that a therapist might experience. It also details typical ways the client might act to engender these coun-tertransference reactions. In real life, those entanglements are far more complex and var-ied, but the table may help to imagine certain general scenarios. Finally, drawing from control mastery theory (Weiss, 1995), the table names some possible ways the client may test the therapist to see if she will act to reinforce the client's core beliefs. These tests are usually calibrated for failure, with the client looking for evidence to support his old beliefs

Table 22.2 Typical Transference and Countertransference Reactions

Character Strategy	Sensitive/Withdrawn	Dependent/Endearing	Self-Reliant	Tough/Generous and Charming/Seductive	Burdened/Enduring	Industrious/Overfocused	Expressive/Clinging
Transference	Therapist seems unwelcoming and unsafe.	Looks to therapist to take the lead.	Does not need therapist's help.	Client doesn't want to be vulnerable.	Client feels stuck and victimized.	Client feels valued only for achievements.	Client feels unheard, unseen, and misunderstood.
Client acts	Withdrawn and analytical.	Helpless and needy. Appeals to therapist to lead; asks many questions.	As if he or she has no needs.	Intimidating, tough, seductive. Must lead and initiate.	Slow and resisting. Automatically disagrees.	Competent, fast-paced, and goal oriented. Mental and fact oriented.	Intense and overwhelming. Dramatizes.
Countertransference	Therapist feels tender toward client or bored because of lack of connection.	Feels important. Feels parental, or repulsed.	Feels useless.	Feels intimidated, admiring, or seduced.	Impulse to push or be sadistic to client.	Not much connection. Feels rushed and pressured.	Feels overwhelmed or entertained.
Test	Is the therapist safe and welcoming?	Can you be patient and tolerant of me? Will you give me room?	Do I have to do it all by myself?	Can I be real and vulnerable without being dominated or manipulated?	Are my impulses and anger acceptable with the therapist?	Will I be valued for myself or only for my accomplishments?	Does the therapist see and hear me? Is therapist interested?
Therapist acts in ways that reinforce the strategy	Therapist uninterested, harsh.	Takes care of client.	Does not provide much support.	Is afraid to confront client or tries to force client to be real.	Pushes or insists on therapist's direction.	Focuses on goals; gets mental, tries to produce as well.	Turns away as a result of feeling overwhelmed.

and ignoring evidence to the contrary. Being able to notice one's own countertransference reactions will provide a key to understanding and assessing the client's characterological predispositions, core beliefs, and historical wounds. In addition, it will provide clues to the preferred types of intervention for each client (Feinstein, 1990).

Therapeutic Response to an Impasse

Most everybody's impulse when noticing being stuck in a system and feeling uncomfortable in it is to try to get out as soon as possible. Very often, the resulting attempts make the situation even worse. That is when the solution becomes part of the problem, as was so beautifully analyzed by Paul Watzlawick and his colleagues (1974). As an example: the client who is slow, helpless, and resistant may trigger a lot of good suggestions and proposals from the therapist. Since the underlying issue is about freedom, though, the client needs to unconsciously sabotage everything that tries to guide him from the outside. This creates an ever-escalating interactional loop with no exit door. The intuitive or even automatic attempt to find a solution for the client makes things worse—as it probably does in the world outside therapy.

Therefore, the first order of business for the therapist is to stay in the system and to study it thoroughly. Trying to jump out too soon is often defeated, as safety and mindfulness need to be well established with the client before such a fine-tuned intervention can work. Tolerating the system, allowing it to show itself fully and deeply, can give both the therapist and the client the time to study and understand the unconscious rules of the game. Jumping out does not mean stopping it, but understanding it first. The jump is foremost a jump of consciousness.

Once the therapist has a sense of the system in which he and the client are engaged, jumping out of the system with the client becomes possible. This kind of intervention contains the risk that the client can feel judged by the therapist's stance of contacting the dynamic that is happening. For success at this juncture, it is critical that the therapist carefully guard against this possibility. Detailed below are a number of steps, both internal and external, that a therapist may go through to intervene on this level.

Steps to Jumping Out of the System

1. The therapist notices some internal discomfort, boredom, frustration, anger, repulsion, fear, feeling overwhelmed, or any other countertransferential experience. He may even feel critical or judgmental toward the client. This can be used as a signal that the therapist and client are caught in a dysfunctional system. At this point, the therapist must sort out what part of his experience is his own issue and what part is engendered by the client. For example, the session may jump from one content area to another, but whenever the therapist tries to focus the exploration, the client jumps to a new topic. The theme in general appears to be the client's longing for understanding, but the session appears to be going nowhere. The therapist notices that he feels frustrated and overwhelmed. The therapist then notices that the client is changing subjects frequently and

refusing to be corralled by his attempted interventions to deepen their exploration together.

2. The therapist becomes aware of and takes responsibility for his part in the system. At first, this is an internal event. The therapist realizes that he is trying to control what the client is presenting, but the effort is futile.

3. The therapist can then begin to assess what the client is actually doing to produce the countertransference reactions. So, for instance, if a therapist feels confused and over-whelmed by the intensity and complexity of his client's expressiveness, and does not usu-ally feel confused by clients, he would begin to look for how the client may be unconsciously attempting to confuse him. It could be a fast pace, sudden shifts, an intense focus on him, or any of a number of other subtle behavioral indicators that may be influencing the therapist.

4. The challenge now is to name what the client is doing, feeling, or perceiving in a way that is nonjudgmental and invites the client's curiosity and willingness to explore further. For example, the therapist says, "I notice that there seem to be so many important things going on at the same time that one chases the next and you hardly get to stay with one. Do you notice that?"

5. The therapist connects the interpersonal issue with the client's presenting problem or theme of the session. He might say, "There's something in you which really needs my com-passionate attention and understanding . . .[?]" In naming the system, in order to avoid sounding judgmental, the therapist must undertake both internal and external activities. Internally, he must find a way to celebrate this trait in the client as inherently creative, intelligent, and adaptive to a difficult situation in the past. In this example, being intense, expressive, and emotional may have been a very good and useful strategy in a family where nobody would pay attention to her if she did not crank up the volume.

6. In order to speak about this, it is sometimes helpful to name the system metaphori-cally, or to initiate the conversation by saying something laudatory or celebratory about the client's role in the system such as, "You're like a butterfly that moves from flower to flower tasting the nectar of each, but never landing and resting" or, with another type of client, "You have a great analytic capacity that you easily lead with, and also something is turning you away from your feelings."

7. A very effective way to address the system while making it okay is to include some-thing that the therapist has already understood about why that behavior makes sense. That can be helpful even if those reasons are as yet unsubstantiated guesses, such as, "When you move so quickly from one topic to the next, it seems like you really want to show me a lot of yourself in a short period of time[?]" or "When you speak about this event in such a factual and even tone, I get a sense that it might help you not to get into a mire of emotions[?]"

8. Once the client's curiosity is engaged (Johanson, 1988), therapist and client together can devise an experiment to be performed in mindfulness that will help bring consciousness to the system so that it no longer exerts an unconscious and covert influence on the client's relationships and behavior. It is critical that experiments are performed with the client's permission, that safety has been established, that there is a strong therapeutic alliance, and

that mindfulness is invoked (Chapter 16). Experiments without prior invocation of mindfulness will be shallow and will yield information only from the neocortex rather than from the deeper structures within the brain in which these narrow patterns are buried. For example, the therapist says, "How about we explore this further? I can try to get you to focus on something in particular, and you can notice your impulse to switch to another topic. As we do that, notice the feelings, thoughts, and sensations in your body, and any images and memories that might arise. Take time to bring your attention inside yourself before we do this, so you can really explore the subtleties of your experience." Once engaged in such an experiment, therapist and client can proceed to explore the issue in their usual ways, using accessing techniques that contact and name the client's present experience, immerse her in it, and get her to study it from the inside instead of discussing or speculating about it. It is critical to have the client immersed in her actual, live experience.

9. Therapist and client can then construct a relationship that is not based on the limiting, old, characterologically driven models embedded in the client's psyche. For example, in the case above where Helen, in her self-reliant way, does all the therapy herself, we eventually explored how to jointly lead and follow in the session. She experimented with allowing herself to notice that I was available to support her as well as with accepting that support. This new relational pattern could then be integrated (Chapter 20) and transferred to her life outside of the session.

Conclusion

While systems may appear to impede the progress of therapy, they are really the very heart of it. Transformation always happens at the barriers. The systems in which clients engage therapists provide keys to the core of their psychological organization. The impact of the aliveness of the moment, and the presence of immediate, direct experience provide an opening that can be deep and impactful. The mindful exploration of how clients engage in a system and how they enroll others in it can help them choose alternatives that are more nourishing in their lives. Working on this level of self-organization is very often the turning point toward success, as the client-therapist team steps out of the unconsciously established roles of interaction and self-management, and discovers a larger and unimagined realm of options.

CHAPTER 23

Hakomi Character-Informed Interventions

Lorena Monda and Jon Eisman

AS CLIENTS EXPLORE their direct experience in mindfulness, core organizing behaviors and beliefs emerge. Some of the basic core patterns that Hakomi therapists assist their clients in uncovering are reviewed in Chapter 8 (cf. Kurtz, 1990a). The goal of Hakomi therapy is to help clients develop effective and satisfying choices beyond these limiting core patterns. The intent is never to take away any valuable lesson or defense clients have learned, but to expand their agency-in-communion (Wilber, 1995) by integrating newer, wider, and deeper connections and possibilities. Character theory is helpful for a clinician to learn because it reviews a number of basic developmental conflicts that everyone goes through, along with the typical ways a characterological issue presents itself (Lowen, 1975). It is a useful map for guiding clinical thinking and therapeutic interventions. It is essential when using this map that every person's developmental uniqueness be kept in mind—as well as every person's formation through multidetermined dispositions (Engler, 1991; Popper & Eccles, 1981) related to internal consciousness, behavioral and biochemical issues (Jean-Didier, 1990), cultural values, and social structures (Erikson, 1963; Paniagua & Yamada, 2013; Wilber, 1995), including pre- and perinatal issues (Grof, 1988; Pesso, 1990).

It is important to remember that character behavior, no matter how dysfunctional, is ultimately meant to be protective—an adaptive defense system that originally arose as the best possible response to less than optimal situations, in a place and time where no better resources were available (Kagen, 1998; Kegan, 1982). The problem is that the client still behaves as if this world of long ago is the world he is living in now. People seek therapy when their internal or external world no longer works for them. Clients' habitual and often unconscious impulses toward avoidance, collapse, protection, seduction, resistance, clinging, mobilization, and so forth feel like existential absolutes and mandates that describe the facts of their world and drive their experiences (Loevinger, 1976). It is the practitioner's job to help the client understand these impulses—where they come from, what habituated and unresourced feelings, thoughts, beliefs, postures, and behaviors accompany them—and how to meet the underlying needs they represent in a more satisfying way.

Unfortunately, the protective nature of character patterns, perceptions, and needs may often be at odds with or in explicit conflict with both the client's desire for transformation and the therapist's pursuit of this goal. The art of Hakomi lies in the therapist's ability to respond successfully to each client's automatic perceptual and behavioral nuances. Because character theory is a map of those nuances, it provides a secondary blueprint for approaching and working through the client's core material. Understanding character theory allows us to respond more effectively to the client. By understanding the unmet needs, woundedness, and adaptations that may underlie habitual behaviors, and by entering a dialogue based on this understanding, modulating the degree or flavor of engagement, therapists can avoid the various projective traps that clients, in their characterological trances, automatically set (see Chapter 22).

In addition to assisting the practitioner to engage successfully with the client, character theory also maps out the developmental needs and missing experiences that Hakomi therapy seeks to provide. Characterological orientation implies and reveals the missing developmental learning experiences (Missildine, 1963). By recognizing the developmental origins of character elements, the practitioner can be more efficient and direct in pursuing a client's specific core needs.

Looking more closely, we can see that a client's character strategy actually creates four kinds of therapeutic avenues for the therapist to explore with the client: (1) the genuine developmental need of the client, often disowned or held in exile; (2) the sense of core hurt from not having the need met (both the internal depletion from the missing experience and the relational betrayal of it not having been provided by others); (3) an organic effort to enlist help, get the need met, and restore relationship; and (4) a protective function constantly seeking to avoid further injury or disappointment.

It is often the case in therapy that as the client gets close to the missing experience or to getting his needs met, the protective strategy is activated, which prevents him from taking in the nourishing experience. In Hakomi we call this the nourishment barrier, a general term for the organizing out of potentially nourishing experience by the client—differentiated from the more specific nourishment barrier (the inability to feel nourished or satisfied) making up one of the four barriers within the sensitivity cycle (see Chapter 17). Studying and working at the client's nourishment barrier is an essential part of Hakomi therapy (see Chapter 19), and each character style approaches this barrier from a unique perspective and with a different strategy. Thus, working with character patterns requires approaching our clients with patience and compassion, embracing whatever they present, and working skillfully to redirect limiting, habitual patterns toward something more nourishing and functional. To see our clients this way, to feel both their genuine humanness and how it is often moderated by learned, protective, and combative instincts, allows us to respond effectively and compassionately.

Kurtz drew from his doctoral studies in experimental psychology to help understand the deep intransigence of characterological dispositions and the deep compassion necessary to work them. He often cited the work of Solomon and Wynne (1953) with their "traumatic avoidance learning" experiments with dogs. They would place a dog in one half of a box, called a "shuttle box," that had a tall divider down the middle that the dog could jump over to shuttle to the other side. Then they would give a signal, followed 10 seconds later by a noxious shock through the floor that would be painful to the dog and would motivate it to jump over the divider to escape. They then studied how many trials were necessary for the dog to learn that the signal indicated an impending shock, which meant the dog should immediately shuttle to the other side of the box to avoid it. They reported that the dogs received only 7 or 8 shocks before reaching the criterion of 10 consecutive avoidance responses. This result was unremarkable.

The truly insidious nature of the experiment was revealed when they turned off the shock and studied how many trials it would take the dog to learn that the signal no longer meant that they would receive a shock. The answer was never. One dog jumped over the barrier 490 times before the experiment was discontinued. Every time the dog's physiological panic reaction at the signal motivated it to shuttle to the other side and find relief, it theoretically thought to itself, "Saved myself again." The tragedy, of course, was that it saved itself from an illusion, since there was no shock. But after hundreds of trials, it was one powerful illusion reinforced by a powerful neural net (Badenoch, 2008; Cozolino, 2010; Porges, 2011).

While it is a theoretical, philosophical jump from animal studies to human studies (Murphy & Brown, 2007), Kurtz could easily imagine instances—appropriate to particular stages of development—such as some kind of need for support from a caretaker being the signal, lack of support serving as a painful experience, and the unconscious decision to be self-reliant a way of shuttling away from the pain of not having one's need met. Then, after years of doing everything oneself to avoid the pain of disappointment, it was easy to imagine that subsequent instances of people actually willing and able to offer support would understandably be met with deep anxiety and distrust.

The following sections provide details about how the character material may be applied to accommodate the client's presentation and to facilitate the therapist's approach—always informed with a compassion and understanding of the client's predicament illustrated by the shuttle box experiment. Of course, space here does not permit a full elaboration of how the information can be used strategically, but the reader should be able to glean a general sense of direction in how to proceed. For each disposition (Popper & Eccles, 1981), we discuss briefly how to recognize the pattern, what issues may need attention, attitudinal and behavioral adaptations the practitioner may need to make, and specific interventions that may be useful for the client. It is essential to remember not only that all of us have combinations of character habits, rendering any merely linear approach ineffective, but also that our clients are whole people, of whom character is one habituated aspect.

In addition, since underlying characterological issues are existential and touch on basic human needs (Maslow, 1943), it could be argued that these issues are alive in us at any time, whether strong at the moment and in the foreground, or sleeping in the background. Marlock and Weiss (2015) proposed understanding character for each individual person as a combination of five great character themes. In this model, every theme is thought to form a polarity of varying degrees of severity. As an example, the theme of safety would form a polarity, with safe/secure/belonging on one end and unsafe/threatened/isolated on the other. The assumption is that a person would have an assigned value for each polarity at any moment. Character would express itself by certain positions a person would inhabit habitually along those polarities, like, in the above example, finding oneself on the unsafe/threatened/isolated end of it a lot of the time. One advantage of looking at character this way is that typecasting can be avoided, and more flexibility and complexity of understanding is offered.

Reading the descriptions of patterns below, the reader may notice the implicit invitation to assign certain patterns to people in their lives. In the Hakomi method, we discourage this tendency and encourage students to use character descriptions to understand the universal psychological needs that lie hidden beneath the surface of complex behavioral patterns. Character descriptions are meant to help us hypothesize and then explore what might actually be the case in a particular person. In truth, if we stay open and curious, we will usually find something unique and unexpected.

The Sensitive/Withdrawn Pattern

The sensitive/withdrawn pattern arises from the developmental need to safely be and belong in the world. Because this need was met with some kind of harshness at a time when the infant had only limited resources for dealing with the world, the child learned to withdraw internally from felt experience and externally from active engagement with life. Life is experienced as overwhelming and potentially annihilating.

We can often recognize the presence of this pattern by structures and behaviors that involve connection and engagement. There is often something noticeable about the eyes: They may appear frozen, startled, intense, or especially wide open. Physically, we may see a sense of contraction toward the core, with the arms pulled in and the chest seeming to constrict in toward the center. The body will have core tension and often elements of asymmetry. There may be an overall sense of delicacy or fragility.

Some of the basic core beliefs of this strategy include: "There's something wrong with me," "The world is harsh and dangerous," "I am not wanted." Behaviorally, the client may seem to be in his own world or, on a deep level, not to connect (inwardly or outwardly). Behavior may seem baffling or incongruent. Strong fear or anxiety is often present. The client may speak in images and metaphors, or in complex, jargony, or abstract terms. Emotions named may not be congruent with their presentation. The client may present as spiritual, creative, or nonconformist, with high integrity and an insistence on honesty.

Therapist Adaptations

Recognizing the underlying fragility of the client, the therapist must proceed especially carefully, slowly, and gently—demonstrating that she is not part of a world that will be harsh, overwhelming, or destroying. The therapist must explicitly create safety, committing herself to respect the client's boundaries, around both physical and psychic space. It is important for the therapist to be sincere, honest, and authentic, as the client will sense and react to any hypocrisy. Because these clients often feel like they were never given the handbook on how to be a person, it is helpful for the therapist to model the value of aliveness and relating, normalize what the client feels, and make clear that there is something inside the client worth gently pursuing.

Equally important are things to avoid. Provocation does not work as an approach with these clients. It is important to avoid dehumanizing them in any way: taking them for granted, assuming or expressing how they are a certain kind of person, not listening to their exact meaning, and so forth. The therapist should not let the intensity of the client's fear keep her from proceeding, but continuously track and gently contact what is happening (Chapter 14).

A friend, Mitch, once spent three hours patiently traversing a small clearing across which a deer stood watching him. At the end of that time, he stood alongside the deer, petting it. Then the deer slowly wandered off into the woods. This is a model of the therapist working with the sensitive/withdrawn pattern (LaPierre & Heller, 2012).

Therapeutic Strategies and Interventions

The main strategy here is to encourage the client's felt experience of her inner world, to help create the ability to engage fully and spontaneously in the outer world, and to develop a sense of the self as whole. Along the way, we may expect to teach the client about aliveness and boundaries, to create a safe container for her to experience her terror and rage, and to assist her to feel alive and welcome in the community of human beings.

Because there are usually strong attachment issues involved, working with the sensitive/withdrawn pattern requires reestablishing limbic resonance and allowing the client's nervous system to ease into dyadic contact while self-regulating. This allows the person to become comfortable in her own skin. Much work can be done around eye gazing and the possibility of, and perhaps eventual embracing of, physical contact. With this pattern, the relationship between the therapist and client is not just a tool for working, it is the work.

In terms of interventions, the most important task is to stay in contact. Track carefully, and teach and encourage careful mindfulness in these clients. Track for signs of the client withdrawing from himself and his felt experience, and withdrawing from the therapist. Some probes that are salient to the sensitive/withdrawn strategy address safety, being welcome, and the naturalness of being alive, such as, "You are welcome/safe here," "What you feel is natural," or "There is nothing wrong with you." Experiment with the eyes and vision: opening and closing them, looking at you and then looking away, and so forth, carefully studying the impact of these seemingly mundane but surprisingly powerful explorations. The same can be done for touch: offering your hand slowly, studying the client's impulses to reach out and retreat. Have the client pay careful attention to the exact quality of experience in all these experiments, searching for the discovery of pleasure in simple engagements—the path from withdrawal to safety and connection.

To help these clients recognize these events, it is often effective to describe their apparent experience as it happens, like a tender parent: "Yeah, you start to reach toward me . . . but now the fear comes up again. . . ." Acceptance is also important; let them know you value their way of operating: "It's okay with me if you want to go a little bit away. . . ."

When, after time, it becomes safe enough, it can be very powerful to take over the physical containment (tension, resistance to connection, and so on). Working with just a small piece (e.g., how the elbow presses against the ribs) or enfolding the client's entire body brings dynamic awareness to the somatic strategy of holding in against feeling. Often such experiments—again, done slowly and carefully with the client in mindfulness— can lead to the client's discovery of his full aliveness. Birth trauma may be revisited and resolved, and the natural desire to have and follow impulses may become available.

Integration for this client comes when he can recognize that the world is sometimes safe and welcoming and sometimes not, and he knows that he has the ability to discern how he organizes himself in relation to what he is experiencing. If a situation is accessed as not welcoming or harsh, there is always the option of withdrawing and taking refuge in music, books, technology, and so forth. If there is a perception of safety where genuine contact and connection might be risked, then the client can consciously choose to experiment with new options.

The Dependent/Endearing Pattern

The dependent/endearing pattern develops when the need to be secure that one's legitimate needs will be met is joined with caregivers that are unreliable, neglectful, not in tune, or distracted. Life is experienced as empty, with a feeling that there will never be enough.

Feeling undernourished and deprived, clients with the dependent/endearing pattern exhibit a tendency to collapse while invoking caring behavior in others. The collapse usually includes a downward, loose posture, as if the puppet strings were slack, with a sunken chest, rounded shoulders, head thrust forward, knees held in a locked position, and overall low energy. Soliciting help, clients may look waiflike with big, soft, puppyish eyes and pouting lips, and an endearing, innocent expression.

Some of the basic core beliefs in this pattern include "I can't get support," "There is nobody there for me," "Everyone will leave me," or "I can't do it." In his interactions, the client disposed toward the dependent/endearing pattern may seem depressed, sad, and/or needy. His participation in the session may be low key, reflecting his low energy. Often the client may want just to talk about himself, with a wistful, "poor me" tone, and will likely have trouble taking in the therapist's offerings of ideas, insights, and experiments. There is a feeling of chronic dissatisfaction. When nourishment is offered, it is difficult for the client to accept it, or to let it be just right or enough.

Underlying these experiences is usually a core sense of loss and abandonment, with deep, insatiable feelings of emptiness and a primal rage at those who were somehow absent. The client will need to find, develop, and apply his own strengths, learn to take in and use nourishment, and decide to trust others in mature and reciprocal relationships.

Therapist Adaptations

Because the dependent/endearing client seeks to indulge dependency while actually needing to become self-sustaining, the attending practitioner needs to balance carefully the genuine need to be nurturing to the client with an unwavering commitment to pursue individuation. Actually being deprived, the client needs some caretaking from the therapist, but eventually must be weaned from such dependency to stand on her own. This requires the practitioner to access his own compassion and generosity while also keeping firm boundaries. It can be easy in this process either to be ensnared by the client's endearing qualities and so become overly nurturing, or to feel drained by demands and so retreat from the client's neediness, replicating the original abandonment events.

The therapist does well to model trustworthiness and the certainty of abundance—demonstrating generosity and confidence in positive outcomes. It's important to avoid rescuing the client and also to avoid abandoning the client in any way, though the client may typically seek to have more and more of the therapist's time and attention. It is also important for therapists to avoid any expression of repulsion at the client's neediness or childishness and, similarly, to resist the impulse to make the client responsible too soon.

Therapeutic Strategies and Interventions

Work with the dependent/endearing client often begins with a period in which the genuinely depleted client needs a certain amount of nurturing, comfort, and reassurance. The therapist must earn the client's trust, demonstrating a heartfelt, no-strings-attached willingness to listen, validate, and respond. Ultimately, however, the therapy will be about not whether the therapist can nourish, but whether or not the client can accept and take in what is offered. The goal of therapy with dependent/endearing clients is to help them discriminate what is nurturing from what is not, and to actually experience the felt sense of being nourished and satisfied, thus creating a foundation for seeing and finding for themselves the abundance available in the world.

Nurturing without rescuing, the therapist can contact lovingly the client's feelings of sadness, loneliness, and helplessness, and have him study their origins, with experiments such as reaching out or placing a hand on the client's heart. Experiment with the ways the client's body surrenders to collapse, such as having him stand and study feeling unsupported, or taking over holding up his shoulders.

Exploring and clarifying the barrier to actually taking in nourishment is central here. It is not enough to offer nourishment; it is also essential to explore the ways in which the client transforms potentially nurturing experiences into toxic or unsatisfying ones (for example, "It won't last," or "Yeah, but you get paid to be nice to me"). Probes that help the client explore this barrier include, "You can get what you need," "I'm here for you now," or "You can do it." Because the dependent/endearing client clings to an empty past and so predicts a bleak future, it is essential to keep her in the present, noticing in the moment if things feel satisfying, and bite-sizing experiences into momentarily acceptable bits of nourishment. Often it will be valuable to provide something nurturing, such as compassionate touch, and then experiment with leaving and then, at the client's request, coming back, so that she learns to trust both abundance and her own ability to obtain it.

Usually there is great rage at the core, and the client's ongoing whininess and complaining are pathways to accessing that deep hurt. Expressing the rage in a safe way (for example, a well-cushioned and supported temper tantrum while in the child state) allows not only catharsis but validation of the client's entitlement to what he needs in life and empowerment for obtaining it. This paves the way for the development of a more firmly grounded adult self who can care for and protect the child, as well as seek and sustain mutual love and support with others.

Integration for people with this pattern will include teaching discernment between situations where it is true that authentic support is not available, and other situations where it is appropriate to practice letting go of their anxiety of there not being enough, so they can take in the actual nourishment that is available. They need to learn the balance between starving in the midst of a banquet and opening themselves to neglectful or toxic relationships sure to confirm their worst fears.

The Self-Reliant Pattern

The self-reliant strategy has an etiology and underlying needs similar to the dependent/endearing pattern, with a different adaptation. Whereas the client with the dependent/endearing pattern responds to lack of support by caving in and imploring assistance, clients with the self-reliant pattern compensate for this lack of support by dismissing help from others and mobilizing against the possibility of collapse. Basic core beliefs of this strategy include: "Nobody is there for me," "I don't need anything," and "I can do it myself."

As with the dependent/endearing strategy, we see the underlying collapse in the self-reliant character structure (sunken chest, locked knees, deep neediness), but with a prominent physical activation layered on top. Shaping the body around the need to handle any physical situation as a matter of survival, the self-reliant client exhibits a gunslinger pose, with elbows crooked and away from the sides, hands energized, and a wide stance. At rest, the energy may seem low or quiet, but with a sturdiness, sense of tension, and readiness to take action.

Behaviorally, people with this pattern are self-attending, operating alone even if others are present. Independent activities like running, biking, mountain climbing, and such are not uncommon. While they can often offer willing, reliable help to others, when help is offered to them, it is turned down with some version of "It's okay—I can do it." With a determination to handle things on their own, these clients will take on challenges, like carrying heavy suitcases, fixing appliances, or taking on the care of others. At the same time, there may be an irritation or weariness about having to do so much—displaying the cost of having to survive without being able to count on anyone but themselves.

In addition, matters of trust will be prominent. The self-reliant client will need not only to allow nourishment in (like the dependent/endearing client), but because he has abandoned the possibility of external support from others (unlike the dependent/endearing person who must rely on others for help), he must find a way to include the realistic support of others—to recognize and trust them as partners and not just parallel presences. In fact, this client may come to therapy at the urging of a partner who feels alone in the relationship, or because the circumstances of his life (illness or job loss, for example) are such that the self-reliant stance no longer works—receiving the support of others is crucial. At the deepest level, others seem moot to the self-reliant client, and the therapy must address this alienation and work to reestablish a trust in the value of genuine connection and support.

Therapist Adaptations

To establish the possibility of a true connection, and to appeal to the genuine need underlying the self-reliance, the therapist must explicitly model the values of trust, abundance, caring, and being loved. The therapist may assume that the client will tend not to allow in much nurturing—heading off instead to work by herself—and so must not succumb to frustration and impatience.

In fact, this tendency for the client to work on herself by herself presents the greatest challenge in trying to proceed in a Hakomi-like manner. The practitioner needs to track carefully for when the client is engaged in therapeutic dialogue, and when she goes off on her own internally to self-process. The therapist must remain diligent in not assuming that he and the client are working together, and invite the client to bring the therapist along as the client works.

Therapeutic Strategies and Interventions

As with the dependent/endearing pattern, the overall therapeutic strategy is to reclaim the ability to be nourished and to trust in the caring of others. In addition, the work must clarify the issues around help being available; uncover the alienated stance of the client and resentment toward others failing him; and develop a view of the world that expects supportive relationships and the ability to engage with others in mutually satisfying ways. In particular, it will be essential to demonstrate attention and consistency, and to continue to offer help, so the client does not have to work on himself alone.

Experimenting with the barrier to taking in nourishment will be central, especially around the client recognizing that nourishment comes from other people. Probes like, "Let me help you," "I will support you," or "You have needs of your own" help the client explore this barrier. Whereas the dependent/endearing process needs to move from dependency to independence, the opposite is true here: the client must learn the value of being dependent—recovering that as a childhood missing experience and integrating it into an option in adult life where appropriate. There will also likely be the need to explore the core rage at this dependency having been unsupported.

Experiments may include working with the posture of mobilization and readiness, studying its purpose, and then, through taking over the shoulders and weight, allowing the client to explore the feeling of being supported and cared for. Trust issues can be explored through falling backward and being caught, or by leading the client on a blind walk (she keeps her eyes closed while you lead her around).

Mindful eye gazing may serve to reestablish connection and dissolve alienation. As you hold eye contact, have the client pay careful attention to when he wishes to look away, and investigate the nuances of what makes him want to leave and what it would require for him to return.

Characterological dilemmas are often based on false choices. Here, it would be between being supported or being self-reliant. The experiment of taking over the weight will often lead to a good feeling of being supported, followed by an anxiety that says, "Okay, that's enough for now," because the person fears living in a perpetual state of needing support. Hakomi never seeks to take away any adaptive strategy from a person but only to integrate new, more encompassing options. The integrative position that transcends the false choice here is: It is okay to be self-reliant and go take care of business yourself when that is right, and it is okay to allow for and take in support when that is what is needed. When the client can embody both positions, he has developed the capacity to make realistic choices that are nourishing and satisfying.

The Tough/Generous Pattern

The tough/generous character strategy arises when the need to be authentic and autonomous in a context of shared intimacy is met with domination, exploitation, or humiliation. The child learns to hide his vulnerability—to toughen up and appear powerful at all costs. People with this strategy see the world as dangerous competition. Core beliefs include, "You can't trust anyone," "People will use you if you let them," "You can't hurt me," "I am special—the rules don't apply to me," "I must get them before they get me." This stance can lead as far as "I must lie, cheat, and use people to survive and succeed."

Feeling invulnerable and superior on the surface, people with this strategy often end up in therapy only at the insistence of others (including the law). Their bodies are bulky and powerful, with large, strong arms and shoulders, and an inflated, "puffed up" chest (as if holding a full inhale with no exhale). Their energy mobilizes upward, to appear larger and more dominating, leaving the lower half of the body thin and stiff by contrast. Their gaze is often direct and challenging.

Behaviorally, people with the tough/generous strategy are often charismatic and generous. They can show great tenderness and sympathy for the underdog and are frequently rescuers, creating dependency in others who are more helpless. They often come across as superior or self-important, needing respect and admiration. They react quickly and impulsively and have difficulty acknowledging their limits. When provoked, these clients can be rageful, blaming, and intimidating. During therapy, tough/generous clients may seem fast-talking, superficial, or glib. They may not take therapy seriously or may want to control the process. They may question the therapist's expertise or try to win the therapist over with flattery or gifts. It is difficult for these clients to open up to the process or to their own feelings, especially those that make them feel vulnerable or out of control. It is common for them to lie to maintain their image.

Underlying these behaviors are great vulnerability and great rage—an abused, fearful, and vengeful child. The missing experience of the tough/generous pattern is to be safely innocent and authentic, without exploitation; to have freedom of action, with realistic boundaries and limits.

Therapist Adaptations

Therapists working with the tough/generous character strategy have the daunting task of working with a client that often does not want to be in therapy, does not want to show or admit vulnerability, tends to blame others for his problems, and whose sense of survival depends on being in control. It is important for the therapist to model honesty and an authentic intimacy and connection not based on image, power, or manipulation. The therapist must avoid expressions of superiority, engaging in power struggles, or being taken in by the client's flattery or generosity.

Tough/generous clients benefit therapeutically from the practitioner's ability to be respectfully direct, honest, consistent, and unintimidated while maintaining warmth, connection, and support. The therapist should be attentive to the client's boundaries (as well as his own) and authentic needs, and make interventions without using coercion or manipulation.

Therapeutic Strategies and Interventions

The therapeutic goal in working with people with the tough/generous strategy is to help them to be vulnerable and honest, to find and express what is real for them—without fear of humiliation, hurt, or manipulation—and to slow down and modulate their impulsivity, so that their reactions can be more thoughtful, deliberate, and reflective of their authentic needs and wants.

Therapists can gain the cooperation of the client's unconscious by tracking boundaries and attending to the therapist's own need to make the client be or act a particular way. Gently and respectfully, uncover the underlying hurts and help the client slow down to discover and study authentic feelings and needs, without the client feeling in a down position because of these disclosures. Some probes that elicit this core material include: "You are important," "It's okay to feel hurt," "You don't need to impress me," "You can be real with me," "I won't take advantage of you."

Experiment at the response barrier, helping clients uncover and explore their impulses and quick reactions. Experiment with closeness, such as slowly walking toward them or placing your hand on their heart, to allow them to see the ways in which they automatically protect themselves. Take over this protection for them. Have them experiment with saying, "I need you" or "You affect me." Allow them to stay with and study the nourishment barrier—what it feels like to be safe while being honest and authentic.

The polarity or false choice for this pattern is being independent and invulnerable versus being close with weaknesses exposed. Since people disposed in this way believe life is all about power, they have chosen the invulnerable position. Much of the therapy work addresses barriers to going the other way: toward opening to vulnerability and intimacy. Though these clients have been deeply entrenched in invulnerability their whole lives before therapy, it is still important to assure them that the therapist has no intention or investment in taking away any of their self-protective strategies. The transparent goal—where there are no secrets—is to help them judge situations where it would also be safe and possible to have more enriching and fulfilling intimacies based on authentic feelings and needs.

The Charming/Seductive Pattern

The charming/seductive character strategy develops in a way similar to the tough/generous pattern, around the same basic needs for autonomy, love, admiration, appreciation, and realistic boundaries and limits. If this is met with narcissism, manipulation, or being used or seduced, rather than becoming tough, dominant, and in control, people in this pattern learn to get what they want by being engaging, seductive, elusive, and "'shape-changing' to suit the other" (Morgan, 2004b). In relationships they are often more interested in the chase (seduction) than in actual, ongoing intimacy. Core beliefs include: "I cannot be open about my feelings or motives," "I will be what others want me to be in order to maintain a feeling of power," "I must make others feel okay, so I'm included where the action is."

Physically, persons with this strategy may appear sensual, with inviting, seductive eyes, and a lithe, hyperflexible body, whose musculature is more balanced than those with the tough/generous pattern. Alexander Lowen, the founder of bioenergetics, used to remark informally, "Show me the person's body and I'll tell you what image of power they are embodying." There can be the biker image, the beauty queen, the Oxford don, and many other images that reflect the arena of power in which the person is operating.

Behaviorally, charming/seductive clients may seem empathic, impulsive, charming, and elusive. They may be ready to please the therapist, to be what the therapist wants them to be, or they may divert the focus of the therapy to the therapist. ("Has this ever happened to you?" "What would you do in this situation?") It is often difficult to pin them down when it comes to their own feelings and needs. As with the tough/generous pattern, they may be deceptive, may believe their own lies, or may have a foggy memory of what they actually did or said.

Underlying this pattern may be a deep inner dissatisfaction, with feelings of emptiness, loneliness, and anger. The missing experience for people with the charming/seductive strategy is to be authentic and intimate—to know and be themselves—to be loved for their real feelings and needs, without being taken advantage of or manipulated. As with the tough/generous strategy, power is the underlying issue. However, not everyone can gain power by being the biggest and scariest person present. Those with charming/seductive strategies choose to find and use power in subtler, seductive ways that do not generate direct confrontation.

Therapist Adaptations

When working with clients with the charming/seductive strategy, it is important for the therapist to be aware of her own expectations of the client, and to track for the client's automatic compliance. It is difficult for these clients to allow the therapy process to deepen toward their authentic experience and needs. Thus, the therapist must be patient and gently persistent (without being challenging or overly directive), and know that as things get real for the client, they become more threatening.

The therapist must also track for signs of being seduced by the client's charm, or of trying to use or manipulate the client in any way.

Therapeutic Strategies and Interventions

As with the tough/generous strategy, the goal of therapy with the charming/seductive client is to facilitate honest, authentic, loving connection in the client with self and others, and to help him explore the ways in which he defends against this. Some probes that can evoke this core material are: "You can be yourself," "You don't have to please me," "I care about what is true for you," "Your feelings are important."

Experiment with closeness, with taking over protection, with creative physical struggling. Explore the client's different personas—making them explicit—so as to discover the underlying need and wants.

As with the tough/generous disposition, the goal of integration is to help the person discern where it can be appropriate and useful to use power—in this case the power of charm and seduction—and where it is appropriate and possible to risk giving up the power game in favor of authenticity, honesty, mutual vulnerability, and intimacy.

The Burdened/Enduring Pattern

The burdened/enduring character strategy arises when the need for self-determination and freedom is met with too much interference or an enduring conflict of wills, ending in defeat or submission for the child. The child sacrifices freedom for closeness. Life is viewed as a constant struggle in which there is no choice but overt obedience, as assertion of one's will is simply not tolerated. Some of the core beliefs of this strategy include: "It's hopeless," "I am loved only if I obey," "I can't express how I really feel," "My life is not my own," "Life is a struggle that I must endure."

Physically, people with this character type look as if they have dug in while being pushed from behind—their bodies are heavy, muscular, and earthbound. Their shoulders are rolled forward as if carrying a heavy burden or in defeat, and their upper back, shoulders, and thighs tend to be overdeveloped. They may move slowly or in a plodding manner. Their complexions are often sallow or ruddy, reflecting energetic and emotional stuckness.

Behaviorally, people with this strategy are often compliant on the surface, but secretly defiant or indignant—with a "Yes, but" or passive-aggressive communication pattern. There may be self-blame, guilt, and low self-worth. They come to therapy often because they feel stuck, frustrated, or depressed. They have difficulty making choices since they are used to deferring to others and are prone to sabotage the positive choices they do make for themselves. They often feel mistreated by others but are unable to speak up for themselves. Because they hold back, they are often passed over by others, and are resentful of people they perceive are treated more favorably. They frequently procrastinate on things they have willingly taken on because they unconsciously project on the boss, teacher, or group the pressure to jump through hoops in order to be loved and accepted.

In therapy, these clients will seem slow and resistant. They will undermine attempts to experiment or to take action that might lead to change because they likewise project on the therapist the approval or disapproval of an external authority. They may become bogged down in hopelessness and in feeling bad about themselves. Although they may be in touch with their own feelings, they have difficulty expressing them to others.

Underlying the burdened/enduring character strategy is a need for love without being controlled by others. They have a strong will to resist this control but have learned that in doing so, in expressing their true feelings, they lose the love they seek. They protect themselves by never fully surrendering to the control of others but never fully expressing themselves—thus creating a huge bind for themselves. The missing experience of people with this strategy is the freedom to be themselves, to express themselves spontaneously and joyfully, and to exercise their will while being loved and supported.

Therapist Adaptations

When working with clients in the burdened/enduring pattern, the therapist must proceed with patience, lightness, and persistence. It is important not to push the client or become impatient or frustrated with the client's slow pace, delays, or automatic resistance. At the same time, it is just as important that the therapist not become bogged down in or weighed down by the client's burdens, negativity, or hopelessness, or take personally the client's frustration or passive aggression. It helps for the therapist to hold compassion for the real suffering of the client, for the genuine bind that he is in, and for how difficult it is for him to change—and to see the client's need for love beneath his indirect expressions of anger and disappointment. This pattern embodies a serious issue of the heart, namely the hurt that arises from being accepted conditionally with multiple strings attached, as opposed to being allowed to discover and express oneself in a life that is one's own.

Thus, it is essential for the therapist to drop any agenda about success and pace—any need to fix anything or to make anything happen—and to track for signs of the client's need to slow down or own what is being done, especially when trying new things. Remember that this strategy was created from the client's feeling controlled or pushed by others and the need to maintain some freedom from this. It is also helpful for the therapist to track for opportunities for spontaneity, humor (but never at the client's expense, as these clients are especially sensitive to humiliation and criticism), and playfulness.

Therapeutic Strategies and Interventions

The goal in working therapeutically with burdened/enduring clients is to allow spontaneous expressions of all kinds—excitement, happiness, and fun, as well as anger, rage, and frustration—in a milieu of loving support; to demonstrate experientially that freedom of expression does not lead to loss of closeness. The therapist can teach the client to balance heavy with light, gloom with joy, and to create habits that build self-worth and self-expression. In the course of therapy, the therapist can assist the client in getting perspective on her automatic "no" and the ways that this manipulates and frustrates others, as well as the ways that she is vulnerable to the control of others. It is helpful to explore and help the client move from passive-aggressiveness to a more direct assertiveness around feelings, needs, and wants.

The cooperation of the unconscious is gained by patiently matching the client's pace, getting permission for experiments, collaborating closely on what moves are in service of the client's own agenda, and contacting the client's self-constraints and the painful bind that they create. Working with core material will uncover the basic conflict between freedom and love, and the barriers to effective expression and action that result. Probes that address freedom of expression and choice and the permission to feel pleasure help to bring core material to the fore, such as: "Your life belongs to you," "It's okay to feel/to be angry/ to say no," "I want to hear what you have to say," "You can do it your way," "You can disagree with me," "You have a choice," "You can play."

Experiment with the response barrier by playing with different facial expressions (contempt, disgust, fear, anger, joy) and other expressions of feeling. Experiment with risk taking—setting boundaries and saying no, making choices. Actively take over muscular tensions, holding patterns, and the resistance to being pushed. Experiment with expression through movement, drawing, writing. Experiment with joining hands, where a client pushes one hand against the therapist's hand while saying "no," and the other hand stays in contact. Take over internalized admonitions against expression and self-worth. Experiment with playfulness and lightness. Explore outrageousness. Contact and experiment with genuine connection and delight around clients' freedom to be themselves.

The integration for this client is to be able to say a genuine "yes" because she can also say a genuine "no." Thus, the person is able to be present with her own hopes, ideas, and preferences, and not simply complying with what she thinks others expect of her. The strengths of this disposition should also be affirmed in the process—the ability to be exquisitely sensitive to heart issues or issues of justice, and to be understanding, loyal, and patient.

The Industrious/Overfocused Pattern

The industrious/overfocused strategy is created when love and a sense of worth and inclusion are conditional on performance. When the child is inevitably excluded from certain contexts by parents, older siblings, or other situations, it is painful. The child answers his own perplexed question, "Why am I excluded?" with "Maybe I am not yet good enough." Persons with this strategy believe that they must earn love and approval by constant effort—working harder, being responsible, being good, or getting better. They are mobilized toward action; they imagine their self-worth is based on what they do, rather than on their intrinsic right to worth as a human being. They may feel unappreciated and ignored by others. Their core beliefs include: "There is always something else to do," "I must try to do better and better," "Life is a problem to be solved," "I can't relax," "I need to earn love and appreciation," "I am not yet good enough."

Physically, these clients seem on alert and ready for action. There may be rigidity throughout their bodies, with square shoulders and a straight back, as if standing at attention like a good soldier, or with an arch in their lower back, as if they are leaning forward into a wind that is blowing against them.

Behaviorally, people with the industrious/overfocused strategy may be tense, focused, and determined. They prefer work over play (or they play seriously and competitively). They may come to therapy to resolve a specific issue, because they are exhausted or lacking in intimacy in their lives (a complaint that often comes from their partners). In therapy, they are oriented toward problem solving—are ready to get at it and work hard to improve. As clients, they are quite cooperative and may be eager to please the therapist. They often present a lot of details about their situation and experiences so that they and the therapist can work toward a good solution, but don't focus much on feelings in general and tend to avoid tender and softer feelings in particular. Industrious/overfocused clients are goal oriented, and as such they may experience frustration or impatience with the process not moving forward toward their goals fast enough.

Underlying the responsible, hard worker in this strategy is often a person who is hurt and longing for tender connection and attention with ease. The missing experience for these clients is the capacity to relax and be loved without having to work to prove their worth—to restore pleasure and connection, rather than effort, as the measure of success.

Therapist Adaptations

When working with the industrious/overfocused character strategy, it is important for the therapist to model a sense of connection through ease and lack of effort. This means considering being as important as doing and avoiding attempts to problem solve, work hard, give praise, or be busy with lots of things to do. It is essential to go slowly, leaving room for the experience itself rather than the goal.

The therapist must also avoid any sense of competiveness or perfectionism with these clients, who may elicit this by their core belief that they must do better in order to be included. The message to embody that is therapeutic for this client is that less is more—no one has to prove anything to anyone. Track for signs of pleasure and joy and help the client stay with them. Track and stay in contact with the client's tender or more vulnerable side—feelings, hurts, and longings—those things that make one authentic and lovable as an ordinary (rather than extraordinary) human being.

Therapeutic Strategies and Interventions

When working with the industrious/overfocused strategy, the aim for therapy is to help clients go from habitual mobilization toward action in order to prove worthiness (effort) to a reclamation of their intrinsic worth through heartful and relaxed connection to life and others. To do this, the therapist must demonstrate acceptance, support feelings of self-acceptance, and help the client surrender constant effort in favor of his deeper feelings within.

This is done through the therapist tracking, contacting, and gently (without pushing or directing toward a goal) staying with feelings and felt experience as they emerge. This brings the client to an exploration of his longing for rest, simple pleasure, and relaxed intimacy—and the core feelings of frustrated inclusion or unworthiness that drive his actions and make it difficult for him to relax or feel complete. Some probes that help this exploration include: "You are perfect just the way you are," "You don't have to do anything right now," "I'm on your side," "It's okay to stop now," "You don't have to prove anything to me."

Experiment at the completion barrier with doing nothing. Another powerful experiment is slowly and tenderly placing a hand on the client's heart. Take over critical voices or the internalized voices that drive the client toward more doing. Do experiments with physical support. An important thing to keep in mind, however, is that any doing should be done mindfully and with ease in order to avoid the feeling of working on something—it is better to do a simple experiment slowly and deeply than to cover a lot of ground by doing too much, which reinforces the client's core beliefs.

Interventions with this pattern are aimed at gently melting the client's rigid and mobilized posture into tender and pleasurable feelings, the deliciousness of ease, and the joy of being accepted and included for just being.

This disposition has a lot of freedom to act, do, and perform that needs to be affirmed. Especially if something is pleasurable, it is good to be able to give good effort and be competent in accomplishing some goal that can theoretically accomplish good in the world. The integration for these clients is to pair this with the capacity to surrender, rest, and participate in nondoing—the freedom to savor, enjoy, and allow others to take delight in them for who they are, whether or not they win the race.

The Expressive/Clinging Pattern

The expressive/clinging pattern arises as a strategy when the need to be heard, understood, and loved is met with rejection or exploitation. Here, there is also the issue of inclusion. In this variation, however, the child does not decide, "I must not yet be good enough," but rather, "I must not yet be interesting enough." The person learns that he must struggle for inclusion and closeness, and does so with attention-getting behavior—being dramatic, expressive, and, in some cases, sexually suggestive. Core beliefs for this pattern include: "No one understands or hears me," "I will not be paid attention to unless I am dramatic," "My father/mother didn't love me for me," "Everyone pushes me away eventually," "My worth depends upon my attractiveness, sexually or in some other way."

Physically, people with this pattern may have mature, evenly proportioned adult bodies or a top/bottom split, with a narrow chest and wide hips—a child's torso on a mature pelvis. They may dress colorfully or exotically. Their movements are energized, dramatic, or sexually suggestive.

Behaviorally, the expressive/clinging person is talkative and energetic and can be an exquisite host. She has a desire to be noticed and attended to, and is full of feelings that she is ready to share. Because the core experience in this pattern is about rejection, the expressive/clinging client is focused on relationships, which are often full of drama or turmoil. In therapy, these clients have a lot of material to present, and revel in dramatic revelations and powerful emotional experiences. It is often difficult to get them to move away from the story into mindfulness, because they feel such a move separates them from contact with the therapist, with whom they crave closeness.

Underlying these behaviors is the missing experience of feeling attended to, understood, and secure in relationship without having to earn it through amping up—the ability to be calm and content both alone and in openhearted connection with others.

Therapist Adaptations

As with the industrious/overfocused strategy, it is important with the expressive/clinging client for the therapist to model being instead of doing: staying away from problem solving or getting caught in the client's drama and panic, and instead offering compassionate and genuine understanding and attention. It is easy to be attracted to an expressive/clinging client, and essential for the therapist to monitor this in himself or herself, as any lessening in the energy of attraction is easily perceived by this client—who experiences it as a rejection—and will trigger her need to capture the therapist's attention again by some escalating dramatic means. Calm, genuine interest is far more therapeutic to the expressive/clinging client than the excitement of attraction.

It is also important for the therapist not to be overwhelmed by the intense, situational feelings of the client, but to orient to the real fear and pain about relating—the broken heart—that underlies the strategy, and to the meaning the client has made of his experience.

The therapist must be willing to gently refocus the client again and again toward mindfulness, meaning, and subtler experience, and away from refuge in intensity.

Therapeutic Strategies and Interventions

The intention of therapeutic interventions with the expressive/clinging client is to help him open to feeling loved—to reach out without expecting rejection—to help him shift from dramatizing to simply speaking the truth about his needs and wants, and to experience being heard and understood at a deep level.

Expressive/clinging clients have barriers to insight (meaning), response (often reacting or acting without thinking), and completion (finding it difficult to let go). Some probes that help these clients study their core organizing beliefs and habits are: "You are lovable just the way you are," "I'm here with you," "I'll listen to you," "I'll pay attention to you."

Experiments can be done with having the client mindfully hold back emotional expression to see what else is there, or pausing periodically to have the client practice getting the meaning of things and then contacting his understanding. Other experiments include taking over, reaching out, letting her hold on, or placing a hand on his heart. Sometimes, especially early in the therapy, persons disposed this way talk so much and so fast that it is hard to get in any kind of word or contact in response. Therapists might have to experiment with raising their hand, politely interrupting the system, and entering into the person's process by saying something along the lines of, "I really want to understand what is happening with you, and to do that, I need us to go a little more slowly." Or "I know you are saying a lot right now, but I'm not sure you know that I am actually hearing you."

When the therapist can really listen to the deep pain and heartbreak of the client, can contact the drama without being seduced or rejecting, and can mindfully explore the creation of a relationship where the client feels listened to and understood without a need for drama, the client disposed to expressive/clinging can experience a genuine opening of the heart. As a result, her creativity and expression can flow into the world from a calm, centered, and informed place. That is the hoped-for integration—not that the client loses her capacity for expressiveness and contact with others, but that it no longer comes from a desperation for inclusion, but from the joy of knowing her fundamental attachments to self and significant others are secure.

Summary

The understanding of character dispositions allows for tailor-made interventions that specifically address clients' particular developmental woundings. When a client's basic conflicts are intuited, they can guide the therapist's informed use of other Hakomi uncovering techniques (see Chapters 14–19), especially jumping out of the system (Chapter 22). After uncovering core organizing beliefs and behaviors, corrective (missing) experiences can be offered in mindfulness, so that the new information, when studied and practiced in the therapeutic milieu, might engender more expansive core beliefs and more satisfying life options for our clients (see Chapter 20).

It is axiomatic in Hakomi that a person is always more than a character type, but rather is disposed toward a particular way of organizing or managing experience. When clients are encouraged to be mindful and study the automaticity of how they are characterologically organized, a constant hope is that they learn more and more about how to rest in a mindful self-state characterized by awareness, curiosity, compassion, and wisdom—beyond the pull of historically influenced ego states—a state of consciousness Schwartz (1995) has called the Self; Eisman (2006) has called the Organic Self; Monda (2000) has called the True Self; Almaas (1986, 1988, 1990) has called the Essential Self; the biblical Paul (Romans 7) has called the Inmost Self; Lossky (1974) has called the Heart Self; and others have called other things in both contemporary psychology and ancient wisdom traditions.

CHAPTER 24

Mindfulness and Trauma States

Manuela Mischke Reeds

EXPERIENCING TRAUMA IS not only a shock in the life of clients, but also an event that alters how they see themselves. Clients categorize their lives in terms of before and after the trauma experience (Herman, 1992; van der Kolk, 2014). "Before my accident I was able to run and go everywhere. Now I am afraid to leave my house." Traumatic events can mark distinctive chapters in one's life or have an ongoing chronic impact on a person's psychoemotional and physical life (van der Kolk, McFarlane, & Weisaeth, 1996).

Much has been written and discovered about trauma, especially since the 1990s. Somatic psychotherapy has been greatly enhanced by the works of Bessel van der Kolk (1987, 1994), Peter Levine (with Frederick, 1997), Pat Ogden (Ogden et al., 2006), Babette Rothschild (2000, 2003), and many others in the field who have advanced our understanding that traumatic events are experienced through the body. Treatment modalities need to include a deep understanding and methodology for resolving trauma on a psychophysiological basis (van der Kolk, 2002, 2014).

We now understand in somatic psychotherapy that work with traumatized clients needs to include working with the sensory experience of the body. Traumatic events cannot be talked away through top-down processing, but need to be carefully renegotiated in the memory and nervous systems of the body through bottom-up processing. The activation levels of the limbic structures of the brain need to be held in an optimum range of neither under- or overactivation, so that the client is able to take in new information on a neocortical level (Ogden et al., 2006). Clients must be able to be alert and focused enough that they can feel, sense, and comprehend what is occurring inside of them, and how they are making sense of their trauma events through a cohesive narrative (Siegel, 2007), so that there is coherent comprehension of what has happened to them.

Like a good story, the event must be understood on all levels of human experience to make sense. Part of trauma is the senselessness of what has occurred. The more loss or life threat clients have experienced, the more they are faced with the senselessness of it all. Making sense requires an intellectual comprehension along with a physical one, with the hippocampus functioning to weave meaning from implicit memory (Schacter, 1992).

Many traumatized clients are not able to mobilize these intellectual and physical requirements for addressing the senselessness of their trauma. They cannot operate within what Ogden and colleagues (2006) term the "window of tolerance," where Porges (2003) says the ventral vagal nerve facilitates our capacity for social engagement, with ourselves (Siegel, 2007) or others. These clients display signs of either hyperarousal (increased sensation, emotional reactivity, hypervigilance, intrusive imagery, and disorganized cognitive processing) or hypoarousal (relative absence of sensation, numbing of emotions, disabled cognitive processing, and reduced physical movement). When these signs are present, it means the person is dissociated to a degree and not really present to the therapy in an effective way (Ogden et al., 2006). Therapists without specific training in working with such indicators of trauma should consider referral or seek the requisite training through the Hakomi Institute, Sensorimotor Psychotherapy Institute, or other qualified training providers.

In this chapter, the focus is mainly on neurological development and trauma therapy from a Hakomi perspective, and how mindfulness can help mediate the comprehension and integration of traumatic experiences. Trauma therapy is a vast topic and here only a few aspects of our unfolding understanding of how to treat trauma symptoms are highlighted. Please see the references for a more in-depth study of this subject.

Meeting the Client, Meeting the Brain

Erikson (1963) helps us understand the trauma to veterans of Vietnam by explaining that key developmental issues such as identity formation happen in late adolescence and early adulthood. However, it also remains true, as object-relations and self-psychologists have researched (Stolorow et al., 1987), that our earliest levels of development leave a foundational footprint that influences how we process later difficulties. Newborn babies are exquisitely sensitive when they arrive in the world. The organ of their skin is taking in every touch as a new experience to be processed throughout their whole body and brain (Schwartz & Begley, 2002). Touch and early sensory stimulations are strong excitations for the young nervous system. They are stressful in the sense that the developing brain of the infant has to process and organize these previously unknown experiences (Siegel, 1999).

The loving orientation of a warm and consistent caregiver provides containment for these arousing experiences. The attuned attention of the caregiver is key as the child learns how to incorporate these strong sensorial activations into an organized pattern of relationship style. For instance, the mother's soft voice and repetitive, gentle strokes along the baby's back as he is crying and arching give rise to a rhythmic and intuitive dance, evolving between caregiver and infant through matching voice tone, eye gazing, smiles, and gentle touch. Over time, the child begins to perceive touch and such stimuli as a nonthreat (Cozolino, 2006).

These experiences are internalized not only as sensory-emotional memory but also as a perception of how the child is being received into the first relationship template. These experiences translate into deep belief structures in the psyche of how one is loved and cared for, and influence one's capacity for loving another (Kurtz, 1990a).

When the touch-care continuum is internalized negatively, many years later, life is perceived and felt as a threat—just as the early template of sensorial stimulation was not matched with the experience of love and care. These deep sensate templates become compounded when trauma is present, and provide a confusing and overwhelming landscape for the trauma client (LeDoux, 1996). The capacity of the trauma client for self-reflection, self-soothing, and basic hope in the face of despair (Shaver et al., 2007) is based on how she is resourced in her foundational years when establishing safety in early relationships is crucial. There is a serious difference between chronic developmental trauma and event-centered trauma such as an accident or war experience.

I am reminded of a Nicaraguan client who was politically tortured, whose capacity for overcoming the most horrific events was admirable. Her reply in one of our sessions to a comment on how well she was doing despite those tragedies was, "They can break my bones, but they can't take my spirit," an idea that could evoke endless hours of contemplation. What we know of trauma survivors, especially those who have been tortured, is that a refugee's unfaltering faith in his or her cause can be a psychological savior in face of such horrifying experiences.

However, there was another truth about this person. As we referenced her statement in the months to come, I discovered in this client's history a very loving and warm family, with a mother who was attuned and caring to my client as a young child. Her foundational relational matrix was intact—despite her injured body, the tragedy of having lost every person she had loved including her child, and the trials of living in a foreign country and having few skills in her new country's language. Still, her internalized mother provided palpable hope in the process of healing her trauma symptoms.

Learning the internalized skill of self-soothing is a delicate exchange between the mother and the infant (Tronick, 1989). The internal state of the mother regulates much of the baby's state and vice versa (Schore, 1994). A colicky baby's cries and fussing can begin to exhaust an already tired parent, setting up an internal chain reaction in the mother (caregiver) and escalating the chain of stimulus until she is overwhelmed. The baby may then experience parental patterns of withdrawal, anger, helplessness, and emotional distancing. Selma Freiberg's famous term "ghosts in the nursery" reflects the entrenched emotional patterns generated in the subtle, moment-to-moment exchange between caregiver and child (Doidge, 2007).

Babies who learn that their cues of distress are not responded to as needed develop a high-activation continuum in the brain stem, diencephalon, and limbic regions of the brain whenever stressful moments are experienced (Perry et al., 1995) and become dysregulated when there is no mediation by the caregiver. The dysregulated internal states of the baby can in turn further dysregulate the mother's internal states, which further dysregulate her infant in a problematic cycle. Infants in this arousal continuum are at great risk for abuse and continuous high stress levels. A prolonged exposure to these high stress levels in the brain can have lasting impact on the developing brain's memory system and capacity for emotional range (Lewis et al., 2000; Schacter, 1996).

The intricate exchange that takes place between mother and child on a moment-to-moment basis is largely nonverbal—gestures, facial expressions, and whole body expressions convey the message of the emotional state. The child becomes masterful in reading these cues and responding to them in ways that preserve and enhance the relationship. These exchanges of subtle cues are, I believe, the same in an in-depth psychodynamic approach to psychotherapy (Lewis et al., 2000; Tronick, 1998).

Psychotherapy as Potentially Overstimulating

The internal states of clients impact psychotherapists a great deal. If a client is highly dysregulated and not making eye contact with the therapist, this can be met in various ways. How therapists respond to the lack of an empathic relationship depends on their own momentary state and their history, as well as their training (Roy, 2007).

For instance, Gerald was unable to look me in the eyes at any time. In fact, he constantly diverted his eyes away from me, staring at the carpet, as if lost in a distant dream. Over time, such somatically embedded behaviors of the client, as well as the basic needs of the therapist, can make even the most compassionate therapist uneasy (this is assuming a Western therapist, and I recognize the cultural bias here; see Foster et al., 1996; Johanson, 1992; Lewis et al., 2000; Sue & Sue, 1990). A subtle rejection might begin to form in the therapist who feels she cannot relate to this client or understand him on a deep level. Feelings of resentment or failure might arise. The loving presence of the therapist begins to alter. This, in turn, fuels the worst fears of the trauma client. Instead of experiencing the delight and consistency of the therapist, he once more experiences a caregiving person not seeing or understanding him, and withdrawing (Feinstein, 1990). The internal arousal of stress is exacerbated.

The intimacy of psychotherapy, and especially somatic psychotherapy such as Hakomi, can easily travel into the terrain of sensory experience (Heckler & Johanson, 2015). This means that although clients might want to discover and transform the core beliefs that are holding them back by impacting their relationships with self and others, the very process of psychotherapy might be adding to their feeling of overwhelm. Activated clients cannot process their core material. The activation level itself prevents clients from bringing the experienced material into the rational and logical part of their brains (the neocortex) for comprehension and processing. The actual experience of the therapy backfires and is experienced as too activating and arousing (Ogden et al., 2006).

This is a crucial point that is often missed by well-meaning verbal and body-inclusive therapists who feel their unconditional positive regard can automatically create a safe place. The arousal states of clients need to be brought down in specific ways in order for them to witness and comprehend what is occurring. Just beginning to experience a high arousal level can bring up learned defense mechanisms, as well as triggering basic survival mechanisms of protection (Morgan, 2006). This is a delicate balance, as the therapist wants to allow and facilitate the client's emotional processing, which in a particular moment can escalate into an activation level or trauma vortex that the client cannot manage. It is often important to begin working on the multiple ways a person can resource herself mentally and somatically before beginning to address the trauma directly. Then client and therapist together can track the ability to go back and forth from the resourced position to a piece of trauma small enough to be titrated and digested by the nervous system.

For more information on how to titrate triggering sensations and how to work without promoting a trauma vortex that can retraumatize a client, we can refer at minimum to the work of Levine (with Frederick, 1997), Ogden and colleagues (2006), and Rothschild (2000, 2003). All somatic psychotherapy that aims to negotiate the arousal of the nervous system in elegant ways seeks to track and address activations and dissociations beyond the client's window of tolerance, so clients can actually be present with their experience and find new ways of relating to their triggers.

Mindfulness and Interruption of Nervous System Patterns

Mindfulness is a state of being, as well as an inner reflection on moment-to-moment experience (Chapter 10). As discussed throughout this book, the use of mindfulness plays a central role in Hakomi therapy in the discovery of internally held beliefs and experiences. The predicament of clients with trauma is that it is a state of disruption of their life force that renders them unable to handle the arousal levels in their body. The coping mechanisms vary with each person according to his or her capacity for self-regulation and function. Nevertheless, in a general sense, the trauma client has lost the capacity for being with himself in a calm, resourced way. Trauma states can be viewed as uninterrupted states of mindlessness. Lower brain functions are in charge as opposed to the thinking brain.

Hakomi therapy can provide a beginning place for meeting the trauma survivor's brain and treating it in a multifaceted way. In Hakomi, we pay attention to present-moment, direct experience, and how the client is relating to it. This direct relationship with time and history has an important function (Pert, 1999). Clients can experience their traumatic past in relationship to multiple parts of themselves (Rowan & Cooper, 1999), as well as to the therapeutic relationship. That the therapist calls the client's attention to what is occurring for him in the moment offers the client the awareness and self-control to interrupt automatic patterns and experience himself in a new way (Siegel, 2007).

> *This might occur in minuscule moments, such as with Sylvia when she glanced up at her therapist with a look worn down by many years of rejection and the chronic emotional pain of trauma. The therapist received her with acceptance and positive regard. She startled. His eyes widened. The Hakomi therapist tracked this and used this moment to gently contact and guide her to noticing that she was surprised not to find the expected hostility. Sylvia's crying deepened as she nodded. A mixture of recognition, pain past and present, were all mixed in a soup of gratitude and aliveness. She had been seen, received, and led into a new state of aware wakefulness. The past did not matter in that moment. The authentic connection with her own pain and the acceptance by another provided a new experience in which her symptoms took a break. She could let in a ray of hope that life need not be as bleak as she had perceived it to be.*

The case above is an example of relating to developmental or chronic trauma, as opposed to the single-incident trauma (accidents, rape, or events related to first-responder work, war, gangs, and so forth, where life is literally at risk) normally diagnosed as PTSD. Though chronic or complex developmental trauma has been identified as a different syndrome than PTSD, it has not yet been included in the diagnostics of the *Diagnostic and Statistical Manual of Mental Disorders* (van der Kolk, 2005).

Hakomi embraces the various ways in which we experience ourselves. No single way is the right one. The discovery of what works organically for a particular person is deeply honored (Germer, 2006). This goes beyond just being respectful of people and their processing preferences. It also includes the way our brains function to come to terms with a traumatic assault of stimuli and sensory inflation that is often hard to decipher (Rothschild, 2000; van der Kolk et al., 1996).

Through my work with trauma clients with many different trauma histories, I have come to view meeting them where their brains are as the best possibility. For instance, new babies need that eye gaze of delight and the gentle adjustable touch that activates the right orbital prefrontal cortex, or joy center, and teaches them that touch and relationship can be a safe haven and a nurturing template for all relationships to come (Doidge, 2007).

Trauma clients, likewise, need that same recognition and understanding of their arousal and fear contingencies—of how their brains have been affected. They also need the initial limbic restructuring experiences with the therapist to help them regulate parts of themselves lost in their instinctual-level coping with traumatic events (Schore, 2003). Or as one of my first clients put it when I was a beginning therapist, "I thought I came here for therapy, but what I really came for was feeling safe and understood and loved." This occurred just as I was taking pride in graduating, complete with my newly acquired therapy skills. It helped me realize that the magic ingredient had not simply been my advanced techniques, but rather the quality of the bond that had developed with my client over time.

A deeply respectful relationship allowed my client to unfold, discover, and transform the sensate and content aspects of his narrative (Johanson, 2015). All my techniques would not have mattered if it had not been for this living connection in which he was held and, in fact, I was held as well (Germer, 2006; Mahoney, 1991). We can call it attunement, limbic resonance, empathy, compassion, or love. The fact is, what heals is a deep relationship with our respective humanities, in all aspects of their being (Lewis et al., 2000).

Uses of Mindfulness With Traumatized Clients

Mindfulness is a powerful tool in aiding the bodymind to understand and integrate traumatic experiences. Mindfulness applied in a manner conscious of traumatic dynamics has several functions:

1. Introducing clients to an ambience of calm and quiet.
2. Slowing down nervous system activity of the brain and settling the body. The middle prefrontal cortex is activated, allowing it to weave connections with the hippocampus—important for the structuring and reconsolidation of memories.
3. Providing an opportunity for clients to engage in listening to themselves as they both witness and are present to their experience in the moment—thus "having" as opposed to "being" traumatic processes.

These three functions are actually difficult for the trauma client to achieve without mindfulness. The internal world of the trauma client is often full of noise, physiological arousal, and constant activation of safety and well-being processes arising from more archaic structures of the brain than the neocortex. The fact that the hippocampus, which is crucial for memory consolidation, is bypassed during traumatic events makes initial narrative memory of events disturbingly unavailable (Schacter, 1992).

> *When my client Sally lay down on the couch, she wanted to relax. As she lay down, she told herself that she was relaxing. In fact, her fists tightened, her jaw clenched, and her breath got shorter and tighter. When I contacted these bodily signs in an observational way, she still maintained her view that she was calming down. It might have seemed that way to her to an extent, since chronic stresses are normally unconscious. A few moments passed. Her body would not calm or release any further. In fact, her body looked like it was becoming even tenser.*
>
> *The spaciousness of my nonjudgmental observing, and the provision of time for her to sense herself, rather than inviting her into a doing mode, allowed for the following: I again contacted her present-moment experience by saying, "You are working really hard on relaxing." With that, she smiled. She said that she could not feel any relaxation at all, but rather she felt a sense of fear in her chest, which she was trying to manage.*

Now we had an opening to work directly with her fear, and with how she was managing herself in that state. This was a precursor to exploring how she was dealing with her trauma experiences, namely pushing through them while excluding feeling. If we had not created a safe atmosphere, with a slowed-down environment for curious, open-ended exploring (Kurtz, 1990a), we would not have had the opportunity to befriend her experience and see it unfold in new psychosomatic patterns.

Another important aspect of introducing mindfulness is interrupting habitual unconscious patterns in favor of providing an emotional holding space where clients can safely experience their high-affect states without spinning off into a trauma vortex. The mindfulness of therapists is also a crucial element, as they become the temporary nervous system that holds the disorganized states of clients—also true in parenting (Siegel & Hartzell, 2003).

Here are some ways to use aspects of mindfulness to interrupt habitual patterns of managing trauma-based states of fear:

1. Therapists actively engage to calm their own levels of racing or triggered thoughts by slowing down and getting mindful distance on their parts being evoked.

2. As therapists become aware of their own "speediness," they calm their own body movements. They then employ simple ways to slow down clients physically. Interventions can include bringing awareness to the quality and rhythm of the breath and introducing a slower, more deliberate breath. Or clients can be encouraged to bring their awareness to the immediate knowledge that they are sitting on a chair, and their attention can be guided to the physical contact points with the chair and their feet on the ground. This attention to breath and to grounding the body helps to bring down the activation levels of the nervous system.

3. If they have not done so already, therapists engage their clients in mindful awareness of multiple ways they can resource themselves through body, images, colors, memories, self-state centeredness, and such (Ogden et al., 2006). This is always a first stage of treatment of trauma issues to ensure that clients always go back into traumatic material resourced, and have resources readily available to counterbalance activation outside their window of tolerance.

4. Therapists use their abilities to track and contact (Chapter 14) to stay closely attuned to the client's experience as it is occurring, thereby enabling the client to bring awareness to the present-moment experience. Trauma is very much about not being congruent with one's own experience, but rather with the past or the future.

5. Therapists support clients in increasing their ability to feel, sense, taste, and experience what is happening directly through the body. Connecting with the here and now enables clients to put thoughts and feelings into perspective. Therapists continually track clients for signs of hyper- or hypoarousal, and move to center, ground, resource, or titrate sensations when signs of dissociation arise indicating the process is going too far, too fast.

6. Therapists can bring mindfulness to bear on the quality of the therapeutic relation-

ship (Fosha, 2000). This can enable the client to become aware of and enriched by the support, understanding, and empathy the therapist is offering, thus breaking the trance of traumatic isolation (Wolinsky, 1991). Directing the client to notice the therapist in the moment can also help break the trancelike quality clients can fall into when recalling traumatic events.

Again, traumatic experiences involve lower regions of the tripartite brain that work before and outside of the influence of the neocortex, thus making clients susceptible to experiencing trauma vortexes that manifest in terms of hyper- or hypoactivation of the nervous system. Hakomi therapists can become skilled in employing mindfulness in the service of bottom-up as opposed to top-down processing to deal with such situations. However, supervision, referral, and further specialized trauma training are all important to avoid putting clients at risk of retraumatization.

CHAPTER 25

Strengths and Limitations of the Hakomi Method: Indications and Contraindications for Clients With Significant Clinical Disorders

Uta Günther

LENDING SUPPORT TO the notion that body-oriented approaches offer opportunities otherwise not available in the treatment of clients with early-onset disorders and weak psychological structures, Maaz (2006) has suggested that the royal road to the preverbal unconscious is the body itself. The application of body-oriented approaches, however, is not without risk. If not appropriately practiced and carried out, body-oriented approaches could lead to retraumatization (van der Kolk, 1989), inappropriate touch (Boadella, 1980; Hunter & Struve, 1998), the collapse of defense mechanisms, or malign regression (Marlock, 1993).

Translated from the German by Hugo Schielke

As a body-centered, experiential approach to psychotherapy, Hakomi incorporates the use of touch alongside the practice of mindfulness. This chapter discusses the indications, contraindications, and risks involved in the utilization of the Hakomi method and Hakomi's use of touch with clients with early-onset, chronic clinical disorders.

For the purposes of discussing clinical disorders, I utilize an approach to developing and discussing clinical diagnostic pictures in terms of (and in relation to) clients' hypothesized psychic structure, an approach that has been described by Maaz (2006) as well as others. Interest in this approach has given rise to a practice-relevant instrument, the Operationalized Psychodynamic Diagnosis (OPD) instrument (OPD Task Force, 2006). The OPD, which serves as the framework for the discussion of clients' psychological organization, is oriented toward looking at disorders and symptoms from within the developmental context from which they are hypothesized to derive. In contrast to the systems of clinical diagnosis that have their roots in Otto Kernberg's (1996) work on character pathology, the OPD "does not limit its focus to a typology of character pathology; instead, it places primary emphasis on the relationship between experience and behavior as expressed in psychic organization, where the deciding factor is the degree to which experience and behavior have come to be integrated in the psychic structure" (Galuska, 2006, p. 586).

The OPD Task Force has put forth a descriptive system to accompany the OPD that describes the axis of structure as follows:

> Psychic structure can . . . be described through the use of four dimensions that can be used to describe both object relationships and the relationship to the self:
>
> Perception (self-and-object relational perception)
>
> - the ability to be self-reflexively aware
> - the ability to accurately perceive others
>
> Regulation (self-and-object relational regulation)
>
> - the ability to regulate one's own impulses, affect, and self-esteem
> - the ability to regulate one's relationships with others
>
> Communication (self-and-object relational)
>
> - the ability to communicate with oneself
> - the ability to communicate with others
>
> Connection (self-and-object relational directed connection)
> - the ability to make use of good inner objects for the purposes of self-regulation
> - the ability to develop and dissolve relationships with others. (1996, p. 118)

The OPD discusses structural disorders in terms of levels of psychological integration along a continuum, describing an inverse relationship between the level of psychological integration and the severity of psychological disturbance, such that the most severe disorders occur within the context of the lowest degree of psychological integration.

> The "structure" axis traces the level of psychological integration from the well-integrated psyche found in a "healthy" individual through decreasing levels of fair, and then low, psychological integration, finally ending in psychological disintegration. The psychological organization of a neurotic represents a fair to good degree of integration; that of a borderline represents a fairly low degree of integration; the psychological structure of a psychotic represents a psychological disintegration. (Galuska, 2006, p. 586)

Within the context of an established therapeutic alliance, the OPD is very helpful in assisting in the process of determining a client's level of structural integration, assessing, for example, a client's ability to both be and remain connected to the experience of reality, and to differentiate self and object, as well as the maturity level of clients' defense mechanisms (Maaz, 2006). As such, the utilization of this type of approach to client work highlights the importance of considering clients' levels of structural organization when considering potential therapeutic interventions. In the case of depression, for example, it is important to utilize therapeutic approaches aimed at specifically targeting the opportunities and strengths available to clients given the coping mechanisms available at their level of organizational integration. Attempting to mindfully immerse clients in their depression prematurely can be contraindicated.

Risks With Clients With Underdeveloped Psychological Structures

An assumption generally held by clinicians is that a relationship experienced by the client as a healing relationship—one that can provide a safe space and a feeling of being accompanied by a competent guide through the processes of self-exploration, as well as the creation, experience, and integration of corrective experiences—is what will make this work possible. The majority of clients that come to us in outpatient settings are generally able to form and maintain therapeutic relationships. However, only fairly well-integrated individuals respond with excitement and relief to therapists' assumptions about these relationships enabling a "cooperation with the unconscious" or connecting with, experiencing, processing, and working through repressed emotional content. For those who have deficits in psychological structure based on difficult experiences very early in life, or for those destabilized by the active experience of trauma, the thought of lowering defenses against difficult content, becoming mindful, willingly opening oneself to inner space, and listening in and allowing oneself to be surprised by what happens is both scary and, in some situations, actually dangerous. For clients on the extreme end of this spectrum, all the steps that lead to mindfully experiencing the present moment are not only difficult but also not necessarily helpful. There is a certain control for safety built into the Hakomi process, however, in that every therapeutic intervention is carefully tracked for signs of dissociation that would signal clients are outside their window of tolerance (Ogden et al., 2006), and defenses are never overridden, but are supported for their wisdom (Chapter 17).

Clients not met at the appropriate level of their deficits may strengthen their intra- and interpersonal defenses in order to protect against a threatening situation, leave therapy, or run the risk of psychologically decompensating. Depending on the client's psychostructural makeup, opening oneself prematurely to emotional experience and the accompanying psychophysiological arousal can be taxing or lead to a partial or complete overwhelming of the client's processing capabilities, or even to an experience of being destroyed, flooded, disintegrated, or extinguished. These clients' original defense and coping mechanisms were able to maintain enough stability in their very fragile inner systems to be able to function under normal circumstances. Typical Hakomi techniques, uncritically employed, could put such clients at risk.

The standard paradigm of uncovering and working through (Chapter 19) has been repeatedly discussed as contraindicated for traumatized clients (Petzold, Wolff, Landgrebe, & Josic, 2002). Major life stressors and experience-activating and defense-weakening interventions have also been discussed as risking the collapse of coping systems leading to a shift to a more significant crisis state or a chronic increase in symptom severity in clients with other forms of structural vulnerability and disturbance (Rudolf, 1996). There is, of course, a large difference between event-driven PTSD and long-term, developmental trauma (van der Kolk, 2014). In either case, the first step in a therapeutic process might well be resourcing. When the trauma has been life threatening, evoking lower brain responses, Hakomi therapy must switch from top-down processing to bottom-up processing of sensations and such (see Chapter 24; Ogden et al., 2006). Relational attachment work might also be a prerequisite to intrapsychic explorations (Fosha, 2003; Lamagna & Gleiser, 2007). For clients with personality disorders, as well as clients who are severely depressed, increased vulnerability is often attributable to deficits in self-determination and affect regulation that also require interpersonal attachment work. "Given that the disordered difficulties are ego-syntonic (that is, not accessible to the self-perception of the individual author of the experience), it is difficult for the patient to see their own contributions to the difficult situations" (Rudolf, 1996, p. 178). Since people with personality disorders tend to blame the environment as opposed to reflecting on their own contributions, patient interpersonal interventions are often required over time until the level of safety is reached that allows intrapsychic Hakomi work. People with phobias might or might not be amenable to more immediate mindfulness-centered interventions.

Given the above cautions, therapeutic work that incorporates experience-activating, experimental, and body-oriented approaches is not suited for immediate implementation with clients that are organizationally or structurally fragile. These clients do not have enough inner structure accessible to be able to process and integrate the meaning of the material that would arise, nor would they be able to tolerate the degree of psychophysiological arousal that would accompany this material. This means that the foundation of the explorative Hakomi method—the mindful exploration of present-moment experience—would not be possible to execute uncritically at the outset of therapy. The practice of mindfulness with closed eyes, and even the invitation to physical relaxation, triggers the fear of having to give up or lose control—a control that is often maintained through the musculature, which requires tension in order to mask sensitivity (Reich, 1949). As always, the Hakomi principles trump the automatic imposition of any techniques. Sometimes intrapsychic mindfulness must be foregone in favor of structure-building mindfulness that helps those who are fragile to connect to reality. For example, asking the client, "Can you hear my voice? How do you know you are hearing it? Can you feel your feet on the ground? What tells you that you are feeling them? Stamp your foot and notice the sensation when it hits the ground."

Another aspect of this discussion relates to the therapeutic relationship itself. The interactional style of early-deficit clients is likely to strain relationships with others, and makes constructive interpersonal relationships difficult, or even impossible (Rudolf, 1996). The countertransference that is evoked can, of course, give the Hakomi therapist clues to how such a person organizes his world, and what kinds of life situations might have created that organization (Stolorow et al., 1987). With the limitations of early, structural-level deficits in mind, the following are examples of scenarios that present challenges to Hakomi-oriented therapists disposed to jump in with classic methods. They highlight the challenges and potential pitfalls to be aware of when engaging in such work.

For individuals with borderline features, defense mechanisms such as splitting, projection, denial, and idealization serve to protect against the disintegration of the self. ("The self" here refers to the psychoanalytic sense of an intrapersonal structure of the ego, or I.) Images of self and other fall into "all-good" and "all-bad" parts, where the negative aspects are projected outside the self. The relationships entered into by someone with these relational habits—splitting, idealization, demonization, or projection—are extremely difficult (Rudolf, 1996). If the severity of the disorder is significant enough, the level of distress, fear, frustration, and so forth leads to unbearable tension and arousal that often prevents clients with these problematic patterns from being able to observe these phenomena within themselves. These clients are in a timeless experience of elevated stress that is made manageable only through dissipation efforts such as movement, self-injury, or the use of soothing substances. To respond to these clients in therapeutically helpful ways presents a special challenge to therapists' own inner stability. However, as Linehan's work has demonstrated (Robins, Schmidt, & Linehan, 2004), mindfulness has an important part to play in the treatment of borderline dispositions when combined with the appropriate structures.

For those with more narcissistically colored personality structures, the fear that a deeper connection with others would expose both feelings of worthlessness and the helpless neediness of a fragile self leads these individuals to protect against deeper relationships. This tendency will also apply to their relationships with their therapists. A client with this type of organizational structure may attempt to devalue and control the therapist in order to "maintain a sense of grandiosity against all attempts at reality testing" (Rudolf, 1996, p. 178). As uncomfortable and difficult as this type of limited relationship is for the therapist striving for a "real connection" with the client, it serves to maintain the "survival" of the client in the narrow sense of the word. This type of protection and stabilization system cannot be jumped out of or exploded—given the client's deficiencies in internal structure, this would lead to the disintegration and decompensation of the client's fragile self. Hakomi therapists must be careful to moderate their own countertransference, as these clients with lack of stable self-structures can bounce back and forth between needs to be independent or in control to the more needy positions that scare them.

Thinking about the above in connection with the classic Hakomi approach to therapeutic process outlined in Chapter 21, the inner logic of Hakomi can suggest where modifications might be necessary in order to continue to be helpful to clients without sufficient access to the resources that are prerequisites for normal work, such as the deficits in perception, regulation, communication, and connection referenced above. An important part of client evaluation is an assessment of how much of a self-state characterized by awareness and compassion they have available, even though they might have had significant developmental traumas (Almaas, 1986; Eisman, 2006; Schwartz, 1995). Borderline and narcissistic personality disorders commonly reveal themselves as disorders of the self.

A special characteristic of the therapeutic relationship in the Hakomi approach, for example, is found in the therapist's interest in making self-awareness accessible to the client when exploring the barriers to growth and transformation associated with the defense mechanisms. Examples of this are seen in a Hakomi therapist creating experiments in mindfulness (Chapter 16) such as, "What happens inside when you hear [pause] . . . 'You are safe here,'" or "What happens inside when you hear [pause] . . . 'You are welcomed with all my heart!'" Individuals who have developed healthy internal structure will be able to understand the experimental setting and make use of the evoked experience to study their own self-organization and relevant inner reactions—thoughts, feelings, images, memories, and impulses.

An individual's psychostructural limitations can become apparent, however, in his or her ability to engage in such imaginative exercises. "As-if" experiments require an understanding on the part of the ego that enables clients to see the meaning of the therapist's offered scenarios as opportunities to study their personal reactions, as opposed to literal interpersonal offerings from the therapist. Often in work with clients with severe structural limitations, invitations to engage in self-observation might not be possible. Some clients cannot understand or experience the experimental "as-if" situation as such, even with additional efforts toward clarification. The Hakomi experiments most easily misunderstood are those stated by the therapist in the first person, such as, "I am here for you." Similar difficulties can be found when taking over an introjected voice, which can trigger significant irritation on the part of the client (such as reacting with "Why are you talking to me like my mother did?"). The client's ability to be mindfully self-reflective is a crucial assessment in the decision to employ Hakomi accessing techniques (Chapter 15).

Nonverbal experiments incorporating touch or body-oriented techniques can make the clients' structural limitation-based difficulties even clearer. For clients with structural deficits, an experimental touch could be interpreted as a direct relationship statement. Utilizing the technique of taking over (Chapter 17) a client's shoulder tension could be interpreted as a relational statement that leads to a habituated response, such as, "That feels good," or "That's awfully nice of you," with the client interpreting the touch as a sign of personal support or compassion, instead of an opportunity for mindful experiential reflection (such as, "Wow, I'm noticing my stomach getting warm and I'm noticing myself beginning to feel joyful"). Thus, Hakomi therapists need to continually track whether the client is reactive or reflective, and whether the client is in fact capable of taking herself under observation.

Similar warnings apply to inner child (Chapter 18) work. On the one hand, when working with possible "missing experiences" in the sense of providing missing parenting or facilitating missing maturation processes, the therapist may take on the ideal role of the protective parent originally not present (Pesso, 1973). In this role, the therapist may, for example, let the "child" attempt to introject the feeling of being physically held and to explore what it is like to be protected. In these situations, there is a danger that instead of integrating the protective parent role into their own structure as a role that they can perform for themselves, a relationship can arise in which clients become dependent on the therapist (as helper-ego) to perform this role. Here, Hakomi therapists must track to make sure clients are always in a dual state of consciousness: sensing the developmental reality of the child alongside their adult consciousness that is aware they are in a therapy process. Sometimes it is helpful to collaborate with the client by asking, "Should I communicate to the child the missing experience or is it good that you do it?" Or, in the integration phase of the work (Chapter 20), after the client has taken in the felt knowledge of the missing experience from without, the therapist can help empower the client's larger self-state from within by saying, "Now how about you say to the child what he heard from me earlier, that he is safe now, and notice if he takes it in."

There is an additional danger, however, in playing the magical stranger role (Chapter 18) when working with significantly traumatized individuals, such as those who were sexually abused as children. If the therapist goes into the role of the good adult prematurely, without resourcing the client and making it clear that she is going to titrate the trauma (Levine with Frederick, 1997) by not operating outside the client's window of tolerance, the process could lead to retraumatization. This could result in the client feeling frighteningly small and powerless, fused or blended with the memories through which the powerless sense of being a victim were originally stabilized. Inner child work and the role of the magical stranger, as originally taught in Hakomi, have been modified over the last 30 years as more about trauma, resourcing, titrating, and having the witness or larger self-states on board has become apparent through both experience and theory arising from current research.

One modified approach to inner child work suggested above that can be helpful is to invite contact with the inner child from the adult part of the client. Sometimes the adult part will know what to say to the inner child, and sometimes this part can give a suggestion on the therapist's behalf. Such an exchange might go as follows:

THERAPIST: Could you ask little Lisa if she wants to show us more today?
ADULT LISA: She says no more for today—but she likes that we believe her!

This, then, is a three-way collaboration between the therapist, inner child, and the adult part or self-state of the client. From the perspective of developing self-empowerment and self-regulation, this approach is one way of keeping the client in control and serves to minimize the risk of a traumatic regression into a feeling of powerlessness.

A final note regarding physical touch. Research has taught us that physical touch can trigger so-called body memories that reside in procedural and implicit memory and have not been made available to meaning-giving explicit memory (Chapter 4). These body memories can, in turn, trigger automated flashbacks that can retraumatize the client (Levine with Frederick, 1997; Yehuda & McFarlane, 1997). Given this, the use of physical touch should be approached with a great deal of caution when therapeutically accompanying traumatized clients through their work. Hakomi assumes the integration of implicit memories and beliefs throughout the spectrum of experience from sensations to tensions, to feelings, to posture and gestures, to thoughts and memories (Caldwell, 1997, 2011; Johanson, 2011c; LeDoux, 1996), knowing that verbal or nonverbal contact can evoke memories at any moment. While the meaning a client makes of touch is always tracked, as is the presence of evoked memories, working with trauma alerts the therapist to be aware of ever-present triggers that neither client nor therapist might know of ahead of time—and of the importance of proceeding with the necessary amount of resourcing so that working with trauma is titrated to a rate that can be assimilated by the client (Chapter 24).

In summary, the defense mechanisms of individuals with structural personality deficits in perception, regulation, communication, and connection should be considered as efforts from their organic wisdom to protect and maintain stability. No defense is ever taken away in Hakomi. The therapy only intends to add new possibilities when a client is able to enter into the transformative process. Defenses should not even be explored for this purpose unless the client is appropriately resourced or until the work has enabled the underlying vulnerable structures to retroactively mature (Rudolf, 1996). The classic Hakomi approach taught in basic training is only applicable when all of the prerequisites below are met by the client in question:

1. An alert, oriented consciousness free of significant distortions or perceptual limitations that would render him unable to take himself under observation is available to the client.
2. The client possesses both the ability for and openness to introspection, self-observation, and mindfulness.
3. The client is capable of disidentifying with particular patterns of experience from time to time in the service of expanding her inner observer or observing ego. (For example, the presence of judgmental, critical parts or overly harsh superego parts must first be dealt with consciously before judgment-free mindfulness can be practiced.)
4. The client is able to enter into a therapeutic relationship, with all that this implies. At a minimum, the client must be able to understand the "as-if" invitations to self-exploration as such.

Further Considerations for Clients With Structural Limitations

Intake and Diagnosis

In order to responsibly proceed with Hakomi's body-oriented, experience-evoking approach in a manner that is mindful of possible destabilizing effects, the pursuit of a thorough intake process is recommended before actively commencing a course of therapeutic treatment. In addition, diagnosis and overall assessment in Hakomi happen as every experiment from saying hello to shaking hands, to offering a seat is tracked for its effect and contacted at the appropriate level of depth. Hakomi therapists are also continually taking in diagnostic bodily information from the person's posture, gestures, breathing, rate of speech, relational characteristics, and so forth (Chapters 4 and 23).

The process of diagnosis will continue in a like manner throughout the course of therapy, such that the diagnosis and core material in play become both more differentiated and more precise as the therapeutic work unfolds. Clinical experience with a client will refine the therapist's perception, as will the therapist's ability to remain in good contact with herself, her client, and the process unfolding in the present moment. By being attentive to all three of these dimensions, the therapist can track the developments in both the intra- and interpersonal fields of the client as well as in the arena of therapist-client countertransference. A continual attentiveness to the development of the client's inner and outer experience, processing, and behavioral possibilities is the deciding factor that enables therapists to respond with interventions that are well attuned to clients' actual psychological states (Siegel, 2007). When in doubt about going forward with an intervention, it is always appropriate to take time to gain more information before doing so. On the other hand, the Hakomi process is self-correcting in that all therapeutic interventions are done experimentally—yielding results that either confirm or disconfirm the therapist's clinical intuition (Marks-Tarlow, 2012), and guiding the next level of contact (Chapter 14) for deepening or repairing the therapeutic alliance (Stolorow et al., 1987).

For some clients, therapy will not progress much beyond providing a stabilizing, supportive effect for some time. This will, however, typically be experienced as a significant improvement in these clients' quality of life. For other clients, once stabilization has taken hold, the goal of psychological maturation and consolidation can be pursued, which in turn can lead to the possibility of pursuing insight-oriented uncovering work. In these cases, it is important to make decisions in a responsible, collaborative manner, such that clients ultimately determine the direction of the work as well as the approaches and interventions utilized in the service of their therapeutic goals (Duncan, 2010).

Anchoring in the Outer World and in Everyday Consciousness

For clients with structural limitations, anything that supports the stable perception of outer reality is helpful. Sometimes this can involve a limited, bounded, and measured shift into using the mind-body interface in a mindful way that the therapist employs cautiously, continuously tracking for the risk of destabilization. For example:

1. Connecting body awareness and emotion through conscious perception.
   The defenses of narcissistic clients often possess an alexithymic quality. According to the results of neurobiological research (Damasio, 2000), the brains of alexithymic individuals are not able to integrate feelings in relation to signals from the body. However, it is possible to create new synaptic connections (such as to the amygdala) through conscious experience of evoked bodily sensations and emotions in the present

moment (Thielen, 2002, 2015). In these cases, mindfulness and accessing can aid in joining right- and left-brain functions.

2. Experiencing the body and its boundaries.

Case example: During a long-term course of psychotherapeutic treatment, a 30-year-old woman who was sexually abused as a child became aware that she would leave her body and become passively permissive whenever her partner was interested in being sexually intimate with her. This was true even when she, too, was interested in being intimate. As an intervention, we explored how she might experience the original traumatic situation in a different way that incorporated her body. Through learning, among other things, a way to tense up her back muscles, open her eyes, and continue to breathe normally, she was able to remain in reality and to pull herself into the physical present when becoming aware of the pull toward her old, defensive behavior.

3. Experiencing and exploring one's own power, resources, and response options.

Case example: When confronted with conflict-laden situations, a young man routinely began to stutter, panic, and dissociate. This client had been physically abused by his father until the age of 18, but now had a powerful physical presence of his own. Given that the client began to dissociate (in connection with a racing heart, shortness of breath, and feeling numb) as soon as he came in contact with difficult memories, an uncovering approach was not feasible. He could not observe his inner world without getting sucked into a painful psychological swamp. He could, however, access his experience in the present moment. As a result, he was capable of realizing how powerless he felt in conflicted situations. In these situations, he experienced himself as a 10-year-old child in relation to his father. We tested his actual current strength through the experiment of him pushing his hands against mine. He began to recognize his own strength and found himself enjoying the moment when my own strength faltered in relation to his power. He was then able to take this experience into conflict-laden scenarios, reminding himself of his own strength through the process of briefly pushing his hands against one another or tensing up his arm muscles. Using these techniques, he was able to prevent himself from slipping into the trauma-driven repetition of his old coping mechanisms. As a result, he learned to improve his breathing and reduce his stuttering.

4. Perceiving and testing reality (such as the meanings of the therapist's reactions).

Case example: Client: "Did you laugh because you're amusing yourself at my expense?" Therapist: "No, I'm just excited about what a good experience you had this weekend at home."

Improving Self-Regulation Through Increasing Self-Awareness

Differentiating the Inner Observer From the Inner Critic

When the ability for self-observation is present to some degree, it can be used in the service of becoming aware of automatic inner and outer reactions as is normal in Hakomi, and perhaps even in the service of changing or regulating them (Schore, 1994). When introducing this method to improve self-regulation, it is important to underscore the difference between the inner observer and inner critic and give the client tools to help avoid confusing the two. Employing the self-state of the client (Eisman, 2006; Schwartz, 1995) in relation to the multiplicity of internal, historically conditioned parts can be helpful in some cases.

> *During a long-term course of psychotherapeutic treatment, a female client in a deep depression became aware of the reason she would repeatedly describe difficult childhood experiences despite the fact that she felt worse afterward. Retraversing the memories of these experiences would always stir her up and lead her to question herself. This repetition, she realized, was focused on the dynamic of being understood—a quality that had not been present in her early life and had been sorely missed. While commenting on her need for understanding, however, she would simultaneously make skeptical comments that served to block its integration. As she became aware of this, she began to get mad at and reprimand herself, which led her to feel even worse. In the end, she would sink into her familiar state of depression. Over time, she became more and more aware of her need for understanding and better able to trust her insights or note when they did not seem to fit. At this point, although further developmental healing work remained to be done, the realization that she was seeking and needing understanding helped her be more understanding of and compassionate with herself. She learned to modify her behavior so as not to be insensitive to those around her. Instead of repeatedly taxing her friends' compassion through repetition of the same stories, she found a way to both ask for and receive what she really needed: compassion and understanding.*

Experiencing and Valuing the Protective Mechanisms

Discussing a client's defense mechanisms is a particularly tricky thing to do. This process of bringing the system into consciousness should be approached and discussed from the perspective that these defenses are valuable and have served a necessary and important purpose, namely, ensuring the client's protection. Failure to do so can put the internal structures that these defense mechanisms have been protecting at risk and destabilize the client. Normally in Hakomi, defense mechanisms are not named and interpreted as in some psychodynamic approaches. They are usually contacted as the process unfolds in a way that invites curiosity and the empowerment of self-discovery: "Oh, anger comes up when someone questions you[?] Are you curious about that? Maybe we can hang out with the anger longer, and see if it can say more about itself." If intrapsychic work is possible, that is, if sufficient structure is present, the client may eventually be able to recognize that these behaviors may no longer always be necessary and can be seen instead as optional approaches along with others that together provide more flexibility and freedom.

Mindfulness

Currently, multiple psychotherapeutic approaches are being introduced and discussed under the name "mindfulness-based therapy." These therapies are discussed in relation to their application for the purposes of stabilizing those with difficult clinical disorders (Grossmann, Niemann, Schmidt, & Walach, 2004; Sonnenmoser, 2005). For each of these approaches, the client must be capable and interested in at least occasional self-reflection, in building up the "reflexive mind" (Aron, 1998b). Mindfulness and the development of an inner observer are important self-regulation techniques in the trauma therapies of Reddemann (2001) and Rothschild (2000, 2003), as well as in Jon Kabat-Zinn's mindfulness-based stress reduction (1990) and in Marsha Linehan's dialectical behavioral therapy (Hayes et al., 2004). With each of these therapies, the goal is for clients to develop the ability to step back and observe themselves from a nonjudgmental stance, such that they are neither overwhelmed nor dissociated, so that they can become more aware of their patterns of action and reaction. In these therapies, mindfulness is one technique employed within the context of other clinical interventions or methods. In contrast, the Hakomi method is the integrated employment of a state of mindfulness throughout its therapeutic approach. This includes assisted meditation (Kurtz, 1990b), staying with and observing one's own experience, and supporting mindful self-study (Johanson & Kurtz, 1993) when a client is structurally capable.

Some experienced therapists have explored using mindfulness with psychotic patients in inpatient settings as a way of helping them introduce a distance between them and voices they hear that can take over the seat of consciousness: "Can you say 'hi' to that jealous voice?" (Coleman & Smith, 2006; Romme & Escher, 2000; Whitehead, 1992). A listing of other resources for working with voices, plus an alternative view of working with psychosis in general that is compatible with Hakomi, can be found in Williams (2012).

The Security-Providing Helper-Ego Function of the Therapist

Because of the number and level of unsettling physical symptoms they are dealing with, structurally deficient clients with anxiety are often not able to engage in mindful observation of their bodies. In these cases, the therapist can provide psychoeducational information about what different physical reactions normally mean.

> *In the closing session of a long-term course of psychotherapeutic treatment, a female client who experienced panic attacks and a number of phobias told me the following: "What was most helpful in the beginning was when you explained that all strong, emotional reactions result in increased heart rate—both in joy and in fear. Learning that this was normal was such a relief."*

In this case, the therapist is not helping the client explore her own self-organization, but is acting as an expert whose information can normalize experiences and help clients better orient themselves and assess their own experience. When this results in a calming response, the therapist can contact it in order to call the client's awareness to it: "It's a relief to know that, isn't it?"

Only a Secure Therapist Can Provide Security

In accompanying clients with structural limitations through their therapeutic journeys—journeys that are challenging for both therapist and client alike—it is the therapist's own internal sense of safety and security that enables a positive therapeutic outcome. The ability of the therapist to successfully provide a holding environment, to be able to create a therapeutic container that can enable clients to share difficult memories and strong emotions while remaining present and not overwhelmed, is largely dependent on how well a therapist knows and is in touch with his own boundaries. In situations in which a therapist is feeling overly challenged, unsure, or threatened by the client's or his own experience in the moment, maintaining the therapeutic framework becomes impossible—and yet, this dyadic regulation (Schore, 2003; Siegel, 2003) is exactly what these clients need most in these moments.

> *In order to feel safe working with a physically imposing client's repressed anger and power, I ensured that our sessions took place while other therapists were present in the practice's office. Knowing that I could call out for help if I needed to enabled me to stay calm and remain present in our work.*

Because therapists working with structurally deficient clients are required to take on responsibility for a great deal of the psychological leadership and regulatory functioning, ongoing supervision is particularly important. It is with supervision, for example, that clarity can be gained around whether feelings of insufficiency are based in countertransference or if they indicate the therapist is up against personal limits or the limits of competence. These types of feelings are important to pay attention to, as is the process of distinguishing the particular meanings they might carry.

Conclusion

The use of the Hakomi method must be approached carefully with clients with structural limitations and those who are more clinically disturbed. Clinical knowledge about disorders and treatment methods is as important as being in touch with oneself, the client, and the process as it unfolds. A diagnostic process that continues throughout the course of therapy in conjunction with supervision will serve the therapist well in this type of work—helping to ensure that the therapist will not come to feel overwhelmed or burned out but will be able to guide even long therapeutic processes with joy and genuine curiosity.

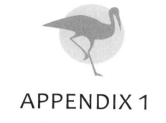

APPENDIX 1

Glossary of Hakomi Therapy Terms

Cedar Barstow and Greg Johanson

THIS GLOSSARY IS provided as a convenience to readers who might not be familiar with all the terms used in the chapters, especially those used earlier in the text that are not more carefully defined until later.

accessing: The process of transitioning from ordinary consciousness through turning a person's awareness inward toward felt present experience in a mindful or witnessing state of consciousness.

barriers: Beliefs that block the normal organic process of attaining sensitivity and satisfaction. Insight barriers block clarity about what is needed. Response barriers block effective action to obtain what is needed. Nourishment barriers block the experience of satisfaction when something is obtained. Completion barriers block the relaxation that functions to savor the need satisfied, release tensions, and give further clarity about what other need the organism is now ready to reorient toward. More generally, barriers are those parts of us that come into play after some sort of wounding that attempts to protect us from the hurt ever happening again.

bottom-up processing: A concept from sensorimotor psychotherapy that contrasts the mindful processing of sensations, tensions, and such generated by lower brain functions as a result of traumatic activation (bottom) with that of the more common mindful processing of thoughts, emotions, and memories available to the cerebral cortex (top-down processing). Premature top-down processing can evoke a harmful trauma vortex, if bottom-up processing of sensations as sensations has not empowered the body to titrate and metabolize such material without being overwhelmed by their normally instantaneous eruptions.

CAS (complex adaptive systems): One of the commonly used terms for the science of living organic systems that informs the Hakomi method's principles and view of human psychology, functioning, and transformation.

character: In a positive sense, a person's stable way of making meaning of life through organizing multiple dispositions from metabolic, psychosocial, and structural factors so that the person displays consistent, predicable behavior. In a therapeutic sense, a way of experiencing and expressing oneself in a rigid way, unaware of or unable to make use of a wider range of realistically available choices.

character process: Any one of a number of characterological ways of being in the world that have been delineated in Hakomi and general psychological literature as having identifiable, predictable components (see character above). Referred to in Hakomi literature by both descriptive and classic terms: sensitive/analytic = schizoid; dependent/endearing = oral; self-reliant = compensated oral; tough/generous = psychopath I; charming/seductive = psychopath II; burdened/enduring = masochist; industrious/overfocused = phallic; expressive/clinging = hysteric.

character strategy: The patterns, habits, approaches to the world a person has developed to achieve pleasure and satisfaction while avoiding perceived painful situations, given the nature of the person's particular core organizing beliefs about the world.

child: A state of consciousness in which one is aware of one's current adult status and at the same time is experiencing the memories, feelings, thought modes, and speech patterns of childhood.

contact: An initial and ongoing technique in which the therapist names the immediate, often emotionally meaningful, experience of the client in a simple way the client can easily confirm or modify. Therapist: "A little sad, huh?" Client: "Uh, it has more of a quality of grief." Level 1 contact is used when the therapist is attempting to build an interpersonal bridge of understanding. Level 2 contact is used as an accessing technique to invite the client to pay mindful attention to his or her intrapsychic experience.

core beliefs: The usually implicit level of consciousness, normally influenced by developmental beliefs and decisions, that organizes and mobilizes experience and response before experience and response happen; the program that is running the computer; the level of creative imagination or filtering that makes reality available to consciousness.

core material: Composed of beliefs, nervous system patterning, sensations, memories, images, emotions, and attitudes about self and the world—and related to (often early) formative experiences—core material shapes our patterns of behavior, our bodily structure, and our experiences. Core material is primarily unconscious until brought to awareness.

deepening: The process of helping a person stay with present experience in a mindful or witnessing state of consciousness long enough for it to lead to information about core organizing beliefs; how reality is being structured or limited.

dispositions: A term from the philosopher of science Karl Popper for describing the unconscious as the result of multiple genetic, metabolic, interpersonal, cultural, and social forces that dispose one's organization of experience in various directions, but do not absolutely determine the result. All persons have at least the ability to be co-creators of how they are organized.

hierarchy of experience: A common shift or progression in the course of the deepening process is from thoughts and ideas, to sensations and tensions, to feelings and emotions, to memories and images, to meanings and beliefs.

holon: A shorthand term from Arthur Koestler in the philosophy of science that describes the most basic building block of life. To be a holon means to be a whole that is made up of parts, which in turn is a part of a greater whole, resulting in an interdependent, participatory universe, one of the implications of Hakomi's unity principle.

intersubjectivity: The assumption that all people, clients and therapists alike, organize their experience in unique ways. The implication for therapy is that no one can claim to experience life cleanly or correctly, so that the process must embrace the humility of curiously collaborating and comparing intuitions of what is happening and what is possible.

jumping out of the system (JOOTS): Going from being in some automatic form of habitual behavior between client and therapist, to noticing the pattern, to the freedom to step outside the normal reactions through nonjudgmentally naming them in a way that brings them under observation.

magical stranger: The therapist as a compassionate adult who appears as if by magic when the client is experiencing a traumatic childhood memory, to support the child through the painful and confusing event.

method: Hakomi therapy as a specific form of psychotherapy that distinctively (in a classic form that always allows for the spontaneous) progresses through a mindful sequence of accessing, deepening, processing, transformation, and integration, with accompanying notions about character, therapeutic approaches, techniques, and so on.

mind-body holism: One of the principles that maintains that mind and body are inseparable in interacting and influencing each other. Core narrative beliefs that can come into mental awareness influence posture, body structure, gesture, facial expression, emotions, and so on through the voluntary musculature, hormone system, and such. Feedback from chronic bodily mobilizations confirms and reinforces belief systems. Hakomi therapy constantly explores the mind-body interface.

mindfulness: A witnessing state of consciousness characterized by awareness turned inward toward live present experience with an exploratory, open focus that allows one to observe the reality of inner processes without being automatically mobilized by them. Also, a principle of the work that maintains the value of being able to step out of the habits and routines that normally control consciousness and behavior to observe the reality and organization of experience without being fused or blended with it, so that choices and change become possibilities.

nonviolence: One of the principles of the work that respects the wisdom of living organic systems to know what they need. A way of working that favors going with the flow, accepting what is, paying attention to the way things "want" to go, supporting rather than confronting defenses, and providing a safe setting in which clients will feel free to explore what is most important from their own perspective.

ordinary consciousness: Normal, everyday, outwardly oriented, goal-directed, narrowly focused awareness ruled by habits and routines in space and time that is appropriate and useful for many tasks.

organicity: One of the principles, the assumption that organic living systems have a "mind" of their own with the capacity to be self-organizing, self-directing, and self-correcting when all the parts are communicating within the whole. Hakomi therapy assumes and nurtures these capacities as central to growing, healing, and transformation processes.

organization of experience: The creative way in which the mind or imagination filters, structures, or transforms the givens of reality in implicit memory to control conscious and unconscious experience and expression in the individual.

principles: The basic, foundational assumptions of Hakomi therapy concerning living systems in general and therapy in particular, taken from contemporary philosophy of science and ancient spiritual traditions. They are unity, organicity, mind-body holism, mindfulness, and nonviolence. What makes any particular method or technique Hakomi is whether it participates in and reflects the principles.

probe: A verbal or nonverbal experiment in mindfulness in which clients are invited to witness whatever spontaneously arises in them in response to potentially nourishing words or actions. The usual form for a probe is, "What do you experience when I say these words . . . [pause] . . . [the words said]?" or "What do you become aware of when I do [or you do] this action . . . [pause] . . . [the action]?" Whatever report issues from the probe then becomes the next part of the deepening thread that is mindfully processed.

process: The general stages Hakomi therapy sessions normally progress through—establishing safety through contact and loving presence, mindfulness, accessing, deepening, processing, transforming around new beliefs, integrating, and completing.

processing: Inviting mindfulness through accessing and maintaining mindfulness through deepening leads to the stage of processing where core material is mindfully discovered, more inclusive core beliefs are experimented with, and barriers to such new transformations are dealt with.

riding the rapids: A state of consciousness characterized by a diminishing of mindfulness, uncontrollable emotional release, spontaneous movements and tensions, and waves of memory and feeling often combined with the use of tension and posture to control the flow of feeling.

self-states: When a person's seat of consciousness is characterized by the grounded bare awareness, compassion, and wisdom of deep mindfulness, he or she can be said to rest or reside in a different neural net than the historically conditioned ego and its multiplicity of parts. This is a state that theorists such as Almaas, Eisman, Monda, Schwartz, and others recommend as healing or whole in itself, and optimal for the healing of wounded ego states.

sensitivity cycle: Stages in the continuing flow of increasingly efficient functioning. Clarity leads to the possibility of effective action, which sets up the possibility of organic satisfaction and nourishment, which may lead to relaxation of tensions mobilized around the original need, and the chance for greater clarity about what the next need may be that the system is ready to orient toward.

taking over: A Hakomi technique in which the therapist takes over or does something as precisely as possible that the client is already doing for himself or herself. Taking over can be physical (taking over the holding in of shoulders), verbal (taking over voices clients hear inside themselves saying things such as, "Don't let others get close"), active (taking over the holding back of an angry punch), or passive (taking over a reaching movement with the arms). The technique is normally an experiment done while inviting mindfulness in the client except during riding the rapids when it is simply used to support spontaneous behavior.

tracking: The therapist pays close attention to spontaneous or habitual physical signs and changes that may reflect present feeling or meaning in the client at each stage of the process.

transformation: In terms of working with the client's transference or organization of experience, transformation is said to occur when the client can organize in some currently realistic aspect of life that he or she has heretofore organized out due to some painful developmental wounding. Nothing is removed from the client's present organization, but new possibilities are added in, thus enhancing the organicity of the person's system while widening his or her perception and expectation of what is possible.

unity: The most inclusive of all the principles that maintains that everything exists within a complex web of interdependent relationships with everything else and that there is a force in life, often called negentropy, that strives to bring about greater wholeness and harmony from component parts and disorganization.

window of tolerance: A concept from the trauma work of sensorimotor psychotherapy that refers to keeping the activation of a client's nervous system within a workable range between hyper- and hypoactivation that precludes the client from dissociating or becoming retraumatized.

witness: That part of mindful consciousness that can simply stand back and observe inner experience without being blended or fused with it. It allows what was once subject to become object and permits growth toward increased complexity.

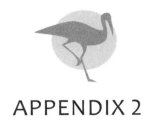

Praxis: Annotated Case Illustrations

Karen A. Baikie, Phil Del Prince, and Greg Johanson

Missing Experience

Karen A. Baikie

Cheryl is a 43-year-old single female. She has never married. She was the firstborn child in her family. When Cheryl was 22 months old, her four-month-old sister died of sudden infant death syndrome. The family was grief stricken, and from what we can ascertain, Cheryl was left alone as her parents grieved. She feels that she carries the family's grief and is always sad. About 18 months later, another daughter, Sharon, was born. Five years ago, there was a family rift between Sharon and Cheryl. Despite Cheryl's efforts to repair the relationship with her sister, Sharon refuses to speak to her. Cheryl still sees her parents, as does Sharon, but the parents do not speak of one daughter to the other. Cheryl carries enormous grief over the loss of her relationship with Sharon, as well as intense grief over the loss of her relationship with her two young nephews. This is particularly painful for Cheryl as she has no children of her own.

We have been working on Cheryl's grief in therapy. Cheryl cries for her lost relationships as well as her "lost life" all the time, but the grief never seems to end. We have observed that as Cheryl begins to touch her sadness, she quickly pulls herself out of it by either going into mental processes or by taking a big breath and interrupting the natural flow of tears. She also feels very alone in her sadness and in her life. Some of her core limiting beliefs include: "It's my fault"; "I'm not good enough"; "I'm all alone"; and "Nobody cares about me." In this session, we find a way to take over the internal voices and physical tension that cut Cheryl off from her feelings. The therapist also provides a missing experience for Cheryl—that of having someone present as she fully experiences her sadness. This enables Cheryl to experience a satisfying, completed grief process for the very first time.

Crossing the Nourishment Barrier

During the week Cheryl had an experience in which she felt exactly the same feeling of deep sadness she felt when she used to walk away from Sharon's house. She would cry all the way to the car. The current experience triggered the belief that no one cared about her. In the session, we explore the sadness and the pattern in which she pulls herself out of the sadness as soon as she touches it by going into thinking. We track the voices that block her sadness each time it hurts too much. She notices that each time she begins to feel sad, she hears words that take her out of the feeling. Cheryl is by now very familiar with mindfulness and Hakomi experiments, so we experiment with Cheryl saying, "It's really sad—no one's here for me," and the therapist taking over the voices that respond, "That's just how it is. . . . You've got to get used to it. . . . You haven't got this yet. . . . You'll never get this." This enables her to begin to stay with the sadness longer. She begins to feel how very sad it was and how deeply alone she felt as a child.

> CLIENT: It's really sad. No one's there for me [tears]. [Hakomi therapists are trained to hear these absolute statements as limiting core beliefs. Presumably the client's neural attractors, or core organizers, are filtering out experiences to the contrary, since life usually offers some opportunities for connection.]
>
> THERAPIST: Yeah. It is really sad. [Nonetheless, the therapist contacts the client's felt sense of sadness, rather than pointing out exceptions or enjoining Cheryl to look on the bright side.]
>
> C: It's just *me*.
>
> T: It's just very alone, huh? Really alone? [In the early part of a Hakomi session, the focus is on establishing a strong therapeutic alliance. Because the client is embedded in a perspective that she is alone, the therapist contacts her words very precisely, in effect, demonstrating, "I'm with you and I get what your experience is like."]
>
> C: I have to keep it that way. It's just *me*. [Child part emerging. The client has started to speak in a higher pitch and sounds more absolute, indicating that she is entering the child state of consciousness.]
>
> T: There's just you, and you're only little, and there's nobody there. [Inflections of the

magical stranger. As the magical stranger, the therapist takes on the quality of a curious and compassionate adult ally who understands and cares about the child's experience. She uses the present tense to help Cheryl stay in the regressed state.]

C: [Big breath.] And I have to be strong and be alone and no one would want to be with me. [Wave of tears, but at the same time trying to pull back from feelings.]

T: Part of you believes that you have to be strong? [The therapist acknowledges that Cheryl has both a young part that feels lonely and very sad, and another part that is trying to be grown up and strong. She hypothesizes that being strong is an adaptive strategy to cope with being alone.]

C: I'm trying . . . [big breath] . . . maybe I don't have to be.

T: So what tells you that? . . . That maybe you don't have to be strong. [The statement "Maybe I don't have to be" indicates that Cheryl is aware that there may be an alternative to her default strategy of being strong. The therapist invites Cheryl to notice how she is getting this information on the inside. This marks an important phase of the work, when the client begins to notice how the solution she devised when she was little made sense back then but is now preventing her from having the support she longs for.]

C: But then what would happen?

T: Part of you is scared about what would happen if you hadn't been strong?

C: Then I'd just be nothing. [The client has now uncovered the fear that keeps the strategy in place: If she stopped being strong, she wouldn't matter. If the therapist had asked, "Why do you have to be strong?" Cheryl would likely have offered a more conceptual answer. Likewise, by encouraging Cheryl to notice what is telling her "maybe you don't have to be strong," the therapist is following Cheryl's intrinsic hunch that there might be a more satisfying alternative to "being strong and alone." If the therapist had tried to persuade Cheryl to accept that possibility before the unconscious fear was made conscious, she would have initiated a subtle power struggle between herself and the part of Cheryl that needs to matter.]

T: It's the kind of strength that makes you feel like you matter, huh? [The therapist's positive and compassionate tone lets Cheryl's strong part know that the therapist understands and respects its intentions. It also helps Cheryl understand herself better.]

C: I know that I just had to be strong. And just be alone.

T: So what if I was to do that part for you? Is that okay? [Therapist extends the verbal taking-over experiment to take over this voice too. Cheryl understands this kind of experiment well, so she sets herself up mindfully. The therapist, after preparing, says] . . . You have to be strong.

C: I don't want to be.

T: You have to be strong. You have to be on your own.

C: I don't want to be. [The therapist is using a verbal taking-over experiment in which she is replicating the words the strong part uses to maintain its dominant position in the client's inner ecology. With this function supported by the therapist, the client is free to experience and give voice to her protest position.]

T: Stay with the energy of that voice for a moment. [After a small pause, the therapist repeats the taken-over words] . . . You have to be strong. You have to be on your own.

C: It's not fair.

T: [Changes tone of voice.] No, it's not fair. . . . See if you can feel that "no" inside you, the sense that it's not fair. [By asking the client to stay with the "no," the therapist is helping Cheryl feel the aspects of her experience that are habitually eclipsed by the strong part.]

C: I feel like I'll burst. Really tired around my neck.

T: A lot of holding, huh? [The client is becoming aware of how much tension she carries in her neck in an effort to be strong and to avoid being in contact with the part that doesn't want to be.]

C: It's unfair, but, oh well.

T: So now the "unfair" collapses, huh? [The client shrugs off the growing awareness that she has made an unfair deal with herself.]

C: Then it goes back to all that, you know, "Deal with it." [Living systems maintain coherence by establishing automatic and rigid responses to new possibilities. As the client starts to unhinge from her strategy, other internal parts convince her that she has to deal with it whether it is fair or not. Notice that the therapist is not talking the client out of her experience. Instead, she is helping Cheryl view and map her system from the inside. The therapist trusts that as the client brings more consciousness to her self-organization, she is making the once automatic and unconscious habit to "be strong," conscious and voluntary. This increases the likelihood that the client will eventually avail herself of other, more satisfying options when it is safe and appropriate to do so.]

T: [Therapist speaks more directly to the child part.] I understand that it was very hard to be angry when everyone around you was sad. Because it was unfair and you were angry about that. [An acknowledgment with the inflection of the magical stranger, and continuing as the magical stranger.]

C: [Crumpling face. Big distress.]

T: . . . Yeah . . . just too much.

C: [Shaking head.] I just never got a look in.

T: Yeah, you never got a look in. There wasn't space for you. Nobody was there for you. That kind of made you mad? [The therapist is offering the child experiences of care and understanding that were needed but unavailable when the client was little. This is the kind of missing experience Hakomi therapists offer to redress developmental injuries.]

C: [More tears.] I don't want to be on my own [child voice].

T: You don't want to be strong on your own anymore? [The therapist is helping the client see that it is not just being alone that is too much, but also being strong as a compensatory strategy.]

C: [Big tears.] I can't be strong anymore. It's just pushing at me everywhere.

T: You're feeling pressure, pushing. . . . How are you feeling that inside? [The therapist is continuing to help the client create a somatic map of the pressure she holds to keep her needs from pressing into consciousness.]

C: Across here [forehead] and here [throat] and across here [back of neck and shoulders]. I just clench up.

T: So there's tightening in your body. Where is it the strongest? [The accessing question "Where is it the strongest?" directs the client's awareness to her present, felt experience and is another way Hakomi therapists manage consciousness. The answer will also help the therapist determine how best to take over the tension later.]

C: Up here [top of neck].

T: Is it all right if I come around and just try something? [As Cheryl nods, the therapist comes around to side, and slowly and cautiously takes over tension and pressure with a hand on the back of Cheryl's neck. Then, as she is holding Cheryl's tension, the therapist adds the words] You have to be strong. You have to do it on your own. [The therapist replicates the client's self-management strategy by using her hand to create pressure on the back of the client's neck.]

C: [Body collapses. With the therapist standing in as a surrogate manager, the client is safe enough to encounter the collapse underneath her compensated strength.]

T: It's kind of like it's all collapsing, huh?

C: [Nods.] There isn't anybody.

T: [Slowly, with pauses that allow the spaciousness for the words to sink in] . . . It's too much for a little girl to be so strong. . . . It's too much to do it on your own when you are only little. . . . You're mad about that. . . . Nobody was there for you. [The therapist guesses the client is circling back to the theme of being alone, of having no support and of having to always be strong.]

C: No, they weren't.

T: No, they weren't. And it's not fair. [The therapist is giving permission for the client to know the full truth of her experience, which supports the unburdening of the grief and anger she has carried all these years.]

C: [Big tears.] It's not fair. [With the support of the therapist—through both words and touch—Cheryl can be in contact with the previously unfelt aspects of her early emotional life.]

T: It's just unfair that they weren't there for you. . . . You had to do it all yourself.

C: Why weren't they there?

T: They weren't there because they had their own stuff. And that's not your fault.

C: What's happened to me?

T: No one's explaining anything to you. No one's telling you what's going on. [Children often conclude that they must be inherently flawed or others would take a greater interest in them. The therapist casts new light on the family situation by saying, "they had their own stuff" to help Cheryl understand why her parents were not there for her. This information is more likely to be integrated because the client is in the original experience.]

C: It's not fair.

T: It's not fair, I agree. Can you feel that, the part that says it's not fair? Can we listen to that part?

C: [Nods.]

T: [The tension in the client's neck is increasing, and she is holding a lot of tension across her whole back and shoulders. So the therapist makes an adjustment to the physical taking over.] Everything's really tight, huh. I'm going to try something else. I've got a sarong. I'm going to put it around the back of you and hold really tight, okay? [The therapist slowly wraps the sarong around the back, enabling better taking over of the upper body tension by pulling on the sarong. As the client accesses the fullness of her grief, her internal protectors create more tension in her body to try to contain the feelings that are now coming into consciousness.]

C: [Immediately the client cries. Something releases; tears start coming more freely now. Big sighs. Big tears. The containment provided by the sarong enables Cheryl to release the feelings that have been managed by the tension in her shoulder and neck.]

T: [Therapist reaches across and gently caresses client's head.] . . . I'm here for you now. I'm here for you—you don't have to do it by yourself. [The client is having strong emotion and experiencing the support of the therapist at the same time. The therapist is using her words to show the client that she is not alone and that she doesn't have to be strong. This is a powerful example of how Hakomi therapists use the therapy relationship to provide a missing experience for the client.]

C: [More tears, starts to sob. When someone finally gets an experience they have waited a lifetime to have, it often elicits grief for having lived so long without it.]

T: [Therapist reaches for a cushion and places it to support the client's head, which is organically leaning over toward the side of the couch. Therapist caresses her head as she cries.] You don't have to do it by yourself. [The statement "You don't have to do it by yourself" is more likely to be integrated because it matches the experience that is happening here and now. The therapist's loving presence, demonstrated through a combination of words and touch, enables Cheryl to actually receive the support she has hungered for both as a child and as an adult.]

C: [She sobs and sobs. Tears coming freely now, with really big breaths. Real crying, not held back—riding the rapids. Having crossed the nourishment barrier, indicated by the client's acceptance of the therapist's support, the client can surrender to the cascade of feelings bound to her core material.]

T: [Slowly, with a lot of long pauses] . . . You don't have to do this by yourself. . . . . It's so sad. It's so sad. . . . It's not fair. . . . Yeah. . . . The sadness just keeps coming, huh? . . . You don't have to do it all alone. [The therapist supports both the management of the feeling and its release, and continues to make contact to indicate she is really with the client.]

C: [Big sigh.] So sad, no one's there [childlike sobbing].

T: I'm here with you. It's okay to be sad. [The reminder that the client is not alone and that things are different now is what makes revisiting the client's past healing rather than rewounding.]

C: [Sobs change, childlike faster breathing; huh-huh-humm. Crying is moving through her body now. As the client gets more and more of what she has always longed for, she surrenders completely to her feelings of grief.]

T: Yeah, it is so sad. So lonely.

C: [Breathing continues as huh-huh-huh-huumm, then a big breath, and starts to become smoother. Therapist continues stroking her forehead. This continues for 3–4 minutes. Big gulp. Easier breathing, body begins to relax. The smooth breathing is an indicator that something is settling on the inside and that the process is nearing completion.]

T: So sad. You're not alone now. . . . I am here. . . .

C: [Moving toward restful state, riding rapids slowing down.]

T: [Continues stroking her head and just being with her for a few more minutes. Touch often communicates presence more powerfully than words, especially when someone is in the child state of consciousness.]

C: I could go to sleep now. [When we have an experience of deep satisfaction, we are able to rest. Having unburdened her grief and surrendered her strategy of being strong, Cheryl now experiences her exhaustion.]

T: Yeah, pretty tired, huh?

C: [Sighs again.]

T: Feeling your sadness when you're not alone. It takes you to a very restful place. [The therapist is linking two formerly irreconcilable things together: having feelings and being supported. The therapist points out that, contrary to the client's belief that she will be nothing if she isn't strong, it is actually taking her to a restful place. If this experience is integrated, it can shift the neural pattern built around the original memory system.]

C: Very restful.

T: Mmm. It's a good place, huh? It's good to not be alone? [Just continuing to be with her, stroking her head, letting her take it in.]

C: [She is integrating this. She moves a little, starts to sit up. Big sighs.] Thank you. So I can cry, but it feels different when I'm not alone with my sadness. [She puts her head back down on the cushion and flops into the side of the couch again. The client is assigning her own meaning to this new experience.]

T: Uh-huh.

C: Because every time I cry, I'm not crying like that. [This is the key missing experience for Cheryl. While she has cried many times in the past, she has never been able to fully release her grief in this way before.]

T: It felt different, huh?

C: [Big sigh, and she sits up.] Yes it does. I could just go to sleep.

T: You may need to do that tonight. Go gently. Take care of yourself.

C: Thank you. Hmm. So I make myself alone too. [Cheryl already recognizes that because she was alone in her sadness as a child, she recreates this aloneness as an adult by not expecting anyone to be there for her when she is sad.]

T: You notice that, huh? . . . Just let yourself rest tonight, holding the good space, not feeling alone. [While it will eventually be important for Cheryl to see how she participates in creating her alone state by being strong, the therapist avoids engaging in a discussion about it at this juncture. Instead, she supports transformation and integration by encouraging Cheryl to savor the experience of being restful and sated. If the client integrates the good space, she will more likely notice future opportunities for support and connection, rather than defaulting to her compensatory strategy.]

C: Okay. [Big sigh.] Yep.

T: [Moving toward finishing up.]

C: Thank you. [She sits up fully, looking brighter in her face. Even though this has been a taxing process, emotionally and physically, the client has integrated possibilities that are ultimately restorative rather than depleting. Her system has received the nourishment it has long been seeking through the therapist's loving presence to her pain. This is exactly the kind of exchange that promotes the neural resculpting needed to experience life in a more accurate and affirming way.]

Working With a Client New to Mindfulness

Phil Del Prince

The following session is offered not as an example of a perfect Hakomi session, but more as a real-world session with a client who has no experience of mindfulness. The client is part of a hard-driving, outer-oriented business world. Though he wants and needs help, he has a hard time joining in the classic Hakomi process. The therapist has to do a lot of work going back and forth between meeting him where he is and inviting him into what for him is a new and strange process.

The client, Mike, is a 38-year-old single male. He works as an executive coach in the corporate world. He is medically healthy except for borderline high blood pressure and is physically active.

His presenting issues involve concern over his inability to sustain intimate relationships over time, and an overreliance on physical exercise to gain an experience of satisfaction in his life.

This is his third session in therapy. I have done some initial education with Mike about mindfulness, bodymind dynamics, and experiential exploration. I've been sensitive to the novelty of these concepts for Mike and have moved slowly in the first two sessions, from building relationship, rapport, and common understanding of Mike's narrative to some initial movement into accessing the mindful state and experimenting with present experience.

This third session marks a more focused exploration of some material possibly underlying Mark's presenting issues. We pick up the session approximately 15 minutes in.

T: I'm wondering how you are with support in your life.

C: Why would you wonder that?

T: Well, I notice that you don't seem to ask very much of me during this session. You seem to work very hard to sense yourself, and then work to get insight from it, and then connect it to the rest of your life, and then plan out a course of action—all pretty much on your own[?] [Here the therapist assumes that there need be no secrets, that the client can better take adult responsibility for his process if an issue is clearly outlined, and that it will promote safety through fostering clear collaboration. The therapist is also naming the dynamics of what he has been tracking in the sessions to this point. It is an example of jumping out of the system in Hakomi, where the transference or organization of experience is now made the focus of mindful exploration. The (?) symbol represents a slight inflection in the therapist's voice that indicates that he is not simply making a declarative statement or interpretation, but is contacting an experience with the implication that the client might want to be curious about it and take it under mindful consideration.]

C: Huh, well, I haven't really considered that before. Let's see. I get a little nervous when you say this to me—I wonder if that means something. Yeah, I'll bet that comes from my dad. He always said, "If you want the right answer, then ask the right person, and that's usually yourself." Maybe I ought to watch that more, or I guess I could have a talk with him about it. Yeah, thanks. [Here the client is partly in mindfulness, noticing his nervousness, but reverts to his default position of figuring things out by himself in ordinary consciousness.]

T: So, right here, in this moment, I have the experience that you're doing this[?] [The therapist maintains focus on the accessing route and contacts the expression of the issue in the present-moment context. By saying "I have the experience," the therapist keeps his contact statement on the ground of his own truth, while promoting the safety inherent in the implication that the client should check it out in his experience.]

C: Doing what? [The client is confused by this unusual intervention of calling attention to present-moment experience of a metalevel dynamic.]

T: Kind of working on your own, while I'm present right here in front of you[?] [The therapist names the dynamic in a gentle, compassionate way without judgment that, again, seeks to evoke the client's curiosity about his own process.]

C: Huh, I've never caught that before. Do you really think that?

T: It sounds surprising to you—like you don't know what to make of it. [Therapist contacts the emotional content of surprise, all the while tracking the client to assess his nonverbal signs of congruence with the words spoken. The therapist does not accept the invitation of expanding on his thinking in ordinary consciousness.]

C: [Nods slowly. The slow nod, as opposed to a quick verbal response, demonstrates that the client is increasingly orienting toward his present-moment experience in a more mindful manner.]

T: It's got you thinking now. [The therapist's contact statement seeks to encourage and stabilize the client's inner exploration.]

C: Yeah, I'm thinking about my father.

T: Tell me a little about your dad. Sounds like he depended on himself a lot. [The therapist makes a judgment that it is still a strange stretch for the client to enter deeply into inner experience. The question allows the client to continue longer in his comfort zone of ordinary analytic conversation and to make some intellectual connections that might help establish the logic for inviting deeper inner exploration later.]

C: [Describes his dad's career as a one-person entrepreneur, primarily a strong and silent type, and being the third child in a household where both Mom and Dad worked much of the time, beginning again to work on making sense of it.]

T: It occurs to me that you kind of got lost in the shuffle somewhat, like it didn't get to be your turn very often[?] [The therapist has an intuition of the emotional meaning of this report by the client, and offers a possible focus for accessing the underlying theme.]

C: [Interrupts.] But they are very good people. They loved us and took care of us and worked really hard and did the best they could—wasn't easy back then, you know. Took a lot to keep things going. [Here the client has a protective reaction and feels called to defend his parents.]

T: It sounds like they really cared about you. And I can easily see how a child could start to feel like the best way to help is not to need very much, and not expect people to be there to help a lot. [The therapist demonstrates understanding of the client's experience through contacting his protective concern with the first sentence. This promotes safety by removing any need for the client to defend his parents. The second sentence returns to the systemic level and adds the frame that the child might have made a choice to be self-reliant as a way to actually help these parents he loves.]

C: Yeah, I guess—I'll think about this.

T: Tell you what—are you willing to do an experiment with this? [The therapist proposes a switch into a mindful state of consciousness that is characterized by an open, receptive, experimental attitude.]

C: With what? [However, the client is still very new to this way of working and has a need to ask more orienting questions.]

T: Well, instead of us just talking and guessing about how you're set up around "your turn" and needs and support, let's see if we can find some ways to know how all of the rest of you, like your feelings and body sense, can join your mind in talking to you about this. [The therapist takes the client's question as a valid safety issue and addresses it directly while doing some brief teaching about the process. Once again, the therapist is collaborating with the client, telling him exactly what he is thinking and proposing.]

C: I really don't know how to go about that. [The client again reacts automatically out of his belief that he is the one who should know how to do everything by himself, but is offering some vulnerability in naming his concern.]

T: Yeah, that's okay. That can be my part of the job. I'll help you into this state of mindfulness that we've been working with a little the last times you were here, where your only job is to watch yourself and notice anything that happens by itself inside you when we do an experiment in mindfulness right in the present moment. You good with that?

The therapist is compassionate with the client's worry, normalizes it, and refers back to previous elements in the therapy that evoke more familiarity and confidence in the client.

By suggesting that he can help and have part of the job, the therapist is not only providing structure and safety, he is setting up an important parallel process between what is happening intrapsychically and in the interpersonal field. The experiment in mindfulness that the therapist is suggesting is an attempt to invoke the reflective awareness or witness of the client and bring it to bear on his own internal process. Hopefully, this will help the client bring his own self-reliance under observation in a freeing and healing way. Since the client is actually allowing the therapist to help guide and support him in this endeavor, there is built in unspoken confirmation that he in truth does not always need to do everything himself. Thus, inner confirmation of new beliefs can be joined with outer confirmation in support of healing transformation. Were this parallel process not congruent, the client's worst fears might end up being confirmed.

> C: Okay, I'm good with that.
> T: [Has Mike close his eyes and turn his awareness inward toward felt present experience.] Find a place where you can just quietly watch whatever happens on its own . . . not concerned with what's true or what anything means . . . just noticing anything that happens inside you automatically, without any effort . . . when you hear a voice that says: [pause] "I'll support you now—it's your turn."

This is a classic Hakomi experiment, in this case a verbal probe. As with many such experiments in Hakomi, the words are put in a theoretically positive form, but are specifically designed to contradict the client's core organizing beliefs. The possibility of support is precisely what has been organized out of this client's experience. If the therapist's hypothesis is correct, it is expected that the experiment will immediately elicit the person's barriers to allowing in the possibility of support, which in turn can be mindfully explored for what the client needs in order to moderate and discriminate situations, or, as Freud put it, enable the person to see new situations as new.

However, if the therapist simply said to the client in ordinary consciousness, "I'll support you now—it's your turn," none of these hoped-for results would be likely since such consciousness is already organized, working unconsciously on automatic. It is only the explicit instructions that lead the client into a mindful state that slows down and suspends theories and judgments in favor of simply bringing bare attention to what is, that allows for distancing from what was subject and making it object.

In conveying the instructions for the mindful experiment, the therapist is careful to model the state being requested by softening his own voice, slowing down his words, and embodying an open, curious, experimental attitude in his inflections.

> C: [Opens eyes.] I really don't know about this whole direction. I mean, come on, I work with people as a coach. I'm all about needs and support. I'm a professional supporter. Good thing I don't work with athletes—they'd call me an "athletic supporter" [laughs]. [The client comes out of mindfulness, which effectively stops the

experiment. Entering into a mindful state of consciousness is entering into a mysterious place of receptiveness and not knowing, and this can be a strange and discomforting experience at first for those accustomed to knowing and being in control. Anxieties or defenses against such a move are predicable.]

T: Quick humor you have there, Mike. So you recognize that on one level you really do respect the whole idea of needing support and having needs. You're actually around these kinds of processes often in your life. Tell me more about how you coach. [The therapist intuits that Mike is not really safe or ready enough to release into deeply watching himself. Since the client has come out of mindfulness to regrasp his normal thinking and humor, the therapist decides not to call attention to the underlying fear, but to support the return to contact and relationship where the client is more comfortable, offering him the invitation to talk about his coaching in ordinary consciousness.]

C: [Relaxing a bit more and becoming animated, Mike enters into a dialogue for a few minutes about his work life and its importance, challenges, and impacts on the rest of his life. Here the therapist decides that it is important to develop a stronger and more connected relationship with the client before entering into the potentially powerful world of mindfully exploring his needs for support. He allows the client to be in the safety of his everyday strength, talking about what he knows well.]

T: So I'm understanding more of how you operate in your life, Mike. You're actually pretty good at picking up the needs of people around you, especially those who are close to you, and you get a lot out of helping out and helping people get what they want. It keeps striking me as we talk that most of what gets you engaged is helping others out. Makes me wonder whether you're "in the club" too. [After talking for a bit in a way that both affirms and normalizes the client's life, the therapist risks contacting the underlying theme again, this time in terms of being "in the club."]

C: What club is that?

T: The "my needs are important" or "let's all help each other" club. I get it that you're good with supporting those around you, but I'm guessing you don't spend that much time getting help or support from them[?] [The therapist once again gently returns to the underlying theme. He is not pushing an interpretation, but hoping to get enough collaborative agreement on the issue that there is a license to move toward mindfully exploring it.]

C: Hmm, you know, I just don't really feel like I need that much. It just doesn't really come up—you're saying something's up with that, aren't you? Like that old Groucho Marx line, "I wouldn't want to join any club that would have me as a member." [Here the client names his every day emotional truth that he is not aware of needing much.]

T: That line pops up, huh—stay with it a little, and when you're ready, tell me more.

"Stay with it a little" is an accessing directive that encourages the client to maintain mindful attention to this piece of his experience, and not automatically skip to the next thought as is normal in ordinary consciousness. Likewise, "when you're ready" is a phrase that implies there is more luxurious, slower, exploratory, spacious time available here than is the case in everyday conversation.

C: It's weird—that line keeps pinging around in my head. [The client is able to witness his internal experience and name it as "pinging" even as other parts of him experience the strangeness of the process.]

T: Tell you what—let's do a little experiment to make it easier for you to deal with the pinging. Close your eyes and just watch. I'll say that statement back to you and you just notice anything that happens in you. [The therapist understands that the pinging phrase has spontaneously emerged. Though it could be considered a defensive or protective emergence, the therapist considers it an organic expression of how the client is organized, something with wisdom that can and should be supported.]

C: Okay. [The client expresses a calmer readiness to experiment.]

T: [Pause] . . . "I wouldn't want to join any club that would have me as a member." [He repeats it again, and then a third time in brief succession. This is a classic Hakomi taking-over experiment where the therapist does for the person what he is already doing for himself (repeating phrases in the head), with the assumption that supporting, as opposed to confronting, defenses provides the safety that enables the client's consciousness to go to a deeper level.]

C: It's funny, I get a little uncomfortable—and then I remember that duck that used to come down during that old Groucho Marx show. What was the name of that show? [The process deepens into a sense of uncomfortableness that has promise, and the more mysterious duck association is evoked.]

T: Yeah, I remember that show—don't remember the name though. Kind of two things come up for you, this slight discomfort and then the idea of the TV show. Can you still feel this uncomfortableness? [The therapist contacts both elements of the client's experience, but decides to go with the uncomfortable sense. While it is an artificial, though informed, decision, the therapist also knows if it is somehow off that he will be able to track signs of that, contact it, and the process will self-correct.]

C: If I focus on it I do. [The "if" indicates a measure of the client's ongoing ambivalence about staying with internal experience.]

T: Just stay with it. [The therapist judges that the ambivalence is not so strong that it needs specific attention and uses another accessing directive for the client to stay with the uncomfortableness. Again, he assumes that if something important is being overridden, it will show up in a way that can be tracked, contacted, and included as necessary.]

C: [Seems to move a little deeper. Therapist tracks nonverbal clues related to mindful state of consciousness.]

T: That's it. Keep turning toward it. [Contacting the client's progress in turning awareness inward toward felt present experience. The accessing directive to stay with the process is more necessary now with a new client than it might be later.]

C: I don't know what it relates to. It's just this little anxiousness.

T: Don't worry about the meaning right now. Just keep sensing your experience. [The therapist again assists the client to understand that mindfulness involves suspending analyses in favor of bare attention to present-moment experience.]

C: [Gets more deeply quiet. Therapist continues to track bodily signs of mindful state.]

T: Does it have a quality of familiarity? [Here the therapist begins to work the mind-body interface. Now that he judges the client has an embodied felt sense of the issue, he moves the process toward meaning by inquiring about familiarity, which might connect with past memories.]

C: Yes, it is familiar. Now I get that I felt the same sensation earlier, when you said that other statement to me. So what are we talking about here? Do you think—uh? [Client mindfully accesses the connection to previous probe, and immediately pops into ordinary consciousness.]

T: Don't work hard to figure it out or make sense of it. We'll just experiment while you stay in touch with that vague sense, and see what it connects to. [The therapist continues to manage consciousness by supporting the client to stay with present experience.]

C: [Nods. The client is increasingly trusting the therapist and process.]

T: Just be quietly watching again, both that sense . . . and for anything else that occurs by itself. . . . You can let my voice be anybody's voice. Notice what happens when you hear a voice that says, [pause] "I'll support you—it's your turn." [He returns to the earlier experiment of the verbal probe. Often clients get additional information when a probe is repeated after further calming, receptiveness, and processing of their initial reactions.]

C: HAH—that's bull! [The client reacts strongly through fusing or blending with the part, as opposed to witnessing it and reporting on it while being present to it.]

T: Strong response[!?] How does that happen for you? Is it a voice in your head, or a sensation that tells you it's bull, or a feeling? . . .

The therapist asks the client to deepen mindfulness through noticing how this reaction happens. The result sought is not acting out the response or talking about the response as a past event, but being present to it and commenting on it without losing the experiential connection.

The accessing questions all have a right-brain form, in that they require the client to reference his experience to check whether it is congruent with the suggestion or not. Thus, the answers to the questions are not as important as their function to keep the client in present-moment awareness longer, which allows the process to deepen. The question list keeps the exploratory field open to many forms of experiencing, as opposed to narrowing the options by asking, "How does it feel?" By ending the list with an implied open-ended "or whatever . . ." the therapist communicates that what is important is the client's own curiosity and discovery.

C: I don't know—what—ask me again. . . . [Spontaneously emergent affect often pushes clients beyond curiosity to being startled, or evokes the issue of allowing out-of-control material to arise.]

T: Don't worry about answering it. Just go back in, and I'll say the same thing again, and you just watch your response again. Notice what happens this time . . . letting any response be okay . . . when you hear: [pause] "I'll support you—it's your turn." [The therapist guides the client back to present experience. The calmness of the therapist communicates trust in the process, that everything that arises has organic wisdom and has a place, and that, again, there is someone present to help. The client does not have to do it all by himself. The therapist is also continuously coming back to one of the most important aspects of mindfulness, namely slowing down.]

C: I hear it in my head—"bull!" . . . and my chest gets tight right in the center. [Here the client offers a truly mindful account that comes from being present to his experience, witnessing it, and reporting on it while maintaining the connection.]

T: You can sense how some place inside you doesn't believe the support at all, huh? [The therapist contacts the barrier to support with the implied suggestion that this could be the next focus in this ongoing curious exploration that is deepening toward core material.]

C: Yeah, man, that's strange, and surprising. Uh, can I open my eyes for a minute? [The client seems to struggle with the strength of his internal response.]

T: Yes, you can open your eyes. We can take some time and talk about how this all happens inside you. [The therapist tracks the struggle. A theoretical possibility here would be to invite mindfulness of what is "strange and surprising." However, the therapist senses that it is best to flow nonviolently with the client's need to open his eyes.]

We talk for a while about automatic behavior (indicators) and how they can relate to information and experience that is below the level of ordinary consciousness; how unconscious beliefs can be different, and sometimes even the opposite of conscious ideas and attitudes; and how sensing these usually unconscious automatic indicators and related information can be surprising and disorienting, best when related to in a space of open and gentle curiosity.

We then connect back to Mike's earlier developmental life, how his parents were basically loving and caring people but were both very busy and somewhat clueless about how to handle and support the high level of sensitivity that Mike was born with in his nervous system. We bridged this to how a child could easily develop the underlying sense of the world as unsupportive and lose confidence and belief in the world literally being there for him.

Mike began talking about the kind of strong self-reliance that he seemed to have and how he was both proud of it and felt constrained by it.

T: So, I'm wondering if you're okay with getting mindful again and checking with how you're responding inside to all the ideas we're generating together here. [The therapist tracks and senses that the integrative conversation in ordinary consciousness has now calmed down the client enough that he is ready again to return to present-moment experience. The therapist asks the client to study how he has organized around the integrative conversation that just occurred.]

C: I'm feeling a little excited and something—I don't know—maybe scared. This is coming together in a whole new way. I feel a little hot. [The client is able to notice and name the spectrum of what he is experiencing.]

T: Take your time. Just get used to being inside and sensing all of this. Don't so much worry about figuring it out or remembering it. Just stay present and have it, like getting used to anything new and unfamiliar. When you can, you can bring me along. [The therapist helps orient the client toward simply staying with present experience. Again, the therapist is modeling the calmness and trust that he is hoping to evoke in the client, thus helping modulate or regulate the client's affect and activation levels. In addition to slowing things down, the therapist asks to be brought along in the process when the client is able, thus allowing the client a new choice of not working alone.]

C: [Client is focused in a quiet way for a couple of minutes, then begins to talk in a slow reflective voice.] It's like a kind of clashing inside me—I can actually see how it fits that I'm good with other peoples' stuff, and don't ask for much back . . . or even think about it really . . . but when I think about that as not being okay with having needs, my head tells me that's nuts. . . . I don't know how to connect the dots.

T: I see that you work hard on trying to connect the dots of what's true here. It might be easier if we explore around for some more dots, and see if they start forming their own picture. [The therapist keeps it an interpersonal, collaborative, therapeutic bubble, while gently moving the client back toward intrapsychic contact with inner experience. The parallel process is maintained. The therapist continues to teach aspects of mindfulness by suggesting that it is not so much a matter of consciously imposing analytic order from above as allowing sometimes precognitive material to emerge effortlessly from below ordinary consciousness. This guidance is only possible because the therapist holds the client in the loving presence of unconditional regard that does not make the client wrong in any way for attempting to figure his experience out.]

T: Yeah, that's it. . . . Just settle into yourself, instead of trying to figure out what's true. . . . Let's go back to that same experiment, and explore some more of what happens in your experience. [The therapist continues to track present-moment experience in the client and contacts what he tracks. This provides a ball bearing that allows the work to progress. Though he is constantly following the client's experience and lead, he also takes charge through proposing experiments and offering directives.]

C: Okay. [The client continues to learn how to rest into trusting the process and implicit support.]

T: So, again, just keep your awareness turned back toward you. Find a place where you can just watch your experience, where any experience is okay, and notice what happens on its own when you hear a voice that says, [pause] "I'll support you—it's your turn." [The therapist maintains focus on the main accessing route that they have been working through repeating the experiment with the verbal probe. It can be tempting for more beginning-level therapists to switch to other experiments when the first attempts don't yield dramatic results.]

C: [Staying inside.] The same thing happens, a little softer but definitely there—the center of my chest tightens, and I hear this one word, "bull." [The client gains increasing facility with studying how he organizes his experience in relation to a particular input.]

T: Stay with it. Notice how the rest of you participates. [The therapist uses another accessing directive that helps broaden the focus to include a larger Gestalt. It is normally the case that an issue brings forth a particular holographic piece of the whole; a sensation, tension, gesture, posture, movement, feeling, attitude, dream, image, symbol, memory, or way of relating. When mindful attention is brought to this aspect of experience, it inevitably draws other threads to itself, which might or might not seem to cohere at the time but eventually reveal the entire creative fabric. Here the therapist makes a judgment that there is sufficient mindfulness of the threads (or dots) so far that it is possible to facilitate the process by asking how the rest of the client participates.]

C: The word faded. My chest relaxed a little but not all the way back, like it was still on guard.

T: I notice you're talking in the past tense. Are there parts of your response that stay or that you can still sense? [The therapist helps facilitate a fuller present-tense focus. A client can easily resort to reporting on past history, even if that history is just seconds previous.]

C: The "on guard" sensation is still here, and I feel something like mad or sad or something.

T: Don't push for anything. Just keep staying with the on-guard sense and the feeling sense. [The therapist helps support the client in staying present to a degree of "not knowing" and promotes nonviolence through cautioning against forcing or pushing for any particular result.] Is it okay to keep exploring this? [The therapist checks out the level of safety present.]

C: [Nods. Even if he feels safe to continue, the client has also received a message that the therapist is concerned for his safety and is ready to honor any hesitation. This helps build safety for the coming stages of the work.]

T: I'll help you explore these responses with as little effort as possible. This time I'll say the same words to you again, and then I'll step into your system and take over the job that these automatic responses are doing by doing those responses for you. You get just to watch where you go when I do the responses for you. Sound okay? [The therapist introduces concept of taking over in a simple way.]

C: Yes.

T: As part of this experiment, I'll be touching your chest a little right in the center to mimic the tension. We've talked about this before, but I want to make sure that's still okay with you. [The therapist engages in a collaborative way that asks for permission and underscores that the client is aware and in charge of the process at every step.]

C: Yeah, thanks, it is. [The client is becoming more accustomed to the therapeutic setting. The proposal that includes touching is a physical variation on the verbal taking over of the voice in the head earlier on. It is clear that the touch is in the service of the client's process. The therapist keeps tracking the client, of course, for any signs of overriding anxieties in the service of being cooperative. Though the process is okay, the client offers explicit thanks that the therapist carries concern for his safety.]

T: So, watch what happens, especially what is evoked spontaneously, when you hear a voice that says, [pause] "I'll support you—it's your turn." [The therapist simultaneously shifts to a position next to Mike, gently tightens the center of Mike's chest with his hand, and then whispers "bull"—a taking-over experiment of both a physical tension and an automatic voice. Since such a procedure is sometimes strange to begin with, which means it introduces some noise of its own into the process, the therapist repeats the experiment of saying the probe and taking over the automatic response two more times while inviting the client to mindfully watch.]

C: [Head dropping forward.] I feel really sad, and tired, man, really tired. [The taking over has been effective in that keeping the normal protection of the client's defenses in place has allowed the client to drop down into the vulnerability protected against underneath.]

T: Goes right to your core. It's okay, man, just let it have you. [The therapist contacts the client's deep experience and offers a reassuring accessing directive that it is okay to enter fully into the experience.]

C: Oh God, man, I'm just so tired of doing everything alone. I just wish someone would help me, for Chrissakes. [Here the client crosses the nourishment barrier from defending against his own need for support to risking letting himself feel it. This is what was protected from consciousness by the automatic habitual chest tightening and the rebuttal voice.]

T: I won't leave you alone here, Mike. Just take your time and get used to feeling this need again. It's been a long time. [The therapist demonstrates deep limbic resonance as he contacts the client's present experience, supporting and stabilizing it.]

C: I feel relieved and sad and good and scared all at the same time. [The client experiences, observes, and names his truth in a mindful way.]

T: You can feel how big a thing this is even though it's happening in a quiet way. It feels totally natural to me. [The therapist stays in supportive contact with the client's unfolding in a way that normalizes it.]

T: Just let your system get used to this, Mike. Don't push through anything. Your whole system knows how to process this at its own rate. Just stay here with yourself and with me. [The therapist uses contact and gently offered support in the service of allowing the organic healing to continue and to stabilize.]

C: I'm not going to go right out onto some street corner with a "help me" sign in the immediate future, but it feels really good right now here with you, like I'm not on my own. [The client begins to make some integrative connections between his historical truth that sometimes people did not support him, and his immediate truth that sometimes some people in some situations can support him.]

T: There's a natural pull to map this into the way you live outside of here, and, ultimately, that's the point. We can talk about this in a little while if you like. Right now, to whatever degree it's okay, just savor the relief you feel a little longer, the feeling of not being on your own and that there's some help around. [The therapist is concerned that bridging into integrative analysis at this point might prematurely interfere with the client taking in the new experience and information at a felt-sense level. He guides the client back to accommodating the new possibility.]

C: [Stays present to the felt sense of his new experience.]

T: Kind of finishing in there, it looks like. [He tracks and contacts signs of client beginning to come back into ordinary consciousness.]

C: Yeah, I'm starting to come back out.

T: Tell you what—you just finish at your own pace and I'll talk to you a little bit as you do. [The therapist actively seeks to integrate the client's experience and hinted-at confusion, so that he can complete his process by not working too hard, and by learning to rest into the support of others, namely the therapist at this point. He invites the client into that in-between space of savoring new experience while also allowing the left brain to start weaving new meaning into its ongoing narrative.]

T: I agree that this experience doesn't cancel out all the experience and learning in your earlier life that led you to decide that there wasn't much support available so you better learn to be on your own. The difference is that up till now, this whole level of little automatic habitual behaviors that run underneath the surface of your awareness has managed your conscious experience so that you no longer even sense your wish and need for support and to not be always on your own. At this moment, you're off automatic, and you can actually feel and sense the way you also really want to be interconnected, giving and receiving support. In some way, this is the first chance in a long time you have to actually explore whether there's more support available in the world you live in now than in the world you originally developed your beliefs in, because now you can again sense and feel that it's important to you. Without sensing the need or desire, there's no drive to explore or fill it. In a way, maybe it's like now the world can possibly have another chance with you. [The therapist is cocreating a narrative that links experience, meaning, and body sense as an integrating tool. Neural networks are integrated—prefrontal, limbic, and posterior.]

C: My head's back online, thinking about where I might check this out in my life, and how to go about it. I don't want to lose it. [The client is completing and returning to an external-world focus, and he is expressing the value of the process and the desire to integrate it in his everyday life.]

T: I really welcome your mind to chew on this and help check out what's available now. We can do some more experiential exploration of this edge in you as we work together, and we can also look at ways to explore this in your family, work, and the rest of the world around you.

C: Thanks, man.

T: Yeah, me too. [The therapist is genuinely touched by engagement in the healing process of this other who is not completely other. The informal language and exchange supports the normalization of the therapy.]

Working With a Veteran and His Family

Greg Johanson

The first two case verbatims here are individual sessions with a wife and husband who both participate in a veteran's program offered by a church-related mental health center with state and county funding.[1] The program offers therapy groups for veterans, support groups for spouse-partners, individual sessions for each, and couples sessions. In this example the vet, Ben, chooses to work on issues in individual sessions because he feels he would have to contain himself too much in a couples session with a nonvet, which is common. However, he is happy for his wife, Trish, to get individual support.

Though both husband and wife are active people by nature, and have never been part of a contemplative tradition, they are relatively easy to work with since they are competent, aware, willing to look at themselves as opposed to blaming the outer world, dedicated to their family, and highly motivated by the effects of the PTSD they experience working on their life together.

Wife, Trish

C: So, I'm really struggling with Ben's wanting to go with me and the kids, alone or separately, wherever we go. It felt, like, caring and protective when he first got home from the deployment. Now it's starting to feel smothering or something. I can feel some angry part of me getting touched. But I don't want to push him away and get him activated, and make him feel like we don't want him. And he is also a bit angry and distant with Ed [four-year-old son]; kind of ordering him around instead of being warm in his communications. [The client is telling the story with appropriate affect in ordinary consciousness.]

T: Okay. So I'd probably need to continue to deal with Ben directly about what's up with Ed. On the smothering thing, it sounds reasonable to feel hemmed in when you are so used to being self-reliant with him away. But you are saying it feels like something in you is cranking up your reaction beyond what might be normal[?] [Sorting out issues in story, and working to collaborate on where the session might focus.]

C: Yeah, it feels like some kind of fire that is ready to react to provocation, even before there is any. [Client is taking responsibility for her part in the couple's interaction

1. Verbatim material was previously published by G. Johanson in two articles: Creative struggling, *Somatic Psychotherapy Today*, 1(2), 2011, pp. 37–38; Mindfulness, emotions, and the organization of experience, *USA Body Psychotherapy Journal*, 10(1), 2011, pp. 38–57.

and expressing a willingness to explore it, knowing Ben is doing the same in his own therapy sessions.]

T: So, exploring more deeply this part of you that is ready to feed the fire seems good, huh? [Proposing an agenda that seems to be where the client's curiosity is. The "huh?" communicates that the therapist is not attached to the agenda and is willing to be corrected or have the proposal be fine-tuned.]

C: Yeah. Let's. I don't want to get into something that ends up being more ugly than it needs to be. [Minicontract confirmed.]

T: Good. Okay. There are a number of ways to get into this. How about you imagine the last time Ben came along that seemed a bit much, and we can slow down and study what that was like for you? [This is an invitation to switch states of consciousness into mindfulness that is fairly brief and straightforward since it is the fourth session and the client has already been exposed to the process.]

C: [Trish closes her eyes, slows down, turns her awareness inward toward her felt present experience. Almost immediately her shoulders shake, and she shows emotion in face and voice.] Oh, it was yucky! But I didn't let myself express it like here. [While the client is observing and reporting her experience, it seems she is fairly fused or blended with the yucky part and doesn't have much distance.]

T: So just remembering that last time is pretty activating, huh? [Tracks for nonverbal assent to contact statement.] How about we get a little more distance on the issue by just imagining you will be calling down the hall to let Ben know you are going out, anticipating he will say, "Oh, I'll come too." But before you actually call, stop and be a witness to whatever is evoked in you prior to calling. As you anticipate his response, notice what comes up for you spontaneously, without you forcing anything—any sensations, muscle tensions, feelings, attitudes, thoughts, memories . . . [?] [The therapist attempts to modulate the energy level by evoking enough of a signal to guide the process, but not so much that the person becomes the emotion as opposed to being present to it. More specific suggestions are offered to support a mindful state of consciousness. Notice the therapist does not limit the study of experience to affect alone, but broadens the range of possibilities.]

C: The anticipation would be more like, "Don't leave! I'll be right there." [It is a good sign for a client to fine-tune the words or process. It is an indication she is immersed in and listening closely to her experience.]

T: Great. Anticipate the "Don't leave!" and study closely what it evokes in you. [The word "study" supports mindfulness in that it invites Trish to be present to her concrete, felt experience, but also a step back where she can notice and be curious about it, as opposed to simply being swept along by it. It is a middle position between talking about her feelings or simply acting them out.]

C: I notice some sense of resentment with my cheeks and arms warmed up, almost hot, but I'm clamped down and feel tension in my face and arm muscles. [Good witnessing by the client, who is both present to her experience and able to comment on it from the position of an observer.]

T: Uh huh. Maybe if you just hang out with the resentment, and be curious about it, you will sense more about it, or it will tell you more about itself[?] [Now that Trish has been invited into a mindful space, the therapist encourages staying in the state longer and deepening into present experience with trust in the organic impulse to unfold toward greater wholeness or complexity.]

C: It seems to be muttering something about "unfair" between clenched teeth, but afraid to really be heard. [More threads or context gather magnetically around the original report of anger as the experiential spaciousness of the mindful process allows the unconscious to lead more deeply into unhealed constraints.]

T: Like really in a bind[?] [A simple contact statement addressed to the present experience facilitates the deepening of the process.]

C: [More emotional, with a younger quality to her voice.] Yeah, like her father loves her but won't let her go play with the other bigger kids, and she is really mad, but can't say so because he is really strict and will punish her right there in front of the other kids, and she would really be embarrassed! [Process spontaneously deepens into a memory.]

T: Oh, a memory comes up. How old does she seem to be? [Contacting details like age helps stabilize the memory, and referring to "she" as opposed to "you" helps maintain the witnessing position. At this point the process has gone from becoming mindful of some aspect of creation—the anger—and has descended close to the level of creation, the memory that informs a core belief about not being able to be liberated to explore in freedom or express displeasure about not being able.]

C: Four, maybe five. [More processing, deepening and stabilizing the memory.]

T: As you simply view the four- or five-year-old from your position of compassionate awareness, what do you sense that she most needs that she is not getting in her situation[?] [Therapist invites both witnessing and compassionate aspects of the client's larger self-state.]

C: She needs to know that it is unfair for her dad to limit her and overprotect her, and then scare her into not even being able to express her feelings about it. And . . . she needs to know, to know, uh . . . it won't be this way forever . . . that sometimes people in power do try to hold you back, . . . that's true, . . . but . . . that there will be times when she finds the freedom to use all her strengths and energies without being held back. [Here the empty, nonagenda space of compassionate awareness releases itself to the situation of the inner child and receives some relevant psychological-emotional information. The slowness and space between realizations is an indicator of a mindful process.]

T: Yes. So go ahead and communicate that to her in any verbal and nonverbal ways that seem right, perhaps having her look in your eyes so she really gets your presence, and check whether she is taking it in or not. [A therapeutic directive that invites her to take the awareness and loving presence of her essential self-state and apply it interpersonally to this inner child, thus, as Daniel Siegel puts it, helping her mindfully become a friend to herself.]

C: Yes, she is getting it. But it is a new thought to get used to, kind of fragile. [Acknowledging both the transformation of organizing in new information previously organized out, as well as the fragility of the process that will need more integration.]

T: That's really important to follow up and keep integrating to foster this new neural network. In particular, ask her if she is willing to have a conversation with you when you go home, directly or through journaling, about how to have a talk with Ben that acknowledges both your knowledge of his care and your need for freedom to use your own strengths. [A directive to help foster this intrapsychic relationship, so the internalized object of the inner child and her larger self-state can dyadically regulate the affect that gets stirred up in these situations with the husband, as well as other situations.]

C: Yes, she wants that . . . and needs that . . . to keep from going into that suppressed rage, and to know more about what is really possible. [Relationship is reinforced, which is an element of integration.]

T: You can really help her grow into a new future by experimenting with this new possibility of freedom in relation to real situations. And do you feel you will be able to have a little distance on the anger when it arises in situations like with Ben, so that it doesn't completely take over and blend and fuse with you? [Reinforcing compassionate intrapsychic relationship and checking for distancing or decentering aspect of mindfulness.]

C: Yes, I think I'm much clearer now about what the anger and fear and holding are about, and if it comes up too hard, too fast, like with Ben, I'll be able to ask for a time-out before we talk more, so I can sit, check with the young one, and get more distance and centeredness before sorting things out with him. I'm not quite clear about what is going on with Ben, but I have a more relaxed sense of compassion for what is going on with me. [Starting to complete and move back into ordinary consciousness.]

T: Awareness and compassion are an ongoing practice we keep learning from. Good luck with this one.

Reflection

Internalized objects such as "self-narratives using stories about experienced events" (Bons-Storm, 1996, p. 437) or inner children frozen in time are ultimately illusion, basically a way of organizing energy and information (Eisman, 1989). To simply allow their manifestations to come into awareness and pass by like clouds in the sky, as in classic meditation practice, is a fine project that enhances spaciousness (Roberts, 2009) and does not give them undue importance and reality. However, when their clouds come continuously into the sky over time and affect the organization of one's experience in the world in unconscious ways, perhaps a little compassion can be helpful in the overall quest to not be at the mercy of unconscious core organizers.

Adding the active elements of compassion to the passive element of the bare attention of awareness can help heal the fragmented ego appreciated in the West. Staying with the practice of simply watching experience arise and move by can help progress toward the unity consciousness esteemed in Eastern psychology. There can be a bridge here, with no need for a false forced choice. Thich Nhat Hahn, the eminent teacher of mindfulness and peace, could come upon a Japanese soldier in the jungle and teach him the value of a witnessing form of meditation. He could also have the active compassion to let the soldier know that the war is over.

Husband, Ben

T: Hey, good to see you. [Promoting positive affect and transference, nourishment, secure attachment, and what Fosha refers to as not just seeking a new ending but also seeking a new beginning.]

C: Uh huh. And what is so good about it? [Trusts therapist enough to challenge—a return greeting in ordinary consciousness.]

T: [Smiling and making eye contact.] Oh, you know. No good reason really. Well, maybe your engaging smile, your dedication to your family, your persistence, your loyalty. Not your good looks, for sure. Well, actually, you are skinnier than me. I wouldn't even be able to deploy. [An attempt at integrating humor into the process. If people are at least cocreators of the meaning of their lives, then the creativity they use to organize their experience in one way is still available to help reorganize it in a new way. Humor affirms this capacity, which would not be appropriate with someone who was an absolute "victim" or "sick." Also an example of the use of self-disclosure (Prenn, 2009).]

C: [Laughs.] Hey, you can be skinny too. Want to join me each morning for a 10-mile run? [Appropriate rejoinder reflecting decent therapeutic alliance, a lot of mutuality, though still asymmetrical. It is important that clients know the therapist appreciates them in their strengths as well as their vulnerabilities.]

T: Pass. Although I am working out a lot. I can now do three laps around the car without needing an oxygen tank! So what is going on that it is not so good to see you today? [Transition from initial nourishing small talk and contact to issues at hand. Important that positive exchanges never gloss over the truth of present experience.]

C: Still having a hard time just relaxing with Ed. End up ordering him round, like I'm trying to whip him into shape or something. Geez! The kid is barely four, and it feels like I'm an E9 [sergeant major]. But the most distressing thing is that I was walking around the village when Trish and Ed were in church; fairly relaxed, taking in the green, starting to feel that maybe I was in a relaxing place when a car backfired and I hit the deck! Jumped back up really quick, but really embarrassing and I haven't been back in town since. [PTSD symptoms: exaggerated startle response, sense of reliving trauma experience, significant social stress, avoiding activities and places.]

T: Wow! Lower brain just took over. Yeah, very disturbing. [Contacting present experience in a way that validates the event. This is the 10th session, and the therapist has been sharing some physiological information with Ben that helps him feel that his reactions are in the ordinary realm in terms of what he has been through, and that it is known, recognizable, and workable.]

C: Seriously. How can I function in the world and think about getting an ordinary job? [More symptoms of detachment, estrangement from the world, and poor sense of future possibilities.]

T: So, just remembering the backfire is activating. Let's stand up together and do some resourcing. Stand in that [baseball] short-stop stance, feel the ground under your feet. . . . Feel the flexibility in your knees. . . . Rock right and left a little bit. Notice the transition between the two. . . . Notice your strength and readiness to do what needs to be done. . . . Put your hand on your lower stomach and breathe into it on the in breath, and make your hand move out. . . . Can you feel your hand there? What tells you it is there? . . . Just notice whatever other signals you are getting from your body. [Because the activation levels are taking the client in a hyperaroused state beyond his window of tolerance, the therapist abandons verbal, top-down processing that could risk setting off a trauma vortex. The client allows him to become very directive, concentrating on the body instead of emotions, since they have done resourcing together before. The therapist does encourage mindfulness of body signals. The instruction to "just notice whatever other signals" is a more general invitation to mindfulness. The therapist is exploring how resourced the client is in relation to being present to experience from the theoretically more safe distancing place of mindfulness.]

C: I feel like I'm on lookout. [The physically ready stance is resourcing but evokes the memory of serving as a lookout.]

T: Yeah, looks like your head is rotating a bit, bobbing and weaving slightly, like you are really vigilant. [Therapist contacts the experience but is a bit worried about not wanting to throw the client back into a traumatizing memory that would overwhelm him.]

C: I can sense my eyes are tightened and squinting. It feels like when I was big into R&S [reconnaissance and surveillance]. I was always good at the Avoid Ambush drills and did a lot of gap work [lining out safe passages through minefields]. [Client is on the dynamic edge of being able to mindfully witness his sensations and tensions, and being in danger of getting flooded and fused with traumatic memories. Kurtz often noted that learning happens on the edge between order and chaos, and the therapist attempts to track the balance here.]

T: Let's just bring your awareness and curiosity to the eyes alone, to the tightening—not what it means, but just study it in terms of muscular tension alone and notice what happens. . . . Report on your experience without coming out of it, and tell me about it. [Therapist feels things are too volatile and chooses to employ what Ogden calls "directed mindfulness," directing mindfulness to lower brain-generated sensations decoupled from emotion, stories, and so on. Reporting without "coming out of it" to tell the therapist about it is a helpful directive for keeping the client's mindful focus on the unfolding of internal experience, which is interrupted when he feels he has to come back to the normally expected realm of interpersonal discourse to report.]

C: As I pay attention to the tightness, it seems to loosen up. . . . Now I'm noticing some kind of fear in my gut. [The process unfolds in this mindful state, with one thing becoming connected to another that fleshes out this procedural tendency.]

T: So, let's pay attention to the fear in the gut simply on a sensation level and follow it wherever it goes. [Continued use of directed mindfulness of sensorimotor processing. The "we" language of "let's pay attention" supports both secure attachment and the dynamic of there always being an interpersonal process parallel to the intrapsychic exploration mindfulness often encourages.]

C: The fear sensation seems to travel up into the throat . . . where it clamps . . . down . . . or clumps up . . . kind of like a ball. [Good witnessing that serves to self-regulate instant, out-of-control fear and maintain a curious, open stance toward it.]

T: I'm just guessing, but it seems like the sensation wants to move, and there is some other part of you that wants to block it for some good reason we don't know right now. How about we experiment with you holding this pillow to your face and mouth and allow it to be the part that is clumping up the movement of the sensation? Don't force anything, but just hold it there and notice what arises spontaneously. [This is an example of a taking-over technique from Kurtz, who finds that when a defense is supported in the state in which it naturally arises, it paradoxically allows the process to go forward. The word "experiment" underscores an experimental attitude that underlies mindful work, which lends itself to more curiosity and allowing, as opposed to forcing or engineering. It fosters the attitude that whatever is evoked in the process is fine and natural and becomes ongoing grist for further processing. Likewise, the phrase "I'm just guessing" makes it crystal clear the client needs to go with the truth of his experience and feel free to ignore the therapist's guess if it is not accurate.]

C: Uh, okay. [Holds pillow close to mouth.] . . . Oh! [Shows signs of increasing agitation. . . . Holds pillow forcefully toward mouth so the sound is quite muffled while screaming into it repeatedly in rhythm with rocking motions of head down and up.] [Spontaneous occurrences such as this that are not the result of directives are usually trustworthy. The pillow muffling the sound has apparently worked in taking over the function of some part of Ben that didn't want people hearing him yelling.]

T: Okay, keep screaming as long as it feels good, feels right. [We are working not with a hydraulic-expressive model here but with an information-processing one, so the therapist is not encouraging simple catharsis or emptying. But tracking pleasure in terms of what feels good, right, or satisfying is often a good indicator of completing some action tendency that has been thwarted.]

C: [Finishes screaming in a semiexhausted but seemingly good state.] Oh man! I got it . . . whew . . . both parts [more heavy breathing, catching breath]. . . . The scream is "Get out! Get out!" I'm so tense being responsible for my men, worrying about their welfare, worrying I'm going to have to call some wife and give her the most shocking f-ing news of her life, and this is no place to be. They need to get out of there, get out of danger. The pillow is duty, mission. [Core Army values—never abandon the mission. The wonderful result of encouraging a mindful, curious process is that clients end up interpreting for themselves, which often allows the therapist to follow more than lead.]

T: Whoa. Yeah. You nailed it. How horrendous being responsible for life and death. No wonder you want to get them out of there. [Basic human confirmation.]

C: God yes! I think this is why I hesitate to go to church. I don't like this God business. [A spontaneous connection arises.]

T: Okay, so we need to check in more about doing God duty. Right now, check in on how your body is doing. Notice if there any other sensations or movement tendencies that are talking to you. [Therapist invites a search for other aspects of the mind-body that might be involved in this procedural tendency to be in hypervigilant duty mode.]

C: There is energy in my legs for sure. [Good witnessing of what is there without slipping into overactivation.]

T: Sense into the energy and notice if it wants to mobilize you into any kind of movement. If so, slowly follow just the beginnings of the movement. [Here the therapist has a hunch and is entraining awareness toward movement, when energy can actually lead to other things as well.]

C: [Slowly, mindfully checks in with energy.] . . . Yeah, it wants to move the legs. . . . IT WANTS TO RUN!

T: Yeah! So in your imagination now, and also allowing your legs to move up and down as much as you want, yell to the squad to get out and *run!* No mission here! Nobody left behind! No reason to be here! Run! Run! Run! [We know from trauma work and recent research in neurobiology that the imagination can stimulate the same neural networks as in real life and can be used to complete action tendencies frozen in time. The instruction here takes into consideration the countermessage of the clumped-up throat that prevented the natural expression of screaming and running in the war zone.]

C: [Takes a few minutes to really get into the running away scene where he shepherds his men like a sheepdog, with his actual legs going up down rapidly while running in place and imagining. Finally collapses on floor in a good way and leans back against the sofa.] Oh, man! Oh, geez. I finally feel relaxed, like I don't have a foot on the gas and brake at the same time. [Natural result of an action tendency taking its course, and an implicit procedural tendency coming into cortical consciousness.]

T: Great. Very nice. So just sit back for awhile and savor what it is like to be in this state of relaxation. Notice in a curious, spacious way what is different in your sensations, tensions, feelings, attitudes, whatever. [Important to savor and integrate the new experience. A large part of mindful processing is simply slowing things down.]

C: [Follows instruction in a slow, mindful way.] . . . I really like looking around with my eyes in a soft way that takes in more information actually than when they are tense and seriously focused.

T: So, from this relaxed state, I would like you to experiment with inviting the on-duty sergeant you that is mobilized to be on mission and worried about his men to come into view. Let me know when you have some kind of visual image or bodily sense that he has come into view. [This is an example of the distancing-while-still-being-present aspect of mindfulness. Saying "visual image or bodily sense" makes room for those who don't get visual images easily.]

C: Okay. He is front and center.

T: Good. So, check if you are in that place of compassionate awareness that can express to him some gratitude and thanksgiving that he can go on this impossible God duty where he takes on a mission while carrying all this concern for his men and just wants to get them out of there. And if you are in that space with him, notice if he can take in the appreciation.

This type of mindful therapy is never about exorcising or fighting against parts of one's internal ecology. Honoring or respecting the benevolent intent behind each part, as Richard Schwartz suggests, helps make each part a harmonious and coherent element of one's narrative.

The compassion of the client's larger self-state that can express appreciation to the God-duty warrior is not necessarily voting for such a position in our war-torn world. The qualifier "if you are in that space" makes room for parts of the client's inner family, team, squad, committee, or tribe to be present that might have objections to thanking the God-duty part, which would then need to be dealt with first.

Here the therapist suggests an interchange. Another option would be to ask the client to sense into what the God-duty part of him needs from him right now in terms of a response, and then offer it.

C: Yes, he is getting it. He appreciates the acknowledgment. [When any member of a team is acknowledged and respected for his or her concerns or perspective, the member tends to relax, trust the leader, and be willing to go along with the team's decision, even if it is not exactly what that member was advocating.]

T: Good. He is an important guy to call on when needed that not everyone has. What I would like us to do next is have you stand up again and slowly, mindfully go back and forth between three positions, really studying the minute differences that go into each position, until you can consciously move between them at will with your mind-body-spirit, which is different than when they just happen to you without your intention. The first is the "war zone God-duty on-mission worried about his squad" guy. There are appropriate times this guy needs to take over things. The second is you at home with your family, safe, behind closed doors, relaxed like you are now, in that place where you can enjoy them and allow them to enjoy you. The third is when you are out with your family in the village, where a little more assessment of danger is called for since you are no longer inside the safety of your home, but normally it is far, far from anything like a war zone. Okay?

Learning to take on these various positions voluntarily in terms of sensations, tensions, thoughts, feelings, attitudes, and so on does not take away the power of lower-brain activation to click in when stimulated by internal or external stimuli.

It does have an empowering effect on vets to do this differentiation practice that consciously reinforces and acknowledges realities such as, "Here I am in the city where cars backfire, vases fall off the ledge and crash, kids light firecrackers, and, yes, sometimes people use guns."

And it is helpful to give both permission and practice to take on the appropriate modes of mobilization for different situations. Being able to take these positions consciously helps enhance awareness and a sense of choice and empowerment, as well as an understanding that it is normal that cars backfiring can evoke startle responses. Going into the city streets with permission to have a measure of vigilance can mitigate the shock of a loud sound.

The session continued with a good amount of time spent integrating this ability to assess and mobilize appropriately and consciously.

Son, Ed (Group Session)

In Hakomi we emphasize that it is important to help clients become mindful in order to get distance on their experience, as opposed to being at the mercy of it. With clients such as Ben who are war veterans this can be problematic, since the bodies of vets can be so stressed from being hypervigilant, holding back impulses, uncompleted action tendencies (Ogden et al., 2006), and such. There is simply too much tension in the system to find that quiet place of consciousness that can be compassionately aware of how one is organized. This was Reich's (1949) main point, that tension or body armor masks sensitivity, and sometimes one does not want to be sensitive to certain signals that are causing distress.

Taking Over and Creative Struggling

Kurtz's taking-over technique called creative struggling (see Chapter 17) can be helpful here with lowering the noise level in the system. With veterans it often means helping them hold back tensions in such a way that they can safely explore them and release them. It is difficult to be both the one who tenses and the one who searches for the meaning of the tension at the same time.

Veterans are often terrified of the thought of becoming uncontained and hurting others, so creative struggling is best done in a group setting where enough physical power is available to provide a safe enough container that allows clients to explore their impulses and fully engage their musculature.

Since holding tensions is normally unconscious, the awareness of the client is focused on the body, and not on verbal meanings, which may or may not come later. What is creative in this process is that one is asked to struggle in a way that feels good, which serves to enjoin mindfulness of large motor muscle groups. The therapist's instructions are constantly directed toward what feels nourishing, right, and positive as opposed to any form of a struggle of wills, of force against force.

If one can struggle in a way that is satisfying on a bodily level, there is a welcome sense of release of tension, as in doing a satisfying stretch. The resultant reduction of stress feels good in itself on a physical level, so no harm has been done, and it often allows the spaciousness for internal emotional signals to arise that want attention.

Ben in Relation to Ed

Ben showed up for a vets' group feeling stressed and wound up, still dealing with his issues of deployment reentry as they affected his wife and four-year-old son.

C: I find myself mad at the kid, nervous about what he is doing, and ordering him around like a recruit. I hate it, but I keep doing it over and over again!

T: So it seems that you are wound pretty tight. How about we use the group to do a little creative struggling, and see where that leads us? [Here the therapist tracks the tension in Ben that interferes with mindfulness practice, and takes charge by suggesting the group exercise. It is nonviolent in the sense that the therapist is helping Ben go where he wants to go at the deepest levels, and it sends a signal of support that he is not totally on his own in his search for healing.]

C: Yeah, getting physical is good. [Ben has already had a taste of the physical satisfaction that this exercise can bring, and knows it is true that he is tense in a way that would make mindful exploration more difficult.]

T: Okay, so let's all stand up. You know the drill. Your buddies here can provide resistance for you in any way that feels right, that feels good. Notice if your body gives you any hunch about how we might start . . . or we can always just do something, and then check to see if it is right, or needs adjusting.

There is no standard protocol for how one should struggle. It is highly unique to each individual. By asking Ben to access what is pleasurable, even though it might involve great effort, the process touches bodily cellular information that is organizing the system and knows what it needs to deal with (Damasio, 1999).

Some participants want to struggle against a force in front of them, or behind them. Some want force coming down vertically on their shoulders that they can struggle up against. For some, it is being pulled in two different directions at once. And others want to move forward with resistance on their legs. It is all quite organic and unpredictable. So the group members who have been trained in this technique stand around and wait for Ben, who also knows the exercise from previous sessions, to give precise instructions.

C: It feels like I want to struggle against something in front of me.

T: Okay. So here is Ted providing resistance to both your right and left shoulders with his arms. Check that out and see if it is right or not.

C: It is close, but I think it would be better with his hands more in the middle of the chest. [It is a good sign that Ben is mindfully involved in the process and listening to the wisdom of his body to be able to fine-tune this adjustment, even though nobody knows what it might mean.]

T: Okay, let Ted do that. [Ted puts his hands more in the middle of Ben's chest, and then Ben moves them with his own hands to be more directly over his heart.]

T: So that is closer to what is needed, huh? Experiment with struggling against the hands now and notice if it feels resonant, or if something else is needed. [The therapist ensures the process is open ended and allows for the emerging wisdom of Ben's system, as opposed to making the exercise into some kind of predictable rote manipulations.]

C: There is something about the arms that needs something.

T: Oh. Would it be more like we could help you hold back from hitting, or hold back from reaching out . . . or . . . ? [Here the therapist introduces an open-ended list of possible moves that function to access Ben's right brain, since he has to check each possibility with his own experience to make a choice or come up with another alternative. Offering some concrete choices is often helpful as opposed to a more open inquiry like, "What do the arms need?"]

C: It is more reaching out.

T: Okay. You are a strong guy, so why don't we get two guys on each arm, and you direct them how it feels best to give you resistance. [Two guys on each arm provides the safety and security for Ben to explore without having to worry about becoming uncontained or hurting someone.]

C: Yeah, it is like I want to reach out, but am holding myself back, so maybe they can do the holding back as I try to move them forward.

T: Sure, let's do that. You adjust their holds so that it feels best, and let yourself move against the resistance when it feels right. [It is all a matter of listening to the wisdom of the body's large muscles in terms of what would feel pleasurable to them. The tensions they normally carry are cortically controlled and thus ultimately carry a sense of meaning.]

C: Oh, yes, this is good. Let me do this some more. [Ben struggles in a satisfying way. Four more vets are involved to provide resistance around both legs to help him feel more safe, more contained, and he finally quits struggling with some satisfying deep breaths, and shows some signs of collapse.]

T: Now it looks like your body wants to go the other way and lean against these guys. Is that okay to do that?

C: Yeah, that's good. Wow. Much more relaxed.

T: So, don't force anything, but just check to see what might be coming into your awareness.

C: It is a vision of my son . . . watching him in a park or something . . . and wanting to go and hug him . . . but holding back . . . struggling against reaching out.

T: [On a hunch.] So as you are hanging out there with that image, would it be okay if Ted put a hand back on your heart where you had it before? [While Hakomi therapists are trained to follow organic impulses within the client, it is okay for them to introduce their own intuitions as well, as long as they are willing to be unattached and deal with what actually arises.]

C: Yeah, that would be good. [Ted puts his hand back on Ben's heart, who adjusts it slightly, while two other vets are supporting Ben from both sides. Therapist and group stand with Ben in silent support and allow his unconscious to lead him where he needs to go. Emotion wells up in Ben's face all of a sudden and he covers his face with both hands. The two vets on each side provide increased support by putting their hands over his.]

C: He could die! The bastard could die! [The other vets nod their heads in the common knowledge that one they love today could be killed in the next moment or next day, and sometimes they just have to steel themselves against caring too much.]

T: Oh, so letting your heart go out to the little guy fully could leave you open to catastrophic heart-wrenching grief, huh?

C: I don't know if I could bear it. I'd die or go crazy. . . . But I don't want to live numb and cheat him out of a father. . . .

The rest of the session dealt with Ben's, and everyone else's in the group, profound and natural ambivalence about being vulnerable to love. The path to this core issue in Ben was facilitated by the body wisdom embedded in the creative struggling exercise that lowered his stress and tension enough to allow his issue to arise into consciousness.

One of the profound advantages of group work here is that Ben now has a built-in support group of brothers and sisters who know, understand, and support him in his life pilgrimage.

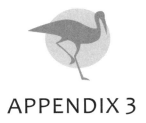

APPENDIX 3

Hakomi in Context: The Large Picture in History and Research

Historical Context

Halko Weiss and Greg Johanson

HAKOMI THERAPY IS a principled and unique approach to human healing and growth that integrates, among other things, mindfulness, the mind-body interface, and nonviolence. It is a paradoxically powerful approach, applicable to both brief and long-term therapy, which participates in the ingenious Eastern principle of nondoing as it applies to trusting the unfolding of living organic systems toward health and healing. It is taught internationally through the faculty of the Hakomi Institute and the Hakomi Educational Network. Since the inception of the Hakomi Institute in 1980, thousands of students have been trained in workshops and comprehensive training courses by a faculty of some 50 worldwide certified trainers and teachers.

The basic Hakomi texts by Kurtz (1990a), Johanson and Kurtz (1991), Fisher (2002), Kurtz and Prestera (1976), and Benz and Weiss (1989) all reflect the clinical wisdom and approach of the Hakomi method—which integrates many sources as well as adding its own unique contributions. However, these volumes do not enter into extensive dialogue with the wider psychotherapeutic tradition. Thus, the current volume is an edited work of international Hakomi faculty members that maps and references the Hakomi approach into the contemporary world of psychology and science. It represents a coherent source of knowledge of how and what is currently taught through the Hakomi Institute.

Practitioners who participate in Hakomi training report there is a unique feel, style, and substance to it that fosters both personal and professional growth in an accepting and creative crucible of learning. However, it is not easy to articulate this uniqueness as it integrates the art and science, the spontaneous and linear aspects of therapeutic processes, weaving in a number of elements held in common with other schools. Perhaps a brief overview of the history of Hakomi can provide some contextual understanding. Though the field of psychology tends to be ahistorical, it is clear that the Hakomi method is a child of its time, arising from a multiplicity of dispositions in its day, which in turn was an emergent product of all that had gone before it (Barratt, 2010; Heller, 2012; Young, 2010).

The World of Psychotherapy

In the 1970s, when eventual Hakomi students and trainers were attracted to Ron Kurtz doing workshops following the publication of his book *The Body Reveals* (with Prestera, 1976), the field of academic and traditional psychological counseling was a mixed bag of promise and disenchantment.

For all the early promise of psychology from the beginning of the 20th century on, the field was no longer looked to by many for answers to humanity's pressing problems of war, violence, economic and cultural disparity, overpopulation, global warming, and such. Mental health specialists were largely on the sidelines during the 1960s in relation to cultural-social issues, outside of advocating for better or more humane treatment of the mentally ill. People intuitively gravitated to novelists more than psychologists to learn what it means to be human (LeShan, 1990).

Much of psychology seemed immersed in an unsuitable endeavor to mimic the physical sciences through attempting to reduce human interactions to quantifiable mechanical interactions that shed little light on actual clinical predicaments (LeShan & Margenau, 1982). In terms of prediction, for instance, LeShan asks, who could pretend to know what Beethoven's Ninth Symphony would be like, even with infinite knowledge of its eight forerunners?

> Human beings are non-predictable in principle. Only papier-mache characters can be predicted. We can make 100 percent accurate predictions that Tom Swift, Tarzan, and James Bond will emerge triumphant from their next adventure, not so for Captain Cook, Al Capone, or Albert Einstein. (1990, p. 56)

To say someone has a one-in-six chance of committing suicide in the next six months is not particularly helpful, since either committing the act or not committing it supports the same prediction (LeShan, 1990). Likewise, statistical analysis of large groups did not shed much light on the individual seeking consultation whose consciousness was not average, quantifiable, or repeatable. And objective situations alone (the stimulus) can rarely predict individual behavior (the response) because the situation is always dependent on one's subjective appropriation of it—which anthropologists teach is highly affected by our cultural-social context.

> Human nature differs to a very considerable extent from place to place and time to time. A Hopi sheepherder, a knight of the First Crusade, a 1980 Wall Street broker, and laboratory psychologist live in different worlds with different definitions of space, time, and honor, different life goals, different views of love and the meaning of death. . . .
>
> [Certainly,] we need different languages for different realms. . . . The "energies" in an electrical battery, a painting by Picasso, an angry crowd, and my hopes for the future are entirely different kinds of meanings and terms. The same word, used in different realms of experience, means something entirely different. (LeShan, 1990, pp. 60, 93)

Though cutting-edge thought in the hard sciences maintained that complex living systems were nonlinear, research in this period (and still today, in most cases) continued to follow a linear paradigm (Thelen & Smith, 2002). Context was largely ignored. Both rats and humans were studied individually in ways that ignored the actual environment within which they lived, until ethnographic work began to make headway. Studies were done, with limited clinical value, that artificially separated out thinking, feeling, willing, and so on, which, in actual life, are all organized together (Siegel, 2009). Family therapy attempted to correct the lack of context in part, but risked jettisoning individual consciousness and agency in the process (Nichols & Schwartz, 1998).

Multicultural, racial, and gender issues were largely ignored, as if one therapy could fit all (Augsburger, 1986). Virtually any spiritual or religious longing in clients was considered suspect within mainline psychology (LeShan, 1990). The human knowledge in thousands of years of wisdom traditions was spurned as premodern. In terms of contemporary knowledge being generated, Wulff (1991) notes that methodological impeccability could yield remarkable triviality and limited applicability. The question about how one quantifies being transformed by a walk in nature, a new relationship, a movie, a song, a lost job, the death of a family member, a military tour of duty, winning the lottery, and so forth was never solved.

The overvaluing of a limited view of objectivity, what Wilber terms "flatland" science (Beutler, 2009; Wilber, 1995), warned, in turn, against the danger of subjective involvements. For instance, when Bowlby reported the result of his attachment research to the United Nations in 1950, specifically that the mother-infant relationship was extremely important and that early separations can hurt growing children, many professionals scorned and ridiculed him (Karen, 1998). There was such an overemphasis on objective materialism that the richness of subjective experience and the hermeneutics of cultural values were underplayed, resulting in an impoverished account of what it means to be human.

Standard therapies such as Freudian, Jungian, behavioral, and humanistic wasted valuable time quarreling with each other, rather than learning from one another. The use of

touch or the body in mainline therapies was inappropriately sexualized and nearly crimi-
nalized through a limited psychoanalytic bias (Peloquin, 1990; Zur, 2007) with no research
to support such a position.

However, the post–World War II era emphasis on self-realization and the strengthening
of a consumer orientation led to new approaches like transactional analysis through popular books such as Erick Berne's (1964) *Games People Play*. The human potential movement of the 1960s led to a great flowering of exotic psychotherapeutic approaches and
experimentation. An openness developed among some to following wherever demonstra-
ble healing seemed to be happening, especially in the experiential therapies such as Gestalt,
body-centered approaches, energy psychology, Buddhist, Taoist, and Eastern approaches
in general.

Distressingly, however, outcome studies had difficulty showing psychotherapy was better than no treatment at all. Trauma issues, especially, were barely recognized and inef-
fectually treated (Herman, 1992; Rothschild, 2000; van der Kolk, 2003). The shift toward
expressive therapies made famous at Esalen in a reaction against incessant and ineffectual
talk therapies did not produce the hoped-for panacea of increased freedom and function.

On the other hand, there were enough anecdotal stories of healing and growth through
therapy that distressed people kept seeking help through various therapists, and therapists
kept seeking more and deeper methods for providing that help. Factors nonspecific to any
particular therapy (Frank, 1986), such as the therapeutic relationship itself, seemed helpful
to a degree (Mahoney, 1991). A general spirit of excitement and experimentation was in
the air. An increasing number of therapists tended toward an eclectic pragmatism and
recognized that help is only helpful when the person being helped acknowledges it as such
(Gibb, 1978).

The Larger World of the 1960s

The situation within psychology, of course, developed within the greater cultural and
social trends of the 1960s and after. Though many, or even the majority, of the World War
II generation still identified with the older values of family, work, religion, and community,
it was a time of cultural turmoil and change that went beyond the radical reactions of a
few estranged youths—in a time when many societal leaders of yesteryear were dying.

Conventional authorities and their wisdom had been shown to be wanting. In politics
there was a credibility gap that followed misinformation about the Vietnam War; manifold instances of corruption; intractable wars in the Middle East, Africa, and Ireland; the
hydrogen bomb tested in a policy of mutually assured destruction (Macy, 1983); the world
population growing at uncontrollable and alarming rates; commandos hijacking airplanes;
former colonies of European powers becoming independent; special interest lobbies frustrating legislation for the common good (Daly & Cobb, 1989; Harrington, 1962); exposing the hidden poor; and much more. These entrenched difficulties and the sometimes
blatant assumption of American and Western moral, political, and economic superiority in
the face of all these issues gave pause to many (Alterman, 2004).

In addition to the unrest and the progress of the civil rights movement in America, women's rights and the feminist movement sought to redefine conventional expectations of where women could participate and lead. In psychology, in particular, feminist self-in-relation theories challenged more male-oriented, grand-autonomous-self theories (Gilligan, 1982; Jordan et al., 1991; Keller, 1986).

In the corporate-economic realm, similar doubts about credibility and efficiency arose (Halberstam, 1986). Corporations came under fire for hiding risk factors and not factoring in issues of sustainability and the effect of what they were doing on the environment. There was a general trend toward an increasing concentration of power in fewer multinational corporations. The question arose of whether the power of science was outstripping our moral ability to use it wisely. A massively litigious society and an economic royalism in America fostered an increasing split between rich and poor. Many worried about crass materialism, utilitarian individualism, and the denigration of indigenous societies (Thurow, 1998; Wallerstein, 1979).

Though religion remained important in the life of the country, it too was going through a notable period of change. Attending a congregation was a common American expectation in the 1950s, but the 1960s morphed into a period termed post-Puritan and post-Protestant. Conservative elements in the church came to consider themselves under fire by the culture (Ahlstrom, 1972). Into this mix came increasing interest in Eastern spiritualities, new religious movements, and cults (Melton & Moore, 1982). Sociologist Robert Wuthnow (1998) notes that there was a movement away from a spirituality of place (neighborhood, denominational congregations) to a spirituality of seeking, which historian Robert Fuller (2001) argues mapped into an enhanced interest in the historic tradition of those who identified themselves as spiritual but not religious.

In Western ethics, the teaching and influence of old schools of thought were found wanting due to many of the events listed above. Authoritative ethics drawn from traditional texts accepted by faith, regular ethics based on rules or principles known by reason, and consequential ethics known by cost-benefit calculations all became suspect as postmodern criticisms arose that exposed underlying relativities and power dynamics that served the political and economic power interests of vested groups (Rosenau, 1992). Tipton (1982) researched the emergence of a new form of expressive ethics that valued the quality of personal feelings and situations known through intuition. The new answer to the ethical question "What should I do?" came from asking, "What is happening?" and then responding with the most suitable act. An act was right because it constituted the most fitting response to a highly specific situation, with the most appropriate or honest expression of one's self. The cardinal virtues of persons considered morally creditable became sensitivity of feeling and intuition of the needed situational response. Resolution of disagreements came through exchanging discrepant intuitions within ongoing relationships until greater empathy, understanding, and consensus emerged (Barstow, 2005). This approach fit well with the emerging influence of feminist ethics emphasizing relationships as opposed to rules (Gilligan, 1982).

The popular media raised critiques of conventional positions through books, movies, songs, clothes, and lifestyles that glorified the emergence of the youth culture, complicated notions of "bad guys," showed aspects of life previously kept in the shadows, and supported values of open sexuality, passion, concreteness, and existential immediacy. Antiestablishment heroes and heroines, violence, and more became standard fare in movies and later in television (Johanson, 2010a; Reich, 1970).

Leaders in education, as holders of the tradition, were discredited as having little to say and little of importance to actually do in relation to the crises all around them. The inherited faith in the American Dream meme (Johanson, 1999b)—that America was part of a divinely ordered millennial movement making sure progress toward perfecting the individual, nation, and world—was weakened and thrown into doubt (McLoughlin, 1978; Wuthnow, 2006). The door had been opened to exploring new alternatives.

The door was kept open through the promise of small groups and support outside the family, and a desire for a unified sense of life stemming from the painful split between a meaningful sense of purpose and a seemingly valueless science and industry that structured the compartmentalization of life and the breakdown of community (Naylor, Willimon, & Oesterberg, 1996). Largely ignored religious fundamentalists (Ammerman, 1993), as well as New Agers of many stripes, sought to weave a larger unity (Ellwood, 1979). Wuthnow notes that the overall thrust of the 1960s was to make individuals work hard to figure out their own lives. There was a new freedom to exercise choice in an open marketplace of ideas and lifestyles where "freedom of choice meant exposing oneself to alternative experiences" (Wuthnow, 1998, p. 83). Overall, in almost every field there was a heightened sense of exploring and experimenting that contrasted with the 1950s' sense of wanting to have order, stability, and economic opportunity following the chaos and devastation of the world wars (Halberstam, 1993).

In Europe, things followed a similar course. After two devastating world wars that consumed almost all cultural resources in many parts of the world, the forces of cultural and political change in the 1960s attempted to give expression and voice to the emerging popular undercurrent. With France at the forefront, the movement was predominantly political at first (the social revolution of 1968). Along with what was happening in America, it became known as the counterculture movement. Even though its political branch, charged by another catastrophe, the Vietnam War, was set to become a powerful force, it was its "soft" face that would forever change the ways of people's lives in the West. To understand its spirit, it is important to realize how authoritarian the social structure had been for centuries, politically, culturally, and spiritually. Feudalistic stratification of European societies had left the individual bereft of much personal expression.

It is also important to note that the spirit of the 1960s described here brought alive a popular undercurrent that had shown its vitality early in the 20th century in central Europe when the "reform movement" tried to shake off the confines of an authoritarian era that didn't attend to basic human and social needs (Marlock & Weiss, 2006; Marlock & Weiss, with Young & Soth, 2015). At that time, a great number of new approaches to communal living, health, body awareness, and personal spirituality had taken hold among the young and well educated. In this climate, Elsa Gindler and Wilhelm Reich, two defining pioneers of body psychotherapy, had each inspired a lineage of schools that are still defining avant-garde resources for many health professionals today.

The popular undercurrent we are describing here was given graphic, exaggerated expression in the 1998 Hollywood movie *Pleasantville*, in which two teenagers of the 1990s miraculously end up in the 1950s as they are watching a TV series from that time. They become members of a lovingly caricatured family and small-town community mirroring "perfect" America when it was still untouched by the extravagant chaotic 1960s. Director Gary Ross illuminates the leap of 40 years from middle-class conformity and uncritical acceptance of standard values to more individuality and personal meanings by initially setting that time in black and white. As the protagonists come alive sexually, emotionally, and mentally with more open possibilities and mysteries before them, color slowly finds its way to the screen.

What gave color to the counterculture as described above was emotionally expressive music, alternate ways of living and relating, sexual and spiritual freedom, personal growth, and personal ethics. The liberation from perceived bonds of orthodoxy was often naive, excessive, and indulgent—for instance, when it came to drugs. Nevertheless a group of social value systems advanced like feminism, ecological awareness, the primacy of love, the freedom to explore one's potential, critical self-reflection, and a philosophical attitude to life that could be called postmodern—meaning the embracing of multiple perspectives—and much more flexibility in meeting life's choices. It indeed shook individuals free to be responsible for their own life and deeds. Scholar Timothy Miller called those swept up in this incoherent and multifaceted movement seekers of meaning and value.

While the media was giving excessive attention to the more sensational manifestations of this phenomenon, like drug consumption and promiscuity, the spirit of the age (Zeitgeist) was creating a more serious and intellectually rigorous base that reflected the substantial shift in consciousness outlined here. An expanding consciousness emerged that Wilber would call "centauric," since it was more clearly a mind-body sensibility, as opposed to the limited rationality of the modern period. It called upon individuals to become aware of their own nature as self-directed organisms, calling forth internal knowledge and consciousness to make personal ethical choices.

While contemporary trends in philosophy were mirroring such developments (structuralism, deconstructionism, postmodernism), those issues were not meant to be kept as mental exercises by the flower-power generation. The new undercurrent of consciousness encouraged real moment-to-moment personal experience. As opposed to Hegelian philosophy, whose idealism was thought to be abstract, general, dispassionate, and objective, this forming new awareness of the Zeitgeist was fundamentally existential in terms of favoring the concrete, the definite, and the passionate where persons as opposed to gods (Absolute Spirit) were considered responsible for their own actions (Johanson, 2010a). One's life or "Existence" was not a given or a state, but a ceaseless striving toward actualization, that is, an act.

Living, let's say, in San Francisco in the 1960s meant being exposed to a torrent of impressions reflecting the changing times. Books, music, art, lifestyles, and the search for ever-more "far-out" experiences invited young people to look at life differently. Among the many experiences available were a number of spiritual and "therapeutic" practices: meditation, Gestalt therapy, dance, encounter groups, and many more. Here, the apprentice would embark on a journey of being in the present and becoming aware of herself.

Therapy was not only for the ones that were suffering anymore, but also for everyone who wished to grow and expand their consciousness. It attracted the attention of a meaningful segment of the counterculture that, in turn, influenced the mainline culture over time.

Hakomi's History

Halko Weiss and Greg Johanson

Into the cultural milieu of the 1960s, stepped Ron Kurtz, with a background in physics, mathematics, electronics, and Eastern wisdom traditions. Ron completed doctoral work in experimental psychology at Indiana University Bloomington with Estes before becoming interested in psychotherapy. Rather than studying in a traditional psychology school, he consulted a variety of master therapists and evaluated and integrated methods on a pragmatic, eclectic basis through the lens of living systems theory.

Likewise, students and future faculty attracted to his early workshops were those post-1960s practitioners disgruntled with status quo psychology and its poor outcomes, primed to be attracted to a way of working that honored both contemporary science and ancient wisdom studies, whether it was in accord with standard protocols or not.

In those early days, experiencing Kurtz's workshops was magical in many ways: The work was alive and experiential, artistic and poetic, as well as scientifically precise. Changing states of consciousness intensified present-moment awareness in a way that transcended tedious talk or emotional acting out. The slowing down and expectant waiting as practiced in the work potentiated experiments in awareness that allowed persons to study how they organized habitually and automatically around various inputs. Verbal and nonverbal experiments were devised, often from bodily clues, to present precisely the opposite of what a client's normally unconscious core organizers believed and employed to control both their perception and response. Thus, barriers to organizing in something previously organized out, like support or intimacy, were evoked and made available for further exploration, often with astonishing speed and grace (Johanson, 2015; Stolorow et al., 1987).

Since experiments were normally set up in a theoretically positive, nourishing form, therapeutic strictures against gratifying were transformed into helping clients study how gratification was defended against. Paradoxically, slowing down, trusting organic wisdom, not pushing for a particular result, supporting defenses as they arose, and encouraging curiosity (Johanson, 1988) and savoring (Kurtz, 1990a; Sundararajan, 2008) moved people along in their process further and faster. A compassionate, nonjudging presence and acute tracking and contacting of present-moment experience, combined with a humor that affirmed one's creative capacities functioned to unlock the cooperation of the unconscious and foster a spontaneous unfolding (Stream, 1994). There was a fresh, nonviolent easiness to the work that pointed to a new paradigm—change without force—a process that helped people go where they wanted to go at the deepest levels (Kurtz, 1990a).

How all this went together in a theoretically coherent way was not immediately clear. A number of those who ended up becoming founding trainers of what later became the

Hakomi Institute recognized that Kurtz was doing something remarkably effective and right. But when asked how he knew what to do, he was not totally clear, as he was working quite spontaneously, drawing on multiple sources. It was obvious that there were influences from Gestalt, bioenergetics, Pesso Boyden system psychomotor (PBSP), Feldenkrais, NLP, Buddhist and Taoist sources, complex linear systems thinking, and more, but the integration was unique. The work could be characterized as psychodynamic because it worked with core organizers that affect transference, or as a form of cognitive therapy, since it accessed and expanded core organizing beliefs, which meant it was also a way of doing narrative therapy. It was humanistic in its embrace of human potentials; transpersonal in its use of a witnessing state of consciousness. It could work through dreams like Jungians, relational material like psychoanalysts, and through the body like many body-centered methods. But it could not be fully understood or taught under any one of these umbrellas.

It was about this time that Bandler and Grinder (1975) published their books, *The Structure of Magic*, that were written after studying master psychotherapists to ascertain if there was any underlying structure to the seeming magic they performed that could be passed on to others. Likewise, we invited Ron to study himself as we also studied him to see if there was any underlying structure we could identify that would help us learn or teach to others. After a number of years of analyzing Ron's talks and verbatim sessions, such a linear structure was discovered, along with underlying principles, and an identifiable method that could be passed on to others. It was at that point that the Hakomi Institute was founded and in 1980 began to offer workshops and training worldwide.

The principles, theory, and techniques of the Hakomi method that were discovered and refined form the bulk of this volume. The linear structure Kurtz developed, which consists of establishing the therapeutic relationship (creating the conditions for mindful exploration), accessing (inviting mindfulness), deepening (sustaining mindfulness), processing (mindfully experimenting with transformation through taking in new options), and integration-completion homework (while transitioning back to ordinary consciousness), represents the first therapeutic method to use mindfulness of the mind as the main therapeutic tool throughout a session. It remains the only one today, though there are some that closely approximate it (Ecker & Hulley, 1996), many that integrate aspects of mindfulness (Bobrow, 2010; Germer, 2009; Germer et al., 2005; Hayes, 2005), a number that use mindfulness practice as an adjunct for therapy (Roberts, 2009), and a wealth of those who experiment with teaching mindfulness practice while dealing with a great number of conditions (Johanson, 2009c; R. Siegel, 2010).

Ron Kurtz's Evolution

After finishing graduate work in experimental psychology and having worked as a technical writer in electronics (he had minored in physics), Kurtz was one of those people diving into the exciting melting pot of ideas and experiences in San Francisco in the mid-1960s. Already familiar with psychotherapy, he joined the crowd of those who would go to workshops and read books, soak up experiences, and then immediately turn around to try their hand at teaching their newly won knowledge to others. At that time, no degrees or licensure were required to do or teach psychotherapy, which, again, had been co-opted by many for the more general cause of personal growth and transformation. If someone could inspire a group through brilliance and effectiveness, he or she could also be accepted as a teacher.

Gestalt therapy was the big thing at the time. Ron's friend Stella Resnick, a clinical psychologist teaching at San Jose State University, whom he had known from his Indiana days, took him under her wing and led "sensitivity groups" with him that were infused with her knowledge about Gestalt therapy processes. Much of what Ron learned at that time, and that still influences the form and spirit of Hakomi work, is based on those first years as he developed his approach.

Through Charlotte Selver and Fritz Perls, the Gindler tradition had survived the war decades and resurfaced with intensity. The work was about being in the moment and being aware. Eastern thought had entered this tradition early in the century during a time of great receptivity for the East (see Hermann Hesse's *Siddhartha*). And here it was again, now with new teachers like Shunryu Suzuki, who also ended up in San Francisco. The present-centeredness of humanistic psychology with its emphasis on experiential elements, emotions in particular, was a powerful assault on classical psychoanalytic approaches that had relied heavily on mental processing, reasoning, and insight. The wake-up cry was, "Lose your mind and come to your senses! Don't talk about experiences—have them!"

Because Gestalt was an obvious heir to psychoanalysis—as it builds on a psychodynamic understanding of self-organization— Freud, Jung, and Reich were also to be found on a seeker's bookshelf.

Ron's great excitement had started with his experiences at a workshop with Will Schutz (1969), one of the godfathers of group encounters, also steeped in the appreciation of moment-to-moment experience, and other workshops that were part of a colorful marketplace of experimental offerings. His exposure to Gestalt had solidified and substantiated his own style. Now he won a teaching job at San Francisco State University that he interpreted as an invitation to open the door to the world of experience for his students.

Buddhism was also leaving its mark on the period. A Vipassana retreat had introduced Ron to mindfulness, which he put to use when teaching at San Francisco State. It was a means for him to help people to "really be in" their experience. With his own long familiarity with his body from doing yoga, Ron had a talent and penchant for translating mindfulness into practical exercises. While the true meaning of what mindfulness has to offer was certainly not yet fully grasped and reflected, it started to set the tone of Ron's style of working: slow, in-the-moment, with detailed attention to internal events and acceptance toward all phenomena perceived inside as reality by the one exploring.

In the early 1970s, Ron moved to Albany, New York, to open a private practice and to teach and work at a 24-hour crisis center, called Refer Switchboard. Just like other large cities, Albany had its counterculture with all its trappings and a lot of therapy in the air.

As he kept experimenting and solidifying his style, Ron continued seeking his own inspirations, like weeks-long workshops with Moshe Feldenkrais and his student Ruthy Alon, seminars with Al Pesso, and many Rolfing sessions, as well as his own therapy. This is when body psychotherapy started to become a major new influence. His therapists were the bioenergetic analyst Ron Robbins and later John Pierrakos, one of the founders of bioenergetic analysis, trained by Wilhelm Reich.

Here again, Ron's work aligned itself with a tradition that had its roots early in the century and held the body in high esteem as a cherished vessel of the self. Elsa Gindler, Wilhelm Reich, and others had taken a stand against the dominance the mind had been given since the Enlightenment. Often intuitively, some therapists had continued to nourish this tradition outside mainstream psychotherapy. They kept listening to the body as a source of truth, healing, and the foundations of self. It would take until the end of the century for the larger psychotherapeutic community to realize the fundamental importance of the body when infant research, neurobiology, trauma work, and other sciences began to challenge long-held mainstream assumptions.

In the 1970s, elements from bioenergetics, aspects of the Feldenkrais method, techniques from Pesso, and other inspirations from body therapy slowly started to show up in Ron's work as they were modified by the defining power of mindfulness and Taoist philosophy. This mindful modification suggested, in contrast to bioenergetic exercises, for instance, that it is a good idea not to oppose powerful forces, but to go along with them and use them. Milton Erickson was one of the therapists who was a master of this strategy through what he called "utilization techniques," and Ron became a great admirer of his creative and unique style of "going with the flow."

These influences led to Ron's unique contribution of taking-over techniques (Chapter 17) that paradoxically serve to help people release their defenses by actually supporting them verbally or nonverbally. Ron also gained experiential and intellectual clarity that this approach was more in line with information-processing models than the older hydraulic or energy ones. In his eyes, clients do not need to yell for 10 years in response to 40 years of frustration once they realize that what was frustrating them is no longer present.

Here we find the beginning of a new therapeutic concept and approach: interventions from bioenergetics, Gestalt, cognitive-behavioral, psychodynamic, and other approaches designed to bring about change and directed toward a specific goal conceived by the therapist had to be rethought. Being directed by specific goals disrupts mindful observation and creates counter forces that make the process more violent and noisy when forces are mobilized to oppose other forces. Lao-tzu suggested as an alternative that one study forces for a long time until they are precisely understood for their functional wisdom (Johanson & Kurtz, 1991). As we see within this book, the general answer and approach that unfolded championed a systemic understanding of internal forces in the spirit of scientific research and experimental attitude (Chapter 11), and toward interventions that would combine an active approach by the therapist with a nonviolent attitude and style (Chapter 12).

The Albany years also brought a surprising change of life's course for someone who was simply enjoying being a local therapist. Ron's friendship with the physician and bioenergetic therapist Hector Prestera produced a book on character styles from the body psychotherapy tradition, called *The Body Reveals*, which turned out to be a huge success (Kurtz & Prestera, 1976).

This led to a life on the authors' circuit, where Ron presented workshops on character structure and how to work with it all over the country and in Europe. He was invited to private practices, event centers, hospitals, and living rooms, traveling more and more and demonstrating a still quite intuitive way of connecting to fundamental layers of personality very quickly. Observing a person precisely, having him or her become mindful, creating an evocative experiment, and processing the ensuing experience worked extremely well and impressed the participants deeply, though it was their unanswered questions about the structure of the method that led to the mutual discovery process mentioned above that resulted in the birth of the Hakomi Institute.

Ron was also a gifted, charismatic, humorous speaker who could inspire an audience through a clear, insightful, relaxed way of presenting that evoked an informal, warm, safe sense of inclusion that transcended artificial divisions between therapists and clients. Consequently, he started to have an appreciative and interested following that continued to grow by word of mouth.

Ron's interest and training in science created another thread that was developed over the years. Math and physics came easily to him, and he continued to nourish his understanding of complex, nonlinear living systems in particular (Chapter 5). Gregory Bateson's groundbreaking final work, *Mind and Nature*, published in 1979, tied together an understanding of self-organization. Bateson proposed that when the parts within the whole of a system are connected and communicating, that the system is self-organizing, and self-correcting. This insight continued to evolve for Kurtz in the works of Erich Jantsch, Ken Wilber, Francesco Varela, Ilya Prigogine, the scientists at the Santa Fe Institute, and many others. It allowed for a psychological theory of human self-organization that reflects an intelligent and sensitive internal ecology integrated by communication between parts and shaped by internal models of reality ("beliefs," Chapter 7) based on powerful emotional experiences and the implicitly remembered meanings that came with them, and that continue to influence the present. Such understanding was later to be supported by neuroscience research.

It is one of the characterizing traits of the last century that the rise of cybernetics and computer sciences made both the search for and the representation of complex systems possible. Von Neumann laid ground for this revolution only after World War II, a revolution that has allowed deeper and more realistic views of many objects of science. In psychology, the trend of moving away from causal thinking toward an understanding of complex and nonlinear systems is still struggling to take hold. Equipped with a keen sense of such important cultural momentum, Ron kept studying and integrating this new way of looking at life through the organic lens of self-organization with its emergent properties.

Here, mindfulness became a means not just of having an experience, but of studying the processes of self-organization as they happen from moment to moment in a way that led to the core organizers that created them. The power of an internal observer (suggested by Buddhist psychology) that holds a metalevel and does not become entangled and drawn into the trances of daily life (Wolinsky, 1991) became a hallmark of the evolving Hakomi method. This aspect marks an especially mature understanding of the power of mindfulness. It also reflects the appreciation of the psychological knowledge of the East, embodied by Ron's guiding figures, such as Meher Baba and Swami Rama. Psychotherapy in the

West, of course, is a little over 100 years old, and began by shunning thousands of years of human wisdom in favor of a limited view of objective and materialistic perspectives (Wilber, 1977, 1995).

The Hakomi Institute Growth and Development

In 1980, after a number of years of creative ferment involving many people in Boulder, Colorado—another meeting place of renowned teachers who inspired Ron, along with a whole generation (Ken Wilber, for instance, or Chogyam Trungpa)—Kurtz found himself in Putnam, Connecticut, with a number of young therapists who were intent on assisting him in organizing his way of working into a teachable method and founding an institute that would offer these teachings. Ron Kurtz was the founder and director, with Dyrian Benz, Jon Eisman, Greg Johanson, Pat Ogden, Phil Del Prince, Devi Records-Benz, and Halko Weiss as founding trainers.

The name "Hakomi" (hah-CO-me) was literally dreamed up by Kurtz's student David Winter in the summer of 1980. At the time, the work was plainly titled "body-centered psychotherapy." In the dream, Kurtz handed David a sheet of stationery with the words "Hakomi Institute" written on it. Trained in anthropology, David discovered it was a Hopi Indian word that meant "How do you stand in relation to these many realms?"—an ancient way of asking, "Who are you?" Since both meanings fit perfectly with helping people study how they organize input from various realms of experience, the name was adopted despite its unfamiliarity to English speakers.

The following years were years of composing and building. Curricula, books, articles, a professional journal, many workshops and training courses, business structures, and a growing number of trained therapists started to spread the method throughout the world.

The Hakomi Institute has since contributed to the field of counselor education through its pursuit of excellence as a training institute. Each time in-depth training is done, the trainers revise the curriculum based on what they see happening with the current students. What part of the theory or techniques are they not getting? What method seems to need a finer breakdown to make the parts explicit? What underlying assumption seems to be missing when the student employs a series of techniques? What questions are students still asking? What balance between theory, experiential learning, and practice needs to be struck? How is the relative emphasis on the personhood of the therapist going in relation to professional skill building? Though the international Hakomi faculty of trainers and teachers has grown to some 50 persons in three decades, there are yearly faculty meetings where such curriculum matters are discussed, and a common core of teachings is affirmed.

Since Kurtz did not come to psychotherapy through any one established school, many of the discoveries and processes of Hakomi (explained within this text) took on unique names, though there might be echoes or parallels in other approaches: riding the rapids, sensitivity cycle, accessing, taking over, burdened-enduring, tough-generous, cooperation of the unconscious, probes, tracking, contact, savoring, nourishment barrier, magical stranger, core organizing beliefs, and so forth. These terms have been retained through the years in recognition of Hakomi as a unique integrative approach, although complementary concepts from the wider field of psychotherapy are also referenced within the training context.

The Hakomi Institute began and continued as a training institute for clinical practitioners and for those who wanted to apply its principles in many fields. In the past 30-plus years, the Hakomi method has expanded rapidly. Workshops and training have been conducted throughout the United States and Europe, as well as Canada, Switzerland, Israel, Mexico, Argentina, Brazil, Japan, Korea, Hong Kong, Russia, Australia, New Zealand, and Inner Mongolia. The Hakomi faculty expanded from the founding trainers to a worldwide faculty who promote and teach the method in their respective localities. In 1993, a professional code of ethics, years in the making, was formally adopted.

In the years following the original development of Hakomi as a teachable method, there were four major sources of inspiration and enrichment. The first is the emergence of additional core concepts. The early and mid-1980s were characterized by the excitement of the (now) senior faculty bringing the work into the world and receiving feedback and insights radiating from the application of the emerging method. Concepts such as the "child" that have since become defining features of Hakomi, were added to the curriculum. With support from the senior trainers, Ron formulated how the work changes when a client moves into the child state of consciousness along with the "magical stranger," the name given to the role the therapist adopts in such instances (Chapter 18). Another development was jumping out of the system (Chapter 22), where the shift of focus from a lower logical level of conscious representation to a higher one became a hallmark of the method.

The second source was collaboration with Richard Schwartz. The guest of honor at the Hakomi International Conference of 1996 was Richard Schwartz (lovingly adopted into the Hakomi community as "Dick"). Dick came to four subsequent conferences and inspired our elaboration of the unity principle (Chapter 5), and systems thinking, since his method, internal family systems, was miles ahead of ours in its understanding of the systemic aspects of an inner ecology of parts in the psyche. He also helped make more explicit that the witnessing and compassionate aspects of mindfulness implied a larger self-state beyond historically conditioned ego states. His ingenious contributions deepened and refined the practice of our method, as he, in turn, absorbed some key features of Hakomi, such as mindfulness and the somatic perspective.

The third source of enrichment was discourse with groundbreaking scientific research. The 1990s and 2000s, now termed "the decades of the brain," were filled with exciting and innovative findings in fields that are foundational to Hakomi therapy: mindfulness, neurobiology, attachment theory, trauma therapy, and infant research in particular. Seminal thinkers in these areas were invited to present at our conferences, and fertile exchanges and collaborative relationships were established with Peter Levine, Bessel van der Kolk, Babette Rothschild, Diana Fosha, Stephen Porges, and Thomas Lewis, many of whom gave keynote addresses at our 16 Hakomi conferences.

These exchanges offered a way to understand the neurological underpinnings and relational dynamics responsible for the dramatic changes witnessed in our clients. It seemed that we had stumbled upon a method that actually did what the research suggested was needed in this current wave of psychotherapy. We now understood how effectively our methodology supports bilateral integration, emotion regulation, and earned secure attachment by going slowly, operating within the nonviolence principle, working with the internal observer, and using mindfulness to access and transform the implicit emotional learning that shapes the schemas and relational templates that carry forward across the life span (Cozolino, 2006).

The fourth source of inspiration is discernment of trauma. The 1990s also brought about the realization that trauma is a very specific kind of experience that needs special procedural attention. When working with regressive states in particular, it became obvious where some limits of our method lay, and how a different way of dealing with trauma was required. Through her alliance with Peter Levine, our senior trainer Pat Ogden became so deeply inspired by this perspective that she formed her own institute and created an approach to trauma, sensorimotor psychotherapy, that builds on Hakomi and is now one of the most respected treatments in the field. Our students today are trained to discern states of trauma and manage them differently than other developmental issues.

While the core Hakomi curriculum is still taught worldwide, individual training weaves in the particular interests faculty members have developed in such areas as movement therapy, internal family systems therapy, psychodrama, music therapy, oriental medicine, the Diamond Approach, accelerated experiential dynamic psychotherapy, and so on. Some faculty delved deeply enough into specific content areas that they developed separate or parallel training courses.

As mentioned above, Pat Ogden synthesized Hakomi with trauma therapy to the extent that she created a new approach that is one of the most cited in the field, sensorimotor psychotherapy (Ogden et al., 2006). It majors in using mindfulness in the service of bottom-up as opposed to top-down processing. Cedar Barstow (2005) created a relational approach to ethics that she termed "the right use of power," which now has a guild that sponsors research, training, and books on the topic.

Jon Eisman's (2010) exploration of self-states resulted in a self-contained approach he titled re-creation of the self, which can be taught alone or integrated with Hakomi. Morgan Holford and Susan McConnell developed a specialized Hakomi training for bodyworkers and Lorena Monda has done likewise for practitioners of oriental medicine. Amina Knowlan's work on group development evolved into the Matrix Leadership Institute. Mukara Meredith developed Matrixworks training, a living systems approach to team building and creativity, now taught in major corporations including the Gap, Procter and Gamble, General Mills, and Mattel. Halko Weiss and Hakomi colleagues in Germany developed a very successful approach to teaching emotional intelligence to corporate executives in companies like Mercedes Benz and Munich Re. Weiss also developed a course called Hakomi Embodied and Aware Relationships Training (H.E.A.R.T.) that teaches a complex approach to conscious relationships. Maci Daye developed Passion & Presence, a course on mindful sexuality for couples in long-term relationships.

Rob Fisher's specialization in couples work resulted in the publication of his 2002 book *Experiential Psychotherapy With Couples: A Guide for the Creative Pragmatist*. Halko Weiss published several books in German, among them two best-selling books on mindfulness, and a thousand-page *Handbook on Body Psychotherapy*, of which an

American version is scheduled to be available in 2015 through North Atlantic Press. Lorena Monda (2000) integrated her background with Hakomi, Thich Nhat Hanh, Yvonne Agazarian, Gabrielle Roth, and oriental medicine, along with research on core transformation, into *The Practice of Wholeness: Spiritual Transformation in Everyday Life* and a specialized training. Richard A. Heckler brought Hakomi sensibilities and curiosity to researching and authoring two books, *Waking Up Alive: The Descent, the Suicide Attempt, and the Return to Life*, and *Crossings: Everyday People, Unexpected Events, and Life-Affirming Change*.

In 1992 Ron Kurtz resigned as director of the Hakomi Institute to form Ron Kurtz Trainings, headquartered in Ashland, Oregon. This enabled him to continue his inventive work of concentrating on the method itself, spontaneously and independently implementing changes as he envisioned them. Kurtz remained a senior trainer in the Hakomi Institute for many years, and remains an ongoing inspiration. Both organizations recognized each other's teaching of Hakomi and certifications of therapists, teachers, and trainers. Before his death in 2011, Kurtz developed a shorter, simplified version of the Hakomi method (outlined in Chapter 3) that he hoped would not only inform professional mental health practitioners but also enhance mutual community, growth, and support for a wide variety of ordinary people. Hakomi Institute students were encouraged to train with him whenever they had the opportunity to benefit from his unique artistry, insight, and humor.

As we look back on all these developments, we can sense how the spirit of the times has formed the very core and feel of the Hakomi method: specifically, its emphasis and trust in the individual's hidden wisdom and freedom, the refusal of practitioners to take a superior position as the all-knowing therapist, the willingness to support each client's highly personal and unique path, the valuing of live felt experience in the body, the appreciation of complexity, the bias toward investigation and curiosity over set goals and treatment plans, and the emphasis on loving presence as foundational for deep healing, all of which reflect the emergent fusion of scientific and spiritual perspectives.

When we look back historically to the 1960s, 1970s, and 1980s, the fruit was all there, waiting to be plucked, processed, and integrated in a unique way by a uniquely gifted person and teacher who has left an ongoing, still unfolding, healing legacy (Johanson, 2011a, 2011b, 2011d).

Hakomi in the Context of Research and Science

Greg Johanson

A unique background foundation in sciences of complex nonlinear systems has served the Hakomi Institute well in its primary functioning as a training institute as opposed to a research institute. Hakomi of Europe, headquartered in Germany, led the way in getting Hakomi approved as a scientifically validated modality within the European Association of Psychology in the European Union (Schulmeister, 2005). As such, the Hakomi Institute is an approved psychotherapy training provider in the European Union. Credits in doctoral programs for studying Hakomi have been obtained through a number of educational institutions worldwide. Likewise, the Hakomi curriculum was approved as an official national training program for psychotherapists in New Zealand through the Eastern Institute of Technology in Napier. Subsequently, chapters on Hakomi therapy have been included in standard textbooks on theories of counseling and psychotherapy (Roy, 2007), as well as being investigated in various theses and dissertations (Benz, 1981; Kaplan, 2005; Myllerup, 2000; Rosen, 1983; Schanzer, 1990; Smith, 1996), other books (Johanson & Taylor, 1988), and articles.

Critical Consumers of Research

Research in general, of course, is a broad topic with numerous aspects. Hakomi, as a training institute consumer of research, has striven to have an engaged, constructive, yet critical relationship with psychotherapy research in particular that remains in tension with its clinical experience.

To begin, Hakomi practitioners have not been willing to wait for positivistic scientific approval of what seemed clearly therapeutically helpful, though we do track a wide range of scientific studies for confirmation or disconfirmation as they arise. For instance, Kurtz realized in the early 1970s the potency of mindfulness in helping clients become aware of and transform the way they organized their experience, something central to depth psychotherapies (Shedler, 2010; Stolorow et al., 1987). The effectiveness of this discovery has been explored and deepened through Hakomi ever since. Most other therapists who were interested in the mindfulness-therapy interface would not allow themselves to speak of it in professional settings until the early 1990s (R. Siegel, 2010). Kabat-Zinn began publishing about the use of mindfulness for working with pain in the mid-1980s (Kabat-Zinn, Lipworth, & Burney, 1985). Linehan (1993) published on the use of mindfulness in treating borderline personality disorders in the early 1990s. Today, there is an ever-growing wealth of studies related to mindfulness and psychotherapy (Johanson, 2006, 2009a). In particular, there is now much exciting knowledge from interpersonal neurobiology about the underlying mechanism of mindfulness (Hanson with Mendius, 2009; D. Siegel, 2007, 2010; Simpkins & Simpkins, 2010).

The example of mindfulness illustrates that experimental psychotherapy research does not generally produce new knowledge so much as evaluate hypotheses generated in clinical practice (Gendlin, 1986; Goldfried, 2009). It is also an example of how Hakomi has maintained "the standard of a respectable minority . . . out of concern that the standard of common practice was insensitive to emerging but not yet popular treatments," a standard that "recognized that the healthcare fields do not always have a consensual view of what is effective" (Beutler, 2009, p. 308).

The Personhood of the Therapist

This stance of a respectable minority has also played out in Hakomi's caution about the supposed gold standard of randomized clinical trials (RCTs) that separate "the person of the therapist from the acts of psychotherapy" (Beutler, 2009, p. 311). Hakomi training always balances concentration on the being or personhood of the therapist with the doing aspects of method and technique, as it has always been obvious that it is the characterological limitations of therapists that restrict their effectiveness in utilizing the process itself. This position is congruent with much research that has built on the investigation of common factors and has underlined the importance of the therapeutic relationship (Ablon & Jones, 2002; Beutler et al., 2003, 2004; Castonguay & Beutler, 2006; Duncan & Miller, 2000; Horvath & Bedi, 2002; Mahoney, 1991; Norcross, 2002, 2005; Orlinsky, Ronnestad, & Willutzki, 2004; Safran & Muran, 2000; Sexton & Whiston, 1991; Shedler, 2010; Tombs, 2001; Vocisano et al., 2004; Wampold, 2001; Whiston & Coker, 2000).

Factors That Comprise Psychotherapy

Along this line, Hakomi practitioners agree with those who argue that we need to "revise our definition of 'research-informed psychotherapy practice' so that it addresses those factors that actually comprise psychotherapy" (Beutler, 2009, p. 302). The Hakomi unity principle agrees that variables must not be ruled out related to "therapist and patient personalities, interpersonal values, therapist and patient gender, socials skills, and attachment levels and the like [which] are not always capable of being randomly assigned" in RCT trials (p. 310). The same applies to cross-cultural issues (Johanson, 1992). And, as Gendlin (1986) has pointed out, it is better not to isolate chemical versus psychological versus social factors, but control for all three and test them together. "They are already always together. . . . Everyone thinks, feels, dreams and imagines; has a body; has a family; acts in situations; and interacts with others" (Gendlin, 1986, p. 135). Likewise, "the practice of therapy often involves more complex clinical cases" with numerous comorbid conditions, which are little dealt with in academic research (Goldfried, 2009, p. 26). Though the *DSM* is purposefully atheoretical, Hakomi continues to see, with others (Blatt & Zuroff, 2005), the connections in character issues related to Axis II that affect many Axis I conditions and, thus, the value of teaching characterology, though in a nonpathologizing way.

Beyond Acute Symptom Alleviation

As a psychodynamic depth psychotherapy, it is significant to Hakomi that "researchers . . . have yet to conduct compelling outcome studies that assess changes in inner capacities and resources," because

> the goals of psychodynamic therapy include, but extend beyond, alleviation of acute symptoms. Psychological health is not merely the absence of symptoms; it is the positive presence of inner capacities and resources that allow people to live life with a greater sense of freedom and possibility. Symptom-oriented outcome measures commonly used in outcome studies . . . do not attempt to assess such inner capacities. (Shedler, 2010, p. 105)

The development of such tools as the Shedler-Westen Assessment Procedure (Shedler & Westen, 2007) that assess "inner capacities and resources that psychotherapy may develop" (Shedler, 2010, p. 105) in support of healthy functioning is important to Hakomi since a main goal of the method is to mobilize a client's capacity to employ mindful or compassionate awareness (Eisman, 2006) with aspects of the self that might be evoked throughout a lifetime, beyond formal therapy. This kind of research could help confirm that it is intrapsychic changes in the organization of a client's experience, something central to Hakomi (Johanson, 2006), that "account for long-term treatment benefits" (Shedler, 2010, p. 103). A change mediated through the neuroplasticity of the brain alters the flow of energy and information and "activates neuronal firing that is integrative and produces the conditions to promote the growth of integrative fibers in the nervous system" (Siegel, 2009, p. 166), the physiological mechanism for effective psychotherapy.

Clinician-Researcher Interface

Many people in the field are aware of the "long standing strain in the alliance between clinicians and researchers" (Goldfried, 2009, p. 25). For one thing, evidence-based treatments don't work as well in actual practice settings as they do in the lab, partly because perfectly and narrowly diagnosed clients do not walk through the treatment door, and it does matter who uses a treatment protocol in what way. Others note "the chasm that exists between science and practice . . . [along with] how weak the evidence is for certain widely held beliefs about the nature of empirically supported treatments" (Beutler, 2009, p. 301; cf. Goldfried, 2009). For instance, it is not true that "psychotherapy would be more effective if everyone practiced an 'empirically supported treatment' . . . [or that] cognitive and cognitive-behavioral therapies are more effective than relational and insight-oriented forms of psychotherapy" (Beutler, 2009, p. 303; cf. Duncan & Miller, 2006; Elkin et al., 1989; Kazdin, 2008; Schulte, Kunzel, Pepping, & Schulte-Bahrenbert, 1992; Shedler, 2010; Wampold, 2001; Wampold et al., 1997).

Likewise, it is now clear that "most manual-driven therapies are equivalently effective and not substantially different from most rationally derived therapies" (Beutler, 2009, p. 310). The effects of cognitive-behavioral interventions tend to fade and require relapse prevention strategies (de Maat, Dekker, Schoevers, & de Jonghe, 2006; Gloaguen, Cottraux, Cucherat, & Blackburn,1998; Westen, Novotny, & Thompson-Brenner, 2004).

Though it is not yet common knowledge in all academic or therapeutic quarters, empirical evidence plainly supports the efficacy of psychodynamic therapy, a characteristic of Hakomi (Ablon & Jones, 1998; Bateman & Fonagy, 2008; Blatt & Auerbach, 2003; Bucci, 2001; Clarkin, Levy, Lenzenweger, & Kernberg, 2007; Fonagy et al., 2002; Jones & Pulos, 1993; Leichsenring, 2005; Leichsenring & Leibing, 2003; Leichsenrinn & Rabung, 2008; Leichsenring, Rabung, & Leibing, 2004; Milrod et al., 2007; Shedler, 2010; Szecsoedy, 2008; Westen, 1998).

Norcross, Beutler, and Levant (2005) note other unexamined assumptions and limitations of research. There is certainly a social construction aspect to validity studies (Kvale, 1995). Linford and Arden (2009) have called into question what they term the Pax Medica of the current three-part standard of therapeutic practice comprising strict *DSM* categories, evidence-based treatments (Blatt & Zuroff, 2005; Duncan & Miller, 2006; Elkin et al., 1989; Kazdin, 2008), and the use of antidepressants (Greenberg, 2010; Kirsch, 2010; Meyer et al., 2001; Turner, Matthews, Linardatos, Tell, & Rosenthal, 2008; Wakefield & Horwitz, 2007).

A Complimentary Model

Based on Hakomi principles (Chapter 5; Johanson, 2009b; Kurtz, 1990a), practitioners recognize the interrelatedness of all things and generally think that psychological science would do well to conceptualize research subjects with a metaphor something like the rhizome suggested by Deleuze and Guattari: "A rhizome has no beginning or end; it is always in the middle between things, interbeing" (1987, p. 25). It embodies an "acentered multiplicity" (p. 17) that is multiply derived or overdetermined, which displays nonlinear emergent properties. Thus, there can be "no dictatorial conception of the unconscious" (p. 17). While hardly anyone will disagree that a human being is a nonlinear system with the possibility of emergent properties that defy easy determinisms, almost all psychotherapy research defaults to a linear setting (Johanson, 2009b, 2009c; Marks-Tarlow, 2011; Thelen & Smith, 2002), and thus builds in constraints and limitations that tend to throw away unexpected results.

The rhizome metaphor would lend itself to adopting Kurtz's preference to work with Popper and Eccles's (1981) conception of unconscious behavioral determinants as "dispositions." We are not absolutely determined, but rather disposed by many factors such as genes, biochemistry, interpersonal relationships, and cultural and social forces in various directions. Since everything is interconnected, each variable will produce a disposition in relation to the others so no one item can remain independent. This approach fosters a healthy degree of humility in psychological research that allows for a pluralistic conception of psychology and a number of types of investigation, something contemporary theorists are calling for (Held, Kirschner, Richardson, Slife, & Teo, 2010; Teo, 2009).

A Model Embracing Awareness and Complexity

Certainly, according to Hakomi and postmodern principles, there is no question that all psychological research and methodologies reflect underlying philosophies and values (Bishop, 2007; Johanson, 1979–1980; Polkinghorne, 1983; Spackman & Williams, 2001), of which one should be as conscious and explicit as possible (Romanyshyn, 2007, 2010). For instance, the pre–World War II period valued the importance of the Freudian differentiated autonomous self as opposed to the self-in-relation concept of postwar feminist therapists (Gilligan, 1982; Jordan et al., 1991). Likewise, Sundararajan, Misra, and Marsella contrast the Western grand atomic self, which considers mental diseases as entities and culture only as an add-on to the self, with multicultural views of a relational or contextual self that affirm that "all mental disorders are culture-bound disorders since no disorder can escape cultural encoding, shaping, and presentation" (2013, p. 75).

Translated into research methodology, the [Western] particle/atomic perspective favors a descriptive model that generates numerous objective lists in psychology—behaviors, personality traits, social cognitions, and so on. By contrast the [multicultural] wave perspective favors the holistic, explanatory models that capitalize on hermeneutics—interpretations and narratives of emergent phenomena such as meaning and subjective experiences. (p. 74)

An Integral Model

Hakomi's unity principle fits most closely with Wilber's (1995, 2000, 2006) AQAL (all quadrants, all levels) integral model of human functioning (see figure 5.1). Here the quadrants are derived from acknowledging the individual and communal aspects of being human, combined with both the objective-outer-monological and the subjective-inner-dialogical aspects. The resultant quadrants represent the inner aspects of individual consciousness and cultural values as well as the outer aspects of individual behavior, biochemistry, and social structures in a nonreductionistic mutual interplay where each quadrant has a science, methodology, and validity appropriate to its field. A danger for research from this integral perspective is overemphasizing variables from one quadrant while ignoring those from the others, which constricts the contextual field and relevance of the research.

This integral, holonic (Koestler, 1967) conception of humanity certainly makes room for the use of qualitative research stemming from phenomenological, existential, hermeneutic perspectives (DeAngelis, 2010; Giorgi, 1970; Giorgi & Giorgi, 2003; Halling & Nill, 1995; Michell, 2003; Moustakas, 1990; Packer & Addison, 1989; Wertz, 2005; Wiggins, 2009). It honors and requires quantitative studies as well. It celebrates developments in neurobiology that demonstrate that mind (inner aspect) and brain (outer aspect) inform each other (Kandel, 2007; Porges, 2011; Schacter, 1992, 1996; Siegel, 1999, 2006, 2007).

Thus, Hakomi affirms the use of mixed-methods research that combines to offer the broadest view of a subject (Creswell & Plano Clark, 2007). Wiggins (2011) writes that there is a dilemma in the use of mixed methods in that every use of the mix tends to come from an underlying positivist or interpretivist worldview that evaluates or subsumes the methods in accord with its privileged viewpoint. Mruk (2010) offers a research approach to an integrated description that carefully conserves overall holistic humanistic concerns and principles, but incorporates traditional positivistic values related to validity, prediction, measurement, control, and real-world utility. The APA Presidential Task Force on Evidence-Based Practice (2006), on the other hand, wanted to endorse "the evidentiary value of a diversity of research methods" (Wiggins, 2011, p. 55). However, in an unacknowledged way, "as Wendt and Slife (2007) observed, the task force proposal places qualitative methods on the bottom of a hierarchy of research methods, ranked according to their rigor and value within a positivistic worldview" (Wiggins, 2011, p. 55).

For Hakomi, the research paradigm wars (Gage, 1989) and dilemmas (Wiggins, 2011) are transcended by the adoption of Wilber's AQAL model that not only honors but invites the "otherness" of methods appropriate to each quadrant. A framework that accounts for, welcomes, and utilizes the most research from the most places is more inclusive than a lesser one, and it is not an arbitrary power move to say this, any more than it is to assert that a molecule has a more inclusive embrace than an atom, or that this paragraph has more significance than a single letter, though atoms and letters are more foundational as building blocks (Ingersoll & Zeitler, 2010; Wilber, 1995). Those espousing the AQAL framework would, however, criticize approaches with a limited viewpoint and methodology such as Baker, Mall, and Shoham (2010), who attempt to be imperialistic or reductionistic in making their partial perspective more than what it is.

Encouraging Developments

With all the above cautions noted, the overall thrust of psychotherapy research in the last 30 years, in conjunction with that of cognate disciplines such as interpersonal neurobiology, trauma, and developmental studies, has been quite substantial and encouraging. It is an exciting time in psychology and psychotherapy. Research now confirms that psychotherapy is actually effective (Seligman, 1995), and the Dodo bird conclusion from comparing therapies that "all have won and must have prizes" has likewise induced some helpful humility in the field, motivating schools to learn from each other, including the delineation of common factors (Bateman & Fonagy, 2008; Beutler et al., 2003; Bohart, 2000; Bucci, 2001; Castonguay, 1993; Frank, 1986; Lambert & Ogles, 2004; Lipsey & Wilson, 1993; Luborsky, Singer, & Luborsky, 1975; Mahoney, 1991; Orlinsky et al., 2004; Sexton & Whiston, 1991; Smith & Glass, 1977; Smith, Glass, & Miller, 1980; Stevens, Hynan, & Allen, 2000; Stiles, Shapiro, & Elliot, 1986; VandenBos & Pino, 1980; Wampold, Minami, Baskin, & Callen-Tirney, 2002; Wampold et al., 1997).

Cautions

At the same time, Lilienfeld (2007) and Cummings and Donohue (2008) have noted the problems of simply following charismatic leaders in the field who circumvent honest dialogue with the research tradition. As Neukrug (2007, p. 384) argues, though it is necessarily true that "all research is biased . . . that does not mean that research is not important." And all research that results in actual data is good, even though the theory that drove the experiment might not hold up (Johanson, 1988). The postmodern quest to know everything contextually in relation to everything else remains and requires that we honor all the pieces of the puzzle available to us (Wilber, 1995).

Levels of Experiencing and More

One of the common factors of therapeutic effectiveness delineated by Castonguay, Goldfried, Wiser, Raue, and Hayes (1996) relates to levels of experiencing. Of the seven levels the study explores, Hakomi therapy operates routinely and preferably at the highest levels of gaining "awareness of previously implicit feelings and meanings . . . [and] an ongoing process of in-depth self-understanding" (p. 499). It has been gratifying that many stock-in-trade elements of Hakomi from its post-1960s beginnings have found mainline psycho-logical support through ongoing research. For instance, Hayes notes that the cognitive-behavioral therapy tradition

> has maintained its core commitments to science, theory, and good practice. In the last 10 years, a set of new behavior therapies has emerged that emphasizes issues that were traditionally less emphasized or even off limits for behavioral and cognitive therapists, including mindfulness, acceptance, the therapeutic relationship, values, spirituality, meditation, focusing on the present moment, emotional deepening, and similar topics. (2004, p. xiii)

Compassion and the Positive

Another gratifying development in psychodynamic work through the influence of attach-ment, developmental, and psychotherapy efficacy studies is research supporting the use of compassion and positive affects in therapy (Baumeister & Leary, 1995; Beebe & Lach-mann, 2002; Bridges, 2006; Davidson & Harrington, 2002; Decety & Jackson, 2004; Fehr et al., 2009; Fosha, 2000, 2004, 2009b; Fredrickson, 2001; Fredrickson & Losada, 2005; Germer, 2009; Gilbert, 2005, 2010; Greenberg & Paivio, 1997; Greenberg, Riche, & Elliott, 1993; Ji-Woong et al., 2009; Johnson, 2009; Keltner & Haidt, 1999; Laithwaite et al., 2009; Lamagna & Gleiser, 2007; Lewis et al., 2000; Panksepp, 2001; Paivio & Lau-rent, 2001; Prenn, 2009; Schore, 2001; Shiota, Keltner, Campos, & Hertenstein, 2004; Trevarthen, 2001; Tronick, 1998; Tugade & Frederickson, 2004). This is something Kurtz (1990a) affirmed from the beginning, though he knew it was not the mainline model of "professional demeanor" (Kurtz, 2008, p. 15) at the time. In training sessions he was often heard to say, "Find something in the client to love."

An Impulse Toward Growth

Something occurs in therapy that seems beyond the control of therapist or client. Growth happens in the face of ignorance, stumbling, and fumbling by therapist and client alike. Growth doesn't happen despite the most highly trained clinician employing the most state-of-the art techniques. Peck (1978) was so impressed that growth happens at all—in the face of so many obstacles working against it—that he posited some spiritual force called grace to account for it in his best seller *The Road Less Traveled*. In Hakomi, Kurtz (1990a) often referred to the concept of "negentropy" as expounded by Bateson (1979), Prigogine and Stengers (1984), and Wilber (1995): the notion that there is a force in life that moves to build wholes out of parts, as well as the more well-known second law of thermody-namics that posits the opposite. By any name ("transformance" for Fosha, 2000; "the life-forward direction" for Gendlin, 1996), there is an organic impulse, which can be expe-rienced phenomenologically, to heal through moving toward increased complexity and wholeness. Hakomi therapists always count on this organic impulse, and it has received increasing research support in recent years (Eigen, 1996; Emde, 1988; Fosha, 2006, 2008, 2009a, 2009b; Ghent, 1999, 2002).

Larger Self-States

There are also core aspects of mindfulness or consciousness—including passive awareness and active compassion—that Hakomi therapists assume are essentially present in all clients. These potentials are there, regardless of the person's object relations history as it shows up on the ego level of past conditioning. Others refer to these essential qualities as comprising the self, core self, heart self, ontological self, and so on. The concept of a larger self, new to Western psychology (Schmidt, 1994), has likewise received research support since Hakomi's beginnings (Almaas, 1988; Fosha, 2005; Kershaw & Wade, 2011; Mones & Schwartz, 2007; Panksepp & Northoff, 2008; Russell & Fosha, 2008; Schwartz, 1995). Eisman (2006) has led the way in Hakomi by developing an entire healing approach called the re-creation of the self that centers on resourcing clients as fast as possible in the non-egocentric transhistorical aspects of this larger self-state.

Resourcing

The emphasis on resourcing through larger self-states is congruent with the more general emphasis on resourcing in Hakomi by helping clients be in touch with their strengths, bodily energies, hopes, positive images and memories, and so forth. Much research supports this emphasis (Gassman & Grawe, 2006). For trauma therapists who work with lower-brain activation, multiple forms of resourcing are absolutely necessary (Ogden et al., 2006). Hakomi in general always begins with fostering qualities of safety, curiosity, and present-moment experiencing, which is a way of resourcing clients to be able to successfully explore inner material (Fogel, 2009). Humor—that Kurtz was so brilliant with—is a hypnotic affirmation of faith communicating to clients that they have what it takes to deal with whatever is afflicting them. Working through barriers to transformation and the introjection of positive "missing experiences" in Hakomi is a way of both unburdening hurtful experiences and expanding a client's toleration of positive experiences (Robbins, 2008). Encouraging clients to move toward the future with hope by integrating more positive experiences in their lives, while dealing mindfully with whatever barriers arise, stimulates the immune system and a more grateful, energized way of meeting life (Johanson, 2010b; LeShan, 1984).

Appropriate Trainees

Although Hakomi therapy training is offered primarily as continuing education for licensed mental health professionals, the central importance of relationship, self-qualities, compassion, and awareness to psychotherapy has led institute faculty to also accept others in training who are assessed as able to benefit from the teaching. An array of bodyworkers, naturopaths, lawyers, teachers, artists, nurses, medical doctors, and others have taken Hakomi training, either to learn Hakomi methods they can incorporate into their work or as a way of tasting the field of psychotherapy before committing to various graduate programs. Is it ethical to train people in therapeutic techniques who are not licensed? What does the research have to say about this?

As it turns out, our commonly held assumptions about what makes better psychotherapists, enshrined in our requirements for licensure and membership in clinical associations, are not faring well in research. Surely, getting advanced degrees and licensure enhances our effectiveness. No, not really. Nyman, Nafzier, and Smith (2010) established that there was no discernible difference in outcome if the therapy was done by a licensed doctoral-level psychologist, a predoctoral intern, or a practicum student. How about professional training, discipline, and experience? It certainly sounds logical, but no, it doesn't hold up (Beutler et al., 2004). Using the right method or the latest evidence-based treatment should help. While we continually keep trying to find the key, any single one has yet to be found, though many seem to work in their own way (Duncan et al., 2010). Plus, no studies support increased effectiveness through continuing education, which is disappointing and hard to believe. What about therapists working on themselves as their own best instrument in therapy? Wonderful subjective benefits are reported here, but they do not show up in terms of affecting effectiveness (Geller, Norcross, & Orlinksky, 2005).

The upshot of this research does not support the necessity of state licensure boards so much as registries of psychotherapists that list one's training and ethical allegiances, and then respects clients' ability to search and find practitioners who provide the help they are seeking. (Hakomi faculty members, due to our tender pride and hubris, might point out that the above research did not study Hakomi training and supervision.)

Collaboration

One bright spot in efficacy outcome studies is that soliciting and responding appropriately to client feedback does improve the outcome for the client and the development of the therapist (Anker, Owen, Duncan, & Sparks, 2010; Duncan, 2010; Duncan, Solovey, & Rusk, 1992). This research finding is fully congruent with training in the Hakomi method. Hakomi's organicity principle states that when all the parts are connected within the whole, the system is self-organizing and self-correcting. This translates into the Hakomi therapist tracking and contacting a client's felt present experience in such a way that the therapist helps the person safely mine the wisdom of his or her own experience in a continuously collaborative way. This fine-tuned collaboration in turn provides a profound safeguard against either licensed or nonlicensed trainees unwittingly committing forms of violence on the client or inducing appropriate resistance. Other aspects of Hakomi training could be explicated that fit in with research findings on how psychotherapists develop and grow (Orlinsky & Roennestad, 2005).

More Encouraging Developments

In contrast to the state of psychology in the 1960s, there is now serious and sustained research dedicated to cross-cultural and social issues (Augsburger, 1986; Foster et al., 1996; Helms & Cook, 1999; Keita & Hurrell, 1994; Marsella, 1998, 2009; Marsella, Bornemann, Ekblad, & Orley, 1994; Marsella, Johnson, Watson, & Gryczyski, 2008; McGoldrick et al.,

1996; Nader, Dubrow, & Stamm, 1999; Pinderhughes, 1989; Ponterotto, Casas, Suzuki, & Alexander, 2010; Sue & Sue, 2010; Vasquez, 2012; Wessells, 1999).

Likewise, though Hakomi has never been presented as a spiritual path or endorsed the path of any other spiritual tradition, it has always been open to the spiritual dimension of clients as an important aspect of their being. This significant facet of many clients' lives (Eisner, 2009; Johanson, 1999b; Mayo, 2009; Monda, 2000; Sperry, 2010; Torrance, 1994), routinely ignored or pathologized in the 20th century (LeShan, 1990), is now being researched in such journals as the American Psychological Association's Division 36 *Psychology of Religion and Spirituality* and the *Journal of Spirituality in Mental Health* from Routledge Press, textbooks such as Miller (2003), numerous APA titles, and myriad contributions of others.

Hakomi-Sponsored Research

Hakomi leaders have encouraged and pursued research wherever possible within Hakomi's context as a training institute. Through the leadership of the Hakomi Institute of Europe, the first major empirical research was done demonstrating the efficacy of body psychotherapy methods in outpatient settings. This multiyear, multicenter investigation was done in Germany and Switzerland, and involved both clinical practitioners and university professors (Koemeda-Lutz et al., 2006). In the United States, Kaplan and Schwartz (2005) provided a methodologically rigorous study of the results of working with two clients within a 12-session protocol.

Further research into body-inclusive psychotherapy was given a major impetus when Halko Weiss, director of the Hakomi Institute of Europe, joined with his colleague Gustl Marlock to edit the *Handbuch der Körperpsychotherapie*, a thousand-page handbook on body psychotherapy published by Schattauer, a highly respected medical publisher in Germany. This well-referenced and positively reviewed work has contributions from 82 international experts. The English translation (Marlock & Weiss, with Young & Soth, 2015) will likewise further the field in many countries and give impetus to the growing literature addressing somatic issues (Aron & Anderson, 1998; Boadella, 1997; Field, 1989; Griffith & Griffith, 1994; Halling & Goldfarb, 1991; Heller, 2012; Kepner, 1993; Leder, 1984, 1990; Matthew, 1998; Ogden et al., 2006; Romanyshyn, 1992; Shaw, 2003, 2004; Stam, 1998; van der Kolk, 1994).

Hakomi faculty have taken leadership positions in the European Association for Body Psychotherapy and the United States Association for Body Psychotherapy, supporting both professional conferences and journals. The Hakomi Institute itself has sponsored numerous professional conferences that have highlighted keynote speakers outside Hakomi, such as Stephen Wolinsky, Peter Levine, Richard C. Schwartz, Thomas Lewis, Stephen Porges, Bessel van der Kolk, Diana Fosha, Susan Aposhyan, Babette Rothschild, Christine Caldwell, and more.

Through 2014, the institute has published 27 editions of its annual journal, *Hakomi Forum*. In the first 10 years of the *Forum*, many contributions concentrated on clinical reports on the use of the method with couples, psychodrama, biofeedback, emotionally disturbed adolescents, values, cancer patients, eating disorders, seniors, the Q-sort technique, storytelling, yoga, curiosity research, neurological correlates, groups, organizations, supervision, adolescents, families, ontological development, transference and countertransference in the here-and-now therapies, touch, pre- and perinatal trauma, laughter, despair, psychotic jail inmates, emotion, grace, boundaries, ethics, multiplicity, self-theory, and more.

As the Hakomi method matured and grew, the editorial board expanded significantly beyond the founding trainers of the institute, and more articles referencing mainline psychology appeared, though the editorial policy continued to accept more experiential, poetic, and clinically informed articles along with scholarly and scientific contributions. A number of colleagues and collaborators outside of Hakomi have contributed to the ongoing dialogue of the *Forum* over the years, including Eligio S. Gallegos, Chogyam Trungpa, Jerome Liss, William S. Schmidt, David Feinstein, Suzanne M. Peloquin, Albert Pesso, Stephen Pattison, Eugene Gendlin, Jack Engler, Richard Schwartz, Stephen Wolinsky, Belinda Siew Luan Khong, Aline LaPierre, David N. Elkins, Martha Herbert, Siroj Sorajjakool, Miriam Greenspan, Carole M. McNamee, Louise Sundararajan, Diana Fosha, and others.

The majority of clinical research by Hakomi therapists has been dedicated to what Gendlin (1986, p. 133) has termed "playing in the laboratory." This is part of the trend in psychotherapy research toward identifying and evaluating small subprocesses of therapeutic interactions, as opposed to evaluating entire therapies in relation to each other (Johanson, 1986). Playing in the lab involves creatively and curiously exploring a subprocess with the rapid feedback in a clinical encounter that can confirm or disconfirm a hunch or open up new trailheads. It eventually leads to promising hypotheses that are worthy of the more extensive time, money, and energy that go into formal research.

The main laboratory settings for Hakomi are private practice, public and private health services clinics, and comprehensive psychotherapy training. Here Gendlin's (1986) suggestion that there be a central data bank of successful cases that can be examined further is carried out. Ron Kurtz left over 400 videotapes demonstrating his work. The Hakomi Institute asks those who have successfully shown enough competency in the method to become certified Hakomi therapists or practitioners to place copies of their certification tapes in a central office archive. These case examples are available for the psychotherapy process Q-sort technique (PQS; Jones, 2000), and other research uses outlined by Goldfried and Wolfe (1996), Jones and Pulos (1993), Kazdin (2007), Nathan and Gorman (2002), and others. There are a number of research studies the Hakomi Institute would like to engage in when possible.

However, on behalf of the many right-brained practitioners drawn to the experiential power of the Hakomi method, it must be said there is much sympathy for the summary of Shedler (2010, p. 107) who asserts:

> Many of the psychotherapy outcome studies . . . are clearly not written for
> practitioners . . . [but] for other psychotherapy researchers. . . . I am unsure
> how the average knowledgeable clinical practitioner could navigate the thicket

of specialized statistical methods, clinically unrepresentative samples, investigator allegiance effects, inconsistent methods of reporting results, and inconsistent findings across multiple outcome variables of uncertain clinical relevance. . . . Psychotherapy research needs to be more consumer relevant (Westen, Novotny & Thompson-Brenner, 2005).

Today, as suggested above, psychology and psychotherapy comprise an exciting and promising field that has grown considerably since Hakomi's beginnings in the post-1960s era. Part of the excitement is the responsibly eclectic expansion of concern to include contributions from developmental studies, interpersonal neurobiology, trauma, and the body (Levine with Frederick, 1997; Ogden et al., 2006; Rothschild, 2000; van der Kolk, 1994, 2003), multicultural values, social structures, and more. All this is being done with a view to better integrate theory and clinical practice while applying the techniques to coaching, teaching, human relationships, groups, corporate situations, and more. Hakomi, as a mindfulness-centered somatic psychotherapy, has a specific and unique contribution to make to the training of healers in today's world. At the same time, the large umbrella of its theoretical principles offers a home base from which research contributions from these many realms of healing can be integrated. A hallmark and value of Hakomi remains the close congruence between theory, method, and technique, always tested and refined through experience in the field.

Final Word

With all that has been said here (and the more that could be said) about Hakomi engaging the ambiguity of the promises and perils of psychotherapy research, it must be noted that the governmental and corporate entities who control third-party payments still look with tunnel vision at hard experimental research yielding quantitative results. It has been hard for psychotherapy in general, let alone somatic psychotherapy (Barratt, 2015; May, 2005; Young, 2010) to meet such requirements in a manner similar to double-blind psychotropic drug research. Given the myriad issues suggested above, more philosophical perspectives that could be brought to bear, political-economic interests, and the overwhelming monetary requirements involved, Hakomi will not likely be producing the requisite research soon, though the institute remains open to finding university, government, or corporate partners who can facilitate such substantial research programs. Though Hakomi can point to over 2,500 research studies on the efficacy of mindfulness in therapy alone, plus so much other research we draw on from interpersonal neurobiology and developmental studies, people in power will still ask, "Where are the studies on Hakomi per se?" This means that prospective Hakomi students will have to make considered choices about training in a method that is subjectively meaningful and effective for clients and therapists, but carries objective costs in terms of finances and official standing beyond private practice settings—another source of ambiguity.

References

Ablon, J. S., & Jones, E. E. (1998). How expert clinicians' prototypes of an ideal treatment correlate with outcome in psychodynamic and cognitive-behavioral therapy. *Psychotherapy Research, 8,* 71–83.

Ablon, J. S., & Jones, E. E. (2002). Validity of controlled clinical trials of psychotherapy: Findings from the NIMH Treatment of Depression Collaborative Research Program. *American Journal of Psychiatry, 159,* 775–783.

Ahlstrom, S. E. (1972). *A religious history of the American people.* New Haven, CT: Yale University Press.

Ainsworth, M. D. S., Blehar, M. C., Waters, E., & Wall, S. (1978). *Patterns of attachment: A psychological study of the strange situation.* Hillsdale, NJ: Lawrence Erlbaum.

Aitkin, K. J., & Trevarthen, C. (1997). Self-other organization in human psychological development. *Development and Psychopathology, 9,* 653–678.

Alexander, F., French, T. M., et al. (1946). *Psychoanalytic therapy: Principles and application.* New York: Ronald Press.

Allen, F. H. (1942). *Psychotherapy with children.* New York: Norton.

Allen, N. B., & Knight, W. (2005). Mindfulness, compassion for self, and compassion for others. In P. Gilbert (Ed.), *Compassion: Conceptualizations, research and use in psychotherapy* (pp. 239–262). New York: Routledge.

Almaas, A. H. (1986). *Essence: The diamond approach to inner realization.* York Beach, ME: Samuel Weiser.

Almaas, A. H. (1988). *The pearl beyond price: Integration of personality into being: An object relations approach.* Berkeley, CA: Diamond.

Almaas, A. H. (1990). *Diamond heart, book three: Being and the meaning of life.* Boston: Shambhala.

Alterman, E. (2004). *When presidents lie: A history of official deception and its consequences.* New York: Viking.

Ammerman, N. (1993). *Bible believers: Fundamentalists in the modern world.* New Brunswick, NJ: Rutgers University Press.

Andersen, P. B., Emmeche, C., Finnemann, N. O., & Christiansen, P. V. (Eds.) (2000). *Downward causation: Minds, bodies and matter.* Aarhus, Denmark: Aarhus University Press.

Anderson, S. (2000). *The journey from abandonment to healing.* New York: Berkley.

Anker, M., Owen, J., Duncan, B., & Sparks, J. (2010). The alliance in couple therapy: Partner influence, early change, and alliance patterns in a naturalistic sample. *Journal of Consulting and Clinical Psychology, 78,* 635–645.

APA Presidential Task Force on Evidence-Based Practice. (2006). Evidence-based practice in psychology. *American Psychologist, 61,* 271–285.

Aposhyan, S. (2004). *Body-mind psychotherapy: Principles, techniques, and practical applications.* New York: Norton.

Arbeitskreis OPD. (1996). *Operationalisierte psychodynamische Diagnostik OPD* (Operationalized Psychodynamic Diagnostics). Bern: Huber.

Ardito, R. B., & Rabellino, D. (2011). Therapeutic alliance and outcome of psychotherapy: Historical excursus, measurements, and prospect for research. *Frontiers in Psychology, 2,* 270.

Aron, L. (1998a). The body in drive and relational models. In L. Aron & F. Anderson (Eds.), *Relational perspectives on the body* (pp. xix–xxviii). Hillsdale, NJ: Analytic Press.

Aron, L. (1998b). The clinical body and the reflexive mind. In L. Aron & F. Anderson (Eds.), *Relational perspectives on the body* (pp. 3–38). Hillsdale, NJ: Analytic Press.

Aron, L., & Anderson, F. S. (Eds.) (1998). *Relational perspectives on the body.* Hillsdale, NJ: Analytic Press.

Augsburger, D. A. (1986). *Pastoral counseling across cultures.* Philadelphia: Westminster.

Badenoch, B. (2008). *Being a brain-wise therapist: A practical guide to interpersonal neurobiology.* New York: Norton.

Baer, R. (2003). Mindfulness training as a clinical intervention: A conceptual and empirical review. *Clinical Psychology: Science and Practice, 10*(2), 125–142.

Baeyer, H. C. v. (2004). *Information: The new language of science.* Cambridge, MA: Harvard University Press.

Baker, T., McFall, R., & Shoham, V. (2010). Current status and future prospects of clinical psychology toward a scientifically principled approach to mental and behavioral health care. *Psychological Science in the Public Interest, 9,* 67–103.

Balint, M. (1992). *The basic fault: Therapeutic aspects of regression.* Evanston, IL: Northwestern University Press.

Bandler, R., & Grinder, J. (1975). *The structure of magic 1: A book about language and therapy.* Palo Alto, CA: Science and Behavior.

Bandler, R., & Grinder, J. (1976). *Structure of magic 2: A book about communication and change.* Los Altos, CA: Science and Behavior.

Barasch, M. (2005). *Field notes on the compassionate life: A search for the soul of kindness.* New York: Rodale.

Bargh, J. A., & Chartrand, T. L. (1999). The unbearable automaticity of being. *American Psychologist, 54,* 462–479.

Barratt, B. (2010). *The emergence of somatic psychology and bodymind therapy.* New York: Palgrave Macmillan.

Barratt, B. (2015). *Research in body psychotherapy.* In G. Marlock & H. Weiss, with C. Young & M. Soth, *Handbook of body psychotherapy and somatic psychology.* Berkeley: North Atlantic Books.

Barstow, C. (2005). *Right use of power: The heart of ethics.* Boulder, CO: Many Realms.

Barton, S. (1994). Chaos, self-organization, and psychology. *American Psychologist, 49,* 5–14.

Bateman, A., & Fonagy, P. (2008). 8-year follow-up of patients treated for borderline personality disorder: Mentalization-based treatment versus treatment as usual. *American Journal of Psychiatry, 165,* 631–638.

Bateson, G. (1979). *Mind and nature: A necessary unity.* New York: E. P. Dutton.

Bateson, G., & Bateson, M. C. (1987). *Angels fear: Towards an epistemology of the sacred.* New York: Macmillan.

Baumeister, R., & Leary, M. R. (1995). The need to belong: Desire for interpersonal attachments as a fundamental human motivation. *Psychological Bulletin, 117,* 497–529.

Baumeister, R., & Sommer, K. L. (1997). Consciousness, free choice, and automaticity. In R. S. Wyer (Ed.), *Advances in social cognition* (Vol. 10, pp. 75–82). Mahwah, NJ: Lawrence Erlbaum.

Beck, A. T., Rush, A. J., Shaw, B. F., & Emery, G. (1979). *Cognitive therapy of depression*. New York: Guilford.

Becker, H. (2006). Körperpsychotherapie, ein Königsweg zum psychosomatisch Kranken (Body-psychotherapy, a royal road to the psychosomatically ill). In G. Marlock & H. Weiss (Eds.), *Handbuch der Körperpsychotherapie (Handbook of body psychotherapy)* (pp. 759–767). Stuttgart: Schattauer.

Beebe, B., & Lachmann, F. (1998). Co-constructing inner and relational processes: Self- and mutual regulation in infant research and adult treatment. *Psychoanalytic Psychology, 15,* 480–516.

Beebe, B., & Lachmann, F. (2002). *Infant research and adult treatment: Co-constructing interactions*. Hillsdale, NJ: Analytic Press.

Begley, S. (2007). *Train your mind, change your brain: How a new science reveals our extraordinary potential to transform ourselves*. New York: Random House.

Beitel, M., Ferrer, E., & Cecero, J. J. (2005). Psychological mindedness and awareness of self and others. *Journal of Clinical Psychology, 61,* 739–750.

Bennett-Goleman, T. (2001). *Emotional alchemy: How the mind can heal the heart*. New York: Harmony.

Benz, D. (1981). *The analysis, description and application of an experiential, body-centered psychotherapy*. (Unpublished doctoral dissertation). Massachusetts School of Professional Psychology, Boston.

Benz, D. (1989). Family: The next larger picture. *Hakomi Forum, (7),* 36–38.

Benz, D., & Weiss, H. (1989). *To the core of your experience*. Charlottesville, VA: Luminas Press.

Berman, M. (1989). The roots of reality. *Journal of Humanistic Psychology, 29*(2), 277–284.

Berman, M. (1990). *Coming to our senses: Body and spirit in the hidden history of the west*. New York: Bantam.

Berman, M. (1996). The shadow side of systems theory. *Journal of Humanistic Psychology, 36*(1), 28–54.

Berne, E. (1964). *Games people play*. New York: Grove.

Berne, E. (1972). *What do you say after you say hello?* New York: Grove.

Bertalanffy, L. von. (1968). *General system theory*. New York: George Braziller.

Beutler, L. E. (2009). Making science matter in clinical practice: Redefining psychotherapy. *Clinical Psychology: Science and Practice, 16*(3), 301–317.

Beutler, L. E., Malik, M., Alimohamed, S., Harwood, T. M., Talabi, H., Noble, S., et al. (2004). Therapist variables. In M. J. Lambert (Ed.), *Handbook of psychotherapy and behavior change* (5th ed., pp. 227–306). New York: John Wiley.

Beutler, L. E., Moleiro, C., Malik, M., Harwood, T. M., Romanelli, R., Gallagher-Thompson, D., et al. (2003). A comparison of the Dodo, EST, and ATI indicators among co-morbid stimulant dependent, depressed patients. *Clinical Psychology and Psychotherapy, 10,* 69–85.

Bishop, R. (2007). *The philosophy of the social sciences: An introduction*. London: Continuum.

Blakeslee, S., & Blakeslee, M. (2007). *The body has a mind of its own: How body maps in your brain help you to do (almost) everything better*. New York: Random House.

Blatt, S. J., & Auerbach, J. S. (2003). Psychodynamic measures of therapeutic change. *Psychoanalytic Inquiry, 23,* 268–307.

Blatt, S. J., & Zuroff, D. C. (2005). Empirical evaluation of the assumptions in identifying evidence based treatments in mental health. *Clinical Psychology Review, 25,* 459–486.

Boadella, D. (1980). Violence in therapy. *Energy & Character, 11*(1), 1.

Boadella, D. (1987). *Lifestreams: An introduction to biosynthesis.* New York: Routledge Kegan & Paul.

Boadella, D. (1997). Embodiment in the therapeutic relationship. *International Journal of Psychotherapy, 2*, 31–44.

Bobrow, J. (2010). *Zen and psychotherapy.* New York: Norton.

Bohart, A. C. (2000). The client is the most important common factor: Clients' self-healing capacities and psychotherapy. *Journal of Psychotherapy Integration, 10*(2), 127–149.

Boorstein, S. (1997*). It's easier than you think: The Buddhist way to happiness.* New York: HarperCollins.

Bons-Storm, R. (1996). *The incredible woman.* Nashville, TN: Abingdon.

Borkovec, T. D. (2002). Life in the future versus life in the present. *Clinical Psychology: Science and Practice, 9*, 76–80.

Bowlby, J. (1969). *Attachment and loss: Vol. 1. Attachment.* New York: Basic Books.

Bowlby, J. (1973). *Attachment and loss: Vol. 2. Separation: Anxiety and anger.* London: Hogarth.

Bradshaw, J. (1990). *Home coming: Reclaiming and championing your inner child.* New York: Bantam.

Brazelton, T. B., Koslowski, B., & Main, M. (1974). The origins of reciprocity: The early mother–infant interaction. In M. Lewis & L. Rosenblum (Eds.), *The effect of an infant on its caregiver* (pp. 49–76). New York: Wiley.

Brefczynski-Lewis, J. A., Lutz, A., Schaefer, H. S., Levinson, D. B., & Davidson, R. J. (2007). Neural correlates of attentional expertise in long-term meditation practitioners. *Proceedings of the National Academy of Sciences, 104*, 11483–11488.

Breslin, F. C., Zack, M., & Mcmain, S. (2002). An information-processing analysis of mindfulness: Implications for relapse prevention in the treatment of substance abuse. *Clinical Psychology: Science and Practice, 9*(3), 275–299.

Breunlin, D. C., Schwartz, R. C., & Mac Kune-Karrer, B. (1992). *Metaframeworks: Transcending the models of family therapy.* San Francisco: Jossey-Bass.

Bridges, M. R. (2006). Activating the corrective emotional experience. *Journal of Clinical Psychology: In Session, 62*, 551–568.

Broderick, P. C. (2005). Mindfulness and coping with dysphoric mood: Contrasts with rumination and distraction. *Cognitive Therapy and Research, 29*, 501–510.

Brown, K. W., & Kasser, T. (2005). Are psychological and ecological wellbeing compatible? The role of values, mindfulness, and lifestyle. *Social Indicators Research, 74*, 349–368.

Brown, K. W., & Ryan, R. M. (2003). The benefits of being present: Mindfulness and its role in psychological well-being. *Journal of Personality and Social Psychology, 84*, 822–848.

Brown, K. W., & Ryan, R. M. (2004). Fostering healthy self-regulation from within and without: A self-determination theory perspective. In P. A. Linley & S. Joseph (Eds.), *Positive psychology in practice* (pp. 105–124). New York: Wiley.

Brown, K. W., Ryan, R. M., & Creswell, J. D. (2007). Mindfulness: Theoretical foundations and evidence for its salutary effects. *Psychological Inquiry, 18*(4), 211–237.

Bucci, W. (2001). Toward a "psychodynamic science": The state of current research. *Journal of the American Psychoanalytic Association, 49*, 57–68.

Caldwell, C. (1997). *Getting in touch: The guide to new body-centered therapies.* Wheaton, IL: Quest.

Caldwell, C. (2011). Sensation, movement, and memory: Explicit procedures for implicit processes. In S. Koch, T. Fuchs, M. Summa, & C. Muller (Eds.), *Body memory, metaphor, and movement* (pp. 255–265). Heidelberg, Germany: University of Heidelberg Press.

Calvin, W. H. (1997). *How brains think: Evolving intelligence, then and now.* New York: Basic Books

Carson, J. W., Carson, K. M., Gil, K. M., & Baucom, D. H. (2004). Mindfulness-based relationship enhancement. *Behavior Therapy, 35*, 471–494.

Cassidy, J., & Shaver, P. R. (Eds.) (2010). *Handbook of attachment: Theory, research and clinical applications.* New York: Guilford.

Castonguay, L. G. (1993). Common factors and non specific variables: Clarification of the two concepts and recommendations for research. *Journal of Psychotherapy Integration, 3*, 267–286.

Castonguay, L. G., & Beutler, L. E. (Eds.) (2006). *Principles of therapeutic change that work: Integrating relationship, treatment, client and therapist factors.* New York: Oxford University Press.

Castonguay, L. G., Goldfried, M. R., Wiser, S. L., Raue, P. J., & Hayes, A. H. (1996). Predicting the effect of cognitive therapy for depression: A study of unique and common factors. *Journal of Consulting and Clinical Psychology, 64*, 497–504.

Castonguay, L. G., & Hill, C. E. (Eds.) (2012). *Transformation in psychotherapy: Corrective experiences across cognitive behavioral, humanistic, and psychodynamic approaches.* Washington, DC: American Psychological Association.

Causey, C. M. (1993). *Touch and pastoral counseling with sexually abused women: An object relationships interpretation.* (Unpublished master's thesis). Southern Baptist Theological Seminary, Louisville, KY.

Chodron, P. (2003). *Comfortable with uncertainty.* Boston: Shambhala.

Clarkin, J. F., Levy, K. N., Lenzenweger, M. F., & Kernberg, O. F. (2007). Evaluating three treatments for borderline personality disorder: A multiwave study. *American Journal of Psychiatry, 164*, 922–928.

Clarkson, P., & Mackewn, J. (1993). *Fritz Perls.* London: Sage.

Clayton, P. (2004). *Mind and emergence: From quantum to consciousness.* New York: Oxford University Press.

Clayton, P., & Davies, P. (Eds.) (2006). *The re-emergence of emergence: The emergentist hypothesis from science to religion.* New York: Oxford University Press.

Coffey, K. (2008). Making Hakomi more transpersonal. *Hakomi Forum, (19–21)*, 85–100.

Cole, J. D., & Ladas-Gaskin, C. (2007). *Mindfulness centered therapies: An integrative approach.* Seattle, WA: Silver Birch Press.

Coleman, R., & Smith, M. (2006). *Working with voices: Victim to victor* (2nd ed.). Lewis, Scotland: P & P Press.

Constantino, M. J., & Westra, H. A. (2012). An expectancy-based approach to facilitating corrective experiences in psychotherapy. In L. G. Castonguay & C. E. Hill (Eds.), *Transformation in psychotherapy: Corrective experiences across cognitive behavioral, humanistic, and psychodynamic approaches* (pp. 121–140). Washington, DC: American Psychological Association.

Cooper, P. C. (1999). Buddhist meditation and countertransference: A case study. *American Journal of Psychoanalysis, 59*, 71–85.

Cowan, G. A., Pines, D., & Meltzer, D. (1994). *Complexity: Metaphors, models, and reality.* New York: Addison Wesley.

Cozolino, L. (2002). *The neuroscience of psychotherapy: Building and rebuilding the human brain.* New York: Norton.

Cozolino, L. (2006). *The neuroscience of human relationships: Attachment and the developing social brain.* New York: Norton.

Cozolino, L. (2010). *The neuroscience of psychotherapy: Healing the social brain* (2nd ed.). New York: Norton.

Craig, A. D. (2003). Interoception: The sense of the physiological condition of the body. *Current Opinions in Neurobiology, 13*, 500–505.

Creswell, J. W., & Plano Clark, V. L. (2007). *Designing and conducting mixed methods research.* Thousand Oaks, CA: Sage.

Crisp, T. (1987). *Mind and movement: The practice of coex.* Essex, England: C. W. Daniel.

Cummings, N. A., & O'Donohue, W. T. (2008). *Eleven blunders that cripple psychotherapy in America.* New York: Routledge.

Daly, H. E., & Cobb, J. B., Jr. (1989). *For the common good: Redirecting the economy toward community, the environment, and sustainable future.* Boston: Beacon.

Damasio, A. (1994). *Descartes' error: Emotion, reason and the human brain.* New York: Putnam.

Damasio, A. (1999). *The feeling of what happens: Body and emotion in the making of consciousness.* New York: Harcourt Brace.

Damasio, A. R. (2000). *Ich fühle, also bin ich* (I feel, therefore I am). Munich: List.

Damasio, A. (2003). *Looking for Spinoza: Joy, sorrow and the feeling brain.* London: Heinemann.

Davidson, R. J., & Begley, S. (2012). *The emotional life of our brain. How its unique patterns affect the way you think, feel and live.* New York: Hudson Street Press.

Davidson, R. J., & Harrington, A. (Eds.) (2002). *Visions of compassion: Western scientists and Tibetan Buddhists examine human nature.* New York: Oxford University Press.

Davidson, R. J., Kabat-Zinn, J., Schumacher, J., Rosenkranz, M., Muller, D., Santorelli, S. F., Urbanowski, F., Harrington, A., Bonus, K., & Sheridan, J. F. (2003). Alterations in brain and immune function produced by mindfulness meditation. *Psychosomatic Medicine, 65*, 564–570.

Deacon, T. W. (2003). The hierarchic logic of emergence: Untangling the interdependence of evolution and self-organization. In B. H. Weber & D. J. Depew (Eds.), *Evolution and learning: The Baldwin effect reconsidered* (pp. 273–308). Cambridge, MA: MIT Press.

Deacon, T. W. (2006). Emergence: The hole at the wheel's hub. In P. Clayton & P. Davies (Eds.), *The re-emergence of emergence: The emergentist hypothesis from science to religion* (pp. 111–150). New York: Oxford University Press.

DeAngelis, T. (2010). Closing the gap between practice and research. *Monitor on Psychology, 41*, 42–45.

Decety, J., & Jackson, P. L. (2004). The functional architecture of human empathy. *Behavioral and Cognitive Neuroscience Reviews, 3*, 71–100.

Deci, E. L., & Ryan, R. M. (1985). *Intrinsic motivation and self-determination in human behavior.* New York: Plenum.

Deikman, A. J. (1996). "I" = awareness. *Journal of Consciousness Studies, 3*, 350–356.

Deleuze, G., & Guattari, F. (1987). *A thousand plateaus: Capitalism and schizophrenia.* Minneapolis: University of Minnesota Press.

de Maat, S., Dekker, J., Schoevers, R., & de Jonghe, F. (2006). Relative efficacy of psychotherapy and pharmacotherapy in the treatment of depression: A meta-analysis. *Psychotherapy Research, 16*, 562–572.

Depraz, N., Varela, F. J., & Vermersch, P. (2000). The gesture of awareness: An account of its structural dynamics. In M. Velmans (Ed.), *Investigating phenomenal consciousness: New methodologies and maps* (pp. 121–136). Philadelphia: John Benjamins.

Doidge, N. (2007). *The brain that changes itself: Stories of personal triumph from the frontiers of brain science.* New York: Viking.

Dornes, M. (1993). *Der kompetente Säugling* (The competent baby). Frankfurt am Main: Fischer.

Dornes, M. (2000). *Die emotionale Welt des Kindes* (The emotional world of the child). Frankfurt am Main: Fischer.

Downing, G. (1996). *Körper und Wort in der Psychotherapy* (Body and words in psychotherapy). Munich: Kösel.

Downing, G. (2015). Early interaction and the body: Clinical implications. In G. Marlock & H. Weiss, with C. Young & M. Soth, *Handbook of body psychotherapy and somatic psychology*. Berkeley: North Atlantic Books.

Duncan, B. (2010). *On becoming a better therapist*. Washington, DC: American Psychological Association.

Duncan, B. L., & Miller, S. D. (2000). *The heroic client*. San Francisco: Jossey-Bass.

Duncan, B. L., & Miller, S. D. (2006). Treatment manuals do not improve outcomes. In J. C. Norcross, L. E. Beutler, & R. Levant (Eds.), *Evidence-based practices in mental health: Debate and dialogue on the fundamental questions* (pp. 140–149). Washington, DC: American Psychological Association.

Duncan, B., Miller, S., Wampold, B., & Hubble, M. (Eds.) (2010). *The heart and soul of change: Delivering what works in therapy* (2nd ed.). Washington, DC: American Psychological Association.

Duncan, B., Solovey, A., & Rusk, G. (1992). *Changing the rules: A client-directed approach*. New York: Guilford.

Dychtwald, K. (1987). *Bodymind*. Los Angeles: Tarcher.

Ecker, B., & Hulley, L. (1996). *Depth oriented brief therapy*. San Francisco: Jossey-Bass.

Ecker, B., Ticic, R., & Hulley, L. (2012). *Unlocking the emotional brain: Eliminating symptoms at their roots using memory reconsolidation*. New York: Routledge.

Edwards, M. (2000). *Future positive: International co-operation in the 21st century*. London: Earthscan.

Eigen, M. (1996). *Psychic deadness*. Northvale, NJ: Jason Aronson.

Eisman, J. (1989). The child state of consciousness and the formation of the self. *Hakomi Forum*, (7), 10–15.

Eisman, J. (2005). Categories of psychological wounding, neural patterns, and treatment approaches. *Hakomi Forum*, (14–15), 43–50.

Eisman, J. (2006). Shifting states of consciousness: The re-creation of the self approach to transformation. *Hakomi Forum*, (16–17), 63–70.

Eisner, T. (2009). Following the footsteps of the soul in research. *Psychological Perspectives, 52*, 24–36.

Eisman, J. (2010). *Responding to life manual*. San Francisco: Hakomi Institute.

Ekman, P., & Rosenberg, E. L. (Eds.) (2005). *What the face reveals: Basic and applied studies of spontaneous expression using the facial action coding system*. New York: Oxford University Press.

Elkin, I., Shea, T., Watkins, J. T., Imber, S. D., Sotsky, S. M., Collins, J. F., Parloff, M. B., et al. (1989). National Institutes of Mental Health Treatment of Depression Collaborative Research Program. *Archives of General Psychiatry, 46*, 971–982.

Ellwood, R. S., Jr. (1979). *Alternative altars: Unconventional and Eastern spirituality in America*. Chicago: University of Chicago Press.

Emde, R. N. (1988). Development terminable and interminable. *International Journal of Psycho-Analysis, 69*, 23–42.

Emmeche, C., Koppe, S., & Stjernfelt, F. (1997). Explaining emergence: Towards an ontology of levels. *Journal for General Philosophy of Science, 28*, 83–119.

Emmons, R. A. (2007). *Thanks! How the new science of gratitude can make you happier.* New York: Houghton Mifflin.

Engler, B. (1991). *Personality theories: An introduction* (3rd ed.). Boston: Houghton Mifflin.

Engler, J. (1986). Therapeutic aims in psychotherapy and meditation. In K. Wilber, J. Engler, & D. Brown (Eds.), *Transformations of consciousness: Conventional and contemplative perspectives on development* (pp. 35–79). Boston: Shambhala.

Engler, J. (2003). Being somebody and being nobody: A reexamination of the understanding of self in psychoanalysis and Buddhism. In J. Safran (Ed.), *Psychoanalysis and Buddhism: An unfolding dialogue*. Boston: Wisdom.

English, H. B., & English, A. C. (1958). *A comprehensive dictionary of psychological and psycho-analytical terms: A guide to usage.* New York: David McKay.

Epstein, M. (1995). *Thought without a thinker: Psychotherapy from a Buddhist perspective.* New York: Basic Books.

Erikson, E. (1963). *Childhood and society* (2nd ed., rev. and enlarged). New York: Norton.

Faucheaux, D., & Weiss, H. (1995). The almost impossible task of just paying attention. *Psychotherapy in Australia, 2*(1), 32–41.

Fehr, C., Sprecher, S., & Underwood, L. G. (2009). *The science of compassionate love: Theory, research and application.* Chichester, UK: Wiley.

Feinstein, D. (1990). Transference and countertransference in the here-and-now therapies. *Hakomi Forum,* (8), 7–13.

Felder, R. E., & Weiss, A. G. (1991). *Experiential psychotherapy: A symphony of selves.* Lanham, MD: University Press of America.

Feldman, B. L., Gross, J., Christensen, T. C., & Benvenuto, M. (2001). Knowing what you're feeling and knowing what to do about it: Mapping the relation between emotional differentiation and emotion regulation. *Cognition and Emotion, 15*, 713–724.

Ferruci, P. (1982). *What we may be: The visions and techniques of psychosynthesis.* Northampton-shire: Turnstone.

Field, N. (1989). Listening with the body: An exploration in the countertransference. *British Journal of Psychotherapy, 5*, 512–522.

Fisher, R. (2002). *Experiential psychotherapy with couples: A guide for the creative pragmatist.* Phoenix, AZ: Zeig, Tucker and Theisen.

Fisher, R. (2011). Case study: Dancing with the unconscious. *Psychotherapy Networker,* July/August.

Fogel, A. (2009). *Body sense: The science and practice of embodied self-awareness.* New York: Norton.

Fonagy, P., Allison, L., Clarkin, J. F., Jones, E. E., Kachele, H., Krause, R., Lopez, D., & Perron, R. (Eds.) (2002). *An open door review of the outcome of psychoanalysis.* London: International Psychoanalytic Association.

Fonagy, P., & Target, M. (1997). Attachment and reflective function: Their role in self-organization. *Development and Psychopathology, 9*, 679–700.

Ford, C. W. (1993). *Compassionate touch: The role of human touch in healing and recovery.* New York: Fireside.

Fosha, D. (1992). Explicit empathy and the stance of therapeutic neutrality. *International Journal of Short-Term Psychotherapy, 7*(3), 193–198.

Fosha, D. (2000). *The transforming power of affect: A model for accelerated change.* New York: Basic Books.

Fosha, D. (2003). Dyadic regulation and experiential work with emotion and relatedness in trauma and disordered attachment. In M. F. Solomon & D. J. Siegel (Eds.), *Healing trauma: Attachment, trauma, the brain and the mind* (pp. 221–281). New York: Norton.

Fosha, D. (2004). "Nothing that feels bad is ever the last step": The role of positive emotions in experiential work with difficult emotional experiences. *Clinical Psychology and Psychotherapy, 11,* 30–43.

Fosha, D. (2005). Emotion, true self, true other, core state: Toward a clinical theory of affective change process. *Psychoanalytic Review, 92,* 513–552.

Fosha, D. (2006). Quantum transformation in trauma and treatment: Traversing the crisis of healing change. *Journal of Clinical Psychology/In Session, 62,* 569–583.

Fosha, D. (2008). Transformance, recognition of self by self, and effective action. In K. J. Schneider (Ed.), *Existential-integrative psychotherapy: Guideposts to the core of practice* (pp. 290–320). New York: Routledge.

Fosha, D. (2009a). Emotion and recognition at work: Energy, vitality, pleasure, truth, desire and the emergent phenomenology of transformational experience. In D. Fosha, D. J. Siegel, & M. F. Solomon (Eds.), *The healing power of emotion: Affective neuroscience, development, and clinical practice* (pp. 172–203). New York: Norton.

Fosha, D. (2009b). Positive affects and the transformation of suffering into flourishing. *Annals of the New York Academy of Sciences, 1172,* 252–261.

Fosha, D., Siegel, D., & Solomon, M. (Eds.) (2009). *The healing power of emotion: Affective neuroscience, development, and clinical practice.* New York: Norton.

Foster, R. P., Moskowitz, M., & Javier, R. A. (1996). *Reaching across boundaries of culture and class: Widening the scope of psychotherapy.* Northvale, NJ: Jason Aronson

Frank, J. (1986). Common features in psychotherapy. *Harvard Medical School Mental Health Letter, 2*(11), 4–5.

Fredrickson, B. L. (2001). The role of positive emotions in positive psychology: The broaden-and-build theory of positive emotions. *American Psychologist, 56,* 211–226.

Fredrickson, B. L., & Losada, M. (2005). Positive affect and the complex dynamics of human flourishing. *American Psychologist, 60,* 678–686.

Freud, S. (1900). Zur Psychologie der Traumvorgänge (On the psychology of dreaming). In *Gesammelte Werke* (Vol. 2/3). Frankfurt am Main: Fischer.

Freud, S. (1912). Recommendations to physicians practicing psycho-analysis. In J. Strachey (Ed. and Trans.), *The standard edition of the complete psychological works of Sigmund Freud* (Vol. 12, pp. 111–120). London: Hogarth.

Freud, S. (1938). An outline of psycho-analysis. In James Strachey et al. (Eds.), *The standard edition of the complete works of Sigmund Freud.* London: Hogarth Press and the Institute of Psycho-analysis.

Freud, S. (1999a). Massenpsychologie und Ich-Analyse (Group psychology and analysis of the ego). In *Gesammelte Werke* (Vol. 13, p. 85). Frankfurt am Main: Fischer.

Freud, S. (1999b). "Psychoanalyse" und "Libidotheorie" ("Psychoanalysis" and the "theory of libido"). In *Gesammelte Werke* (Vol. 13, p. 215). Frankfurt am Main: Fischer.

Fuchs, T. (2004). Neurobiology and psychotherapy: An emerging dialogue. *Current Opinions in Psychiatry, 17,* 479–485.

Fuller, R. C. (2001). *Spiritual, but not religious: Understanding unchurched America*. New York: Oxford University Press.

Fulton, P. R., & Siegel, R. D. (2005). Buddhist and Western psychology: Seeking common ground. In G. K. Germer, R. D. Siegel, & P. R. Fulton (Eds.), *Mindfulness and psychotherapy* (pp. 28–54). New York: Guilford.

Gabbard, G. (1994). *Psychodynamic psychiatry in clinical practice*. Washington, DC: American Psychiatric Press.

Gage, N. L. (1989). The paradigm wars and their aftermath: A "historical" sketch of research on teaching since 1989. *Educational Researcher, 18*(7), 4–10.

Gallese, V. (2001). The "shared manifold" hypothesis: From mirror neurons to empathy. *Journal of Consciousness Studies, 8*, 5–7.

Gallistel, C. R. (1980). *The organization of action*. Hillsdale, NJ: Erlbaum.

Galuska, J. (2006). Körperpsychotherapie im Spektrum des Strukturniveaus (Body psychotherapy through the spectrum of psychic structure). In G. Marlock & H. Weiss (Eds.), *Handbuch der Körperpsychotherapie* (pp. 585–597). Stuttgart: Schattauer.

Gassman, D., & Grawe, K. (2006). General change mechanisms: The relation between problem activation and resource activation in successful and unsuccessful therapeutic interactions. *Clinical Psychology and Psychotherapy, 13*, 1–11.

Geller, J., Norcross, J., & Orlinsky, D. (Eds.) (2005). *The psychotherapist's own psychotherapy: Client and clinician perspectives*. New York: Oxford University Press.

Gendlin, E. T. (1982). *Focusing* (2nd ed.). New York: Bantam.

Gendlin, E. T. (1986). What comes after traditional psychotherapy research? *American Psychologist, 41*, 131–136.

Gendlin, E. T. (1992). On emotion in therapy. *Hakomi Forum, (9)*, 15–29.

Gendlin, E. T. (1996). *Focusing-oriented psychotherapy: A manual of the experiential method*. New York: Guilford.

Gerhardt, S. (2004). *Why love matters: How affection shapes a baby's brain*. New York: Brunner-Routledge.

Germer, C. (2005). Mindfulness: What is it? What does it matter? In C. K. Germer, R. D. Siegel, & P. R. Fulton (Eds.), *Mindfulness and psychotherapy*. New York: Guilford.

Germer, C. (2006). You gotta have heart. *Psychotherapy Networker, 30*(1).

Germer, C. (2009). *The mindful path to self-compassion*. New York: Guilford.

Germer, C. K., Siegel, R. D., & Fulton, P. R. (Eds.) (2005). *Mindfulness and psychotherapy*. New York: Guilford.

Ghent, E. (1999). Masochism, submission, surrender: Masochism as a perversion of surrender. In S. A. Mitchell & L. Aron (Eds.), *Relational psychoanalysis* (pp. 211–242). Hillsdale, NJ: Analytic Press.

Ghent, E. (2002). Wish, need, drive: Motive in light of dynamic systems theory and Edelman's selectionist theory. *Psychoanalytic Dialogues, 12*, 763–808.

Gibb, J. R. (1978). *Trust*. Los Angeles: Guild of Tutors Press.

Gilbert, P. (Ed.) (2005). *Compassion: Conceptualizations, research and use in psychotherapy*. London: Routledge.

Gilbert, P. (2010). *Compassion focused therapy*. New York: Routledge/Taylor and Francis.

Gill, M. M. (1983). The interpersonal paradigm and the degree of the therapist's involvement. *Contemporary Psychoanalysis, 19*, 200–237.

Gilligan, C. (1982). *In a different voice: Psychological theory and women's development.* Cambridge, MA: Harvard University Press.

Gilligan, S. (1997). *The courage to love.* New York: Norton.

Giorgi, A. (1970). *Psychology as a human science: A phenomenologically based approach.* New York: Harper and Row.

Giorgi, A. P., & Giorgi, B. M. (2003). The descriptive phenomenological psychological method. In P. Camic, J. E. Rhodes, & L. Yardley (Eds.), *Qualitative research in psychology* (pp. 242–273). Washington, DC: American Psychological Association.

Gladwell, M. (2005). *Blink.* New York: Little, Brown.

Gleick, J. (1988). *Chaos: Making a new science.* New York: Penguin.

Gloaguen, V., Cottraux, J., Cucherat, M., & Blackburn, I. (1998). A meta-analysis of the effects of cognitive therapy in depressed patients. *Journal of Affective Disorders, 49,* 59–72.

Gold, T. (2004). *Living Wabi Sabi: The true beauty of your life.* Kansas City, MO: Andrews McMeel.

Goldfried, M. R. (1980). Toward the delineation of therapeutic change principles. *American Psychologist, 35,* 991–999.

Goldfried, M. R. (2009). Making evidence-based practice work: The future of psychotherapy integration. *Psychotherapy Bulletin, 44*(3), 25–28.

Goldfried, M. R., & Wolfe, B. E. (1996). Psychotherapy practice and research: Repairing a strained alliance. *American Psychologist, 51,* 1007–1016.

Goleman, D. (1996). *Emotional intelligence: Why it can matter more than IQ.* New York: Bantam.

Goleman, D. (2003). *Destructive emotions: How can we overcome them?* New York: Bantam.

Goleman, D. (2004). *Destructive emotions: A scientific dialogue with the Dalai Lama.* New York: Bantam Books.

Gottman, J. (1998). *Why marriages succeed or fail.* London: Bloomsbury.

Gottman, J. M., Murray, J. D., Swanson, C. C., Tyson, R., & Swanson, K. R. (2005). *The mathematics of marriage: Dynamic nonlinear models.* Cambridge, MA: MIT Press.

Graves, M. (2008). *Mind, brain and the elusive soul: Human systems of cognitive science and religion.* Burlington, VT: Ashgate.

Grawe, K. (2001). *Psychotherapie im Wandel* (Psychotherapy in transition). Göttingen: Hogrefe.

Grawe, K. (2002). *Consistency theory: A neuroscientific view of symptom formation and therapeutic change.* Paper presented at the annual meeting of the Society for Psychotherapy Research, Santa Barbara, CA.

Grawe, K. (2004). *Psychological therapy.* Seattle: Hogrefe.

Grayson, H. (2003). *Mindful loving.* New York: Gotham.

Greenberg, G. (2010). *Manufacturing depression: The secret history of a modern disease.* New York: Simon and Schuster.

Greenberg, L. S., & Paivio, S. C. (1997). *Working with emotions in psychotherapy.* New York: Guilford.

Greenberg, L. S., & Rhonda, L. (1988). Training in experiential therapy. *Journal of Consulting and Clinical Psychology, 56*(5), 696–702.

Greenberg, L. S., Riche, L. N., & Elliott, R. (1993). *Facilitating emotional change: The moment-by-moment process.* New York: Guilford.

Greenberg, L. S., Watson, J. C., & Lietaer, G. (1998). *Handbook of experiential psychotherapy.* New York: Guilford.

Grepmair, J. L., & Nickel, M. K. (2007). *Achtsamkeit des Psychotherapeuten* (The mindful psychotherapist). Wien: Springer.

Grepmair, L., Mitterlehner, F., Loew, T., Bachler, E., Rother, W., & Nickel, M. (2007). Promoting mindfulness in psychotherapists in training influences the treatment results of their patients: A randomized, double-blind, controlled study. *Psychotherapy and Psychosomatics, 76*(6), 332–338.

Griffith, J. L., & Griffith, M. E. (1994). *The body speaks: Therapeutic dialogues for mind-body problems.* New York: Basic Books.

Grof, S. (1975). *Realms of the human unconscious: Observations from LSD research.* New York: Viking.

Grof, S. (1988). *The adventure of self-discovery.* Albany: State University of New York Press.

Grossman, P., Niemann, L., Schmidt, S., & Walach, H. (2004). Mindfulness based stress reduction and health benefits: A meta-analysis. *Journal of Psychosomatic Research, 57*(1), 35–43.

Gunaratana, H. (1991). *Mindfulness in plain English.* Boston: Wisdom.

Guntrip, H. (1968). *Schizoid phenomena, object relations and the self.* London: Hogarth.

Habermas, J. (1979). *Communication and the evolution of society.* Boston: Beacon.

Halberstam, D. (1986). *The reckoning.* New York: William Morrow.

Halberstam, D. (1993). *The fifties.* New York: Fawcett Columbine.

Hall, J. (1993). *The reluctant adult: An exploration of choice.* Dorset: Prism.

Halling, S., & Goldfarb, M. (1991). Grounding truth in the body: Therapy and research renewed. *Humanistic Psychologist, 19,* 313–330.

Halling, S., & Nill, J. D. (1995). A brief history of existential-phenomenological psychiatry and psychotherapy. *Journal of Phenomenological Psychology, 26,* 1–45.

Hanh, T. N. (1976). *The miracle of mindfulness.* Boston: Beacon.

Hanh, T. N. (1987). *Being peace.* Berkeley, CA: Paralax.

Hanson, R., with Mendius, R. (2009). *Buddha's brain: The practical neuroscience of happiness, love and wisdom.* Oakland, CA: New Harbinger.

Harrington, M. (1962). *The other America: Poverty in the United States.* Baltimore: Penguin.

Harvey, D. (1989). *The condition of postmodernity: An inquiry into the origins of cultural change* (2nd ed.). Oxford: Blackwell.

Hayes, A. M., & Feldman, G. (2004). Clarifying the construct of mindfulness in the context of emotion regulation and the process of change in therapy. *Clinical Psychology: Science and Practice, 11,* 255–262.

Hayes, S. C. (2004). Acceptance and commitment therapy and the new behavior therapies: Mindfulness, acceptance, and relationship. In S. C. Hayes, V. M. Follette, & M. M. Linehan (Eds.), *Mindfulness and acceptance: Expanding the cognitive-behavioral tradition* (pp. 1–29). New York: Guilford.

Hayes, S. C., Follette, V. M., & Linehan, M. M. (Eds.) (2004). *Mindfulness and acceptance: Expanding the cognitive-behavioral tradition.* New York: Guilford.

Hayes, S. C., with Smith, S. (2005). *Get out of your mind and into your life: The new acceptance and commitment therapy.* Oakland, CA: New Harbinger.

Hayes, S. C., Strosahl, K., & Wilson, K. G. (1999). *Acceptance and commitment therapy: An experiential approach to behavior change.* New York: Guilford.

Heckler, R., & Johanson, G. (2015). Enhancing the immediacy and intimacy of the therapeutic relationship through the somatic dimension. In G. Marlock & H. Weiss, with C. Young & M. Soth, *Handbook of body psychotherapy and somatic psychology.* Berkeley: North Atlantic Books.

Heidegger, M. (1966). *Discourse on thinking.* New York: Harper Torchbooks.

Held, B., Kirschner, S. R., Richardson, F., Slife, B., & Teo, T. (2010). *Uses and misuses of critical thinking in psychology*. Symposium presentation at the American Psychology Association meeting at the San Diego Convention Center, August 13.

Heller, M. C. (2012). *Body psychotherapy: History, concepts, and methods*. New York: Norton.

Helms, J. E., & Cook, D. A. (1999). *Using race and culture in counseling and psychotherapy: Theory and process*. Boston: Allyn and Bacon.

Hendricks, G., & Hendricks, K. (1993). *At the speed of life: A new approach to personal change through body-centered therapy*. New York: Bantam.

Herlihy, B., & McCollum, V. (2007). Feminist theory. In D. Capuzzi & D. R. Gross (Eds.), *Counseling and psychotherapy: Theories and interventions* (4th ed., pp. 338–368). Upper Saddle River, NJ: Pearson, Merrill/Prentice Hall.

Herman, J. L. (1992). *Trauma and recovery*. New York: Basic Books.

Hick, S. F. (2008). Cultivating therapeutic relationships: The role of mindfulness. In S. F. Hick & T. Bien (Eds.), *Mindfulness and the therapeutic relationship* (pp. 3–18). New York: Guilford.

Hick, S. F., & Bien, T. (Eds.) (2008). *Mindfulness and the therapeutic relationship*. New York: Guilford.

Hirsch, I. (1987). Varying modes of analytic participation. *Journal of the American Academy of Psychoanalysis, 15*(2), 205–222.

Hobson, A. (1996). *The chemistry of conscious states*. New York: Little, Brown & Co.

Holland, J. H. (1995). *Hidden order: How adaptation builds complexity*. Cambridge, MA: Perseus.

Holland, J. H. (1998). *Emergence: From chaos to order*. New York: Oxford University Press.

Horner, A. J. (1974). *Object relations and the developing ego in therapy*. New York: Jason Aronson.

Horvath, A. O., & Bedi, R. P. (2002). The alliance. In J. C. Norcross (Ed.), *Psychotherapy relationships that work: Therapist contributions and responsiveness to patients* (pp. 37–61). New York: Oxford University Press.

Hoyt, M. (Ed.) (1998). *The handbook of constructive therapies: Innovative approaches from leading practitioners*. San Francisco: Jossey-Bass.

Hubble, M. A., Duncan, B. L., & Miller, S. D. (1999). *The heart and soul of change*. Washington, DC: American Psychological Association.

Hunter, M., & Struve, J. (1998). *The ethical use of touch in psychotherapy*. Thousand Oaks, CA: Sage.

Hycner, R. (1991). *Between person and person*. Highland, NY: Gestalt Journal.

Ingersoll, R. E., & Zeitler, D. M. (2010). *Integral psychotherapy: Inside out/outside in*. Albany: State University of New York Press.

James, W. (1890). *Principles of psychology, vol. 1*. New York: Holt.

Jean-Didier, V. (1990). *The biology of emotions*. Oxford: Basil Blackwell.

Ji-Woong, K., Sung-Eun, K., Jae-Jin, K., Bumseok, J., Chang-Hyun, P., Ae Ree, S., et al. (2009). Compassionate attitude towards others' suffering activates the mesolimbic neural system. *Neuropsychologia, 47*, 2073–2081.

Johanson, G. (1979–1980). The psychotherapist as faith agent. *Journal of Pastoral Counseling, 14*(2), 71–75.

Johanson, G. J. (1984). Editorial: Watzlawick, Wilber, and the work. *Hakomi Forum*, (1), 1–5.

Johanson, G. J. (1986). Editorial: Taking it home with you. *Hakomi Forum*, (4), 1–6.

Johanson, G. J. (1988). A curious form of therapy: Hakomi. *Hakomi Forum*, (6), 18–31.

Johanson, G. J. (1992). A critical analysis of David Augsburger's Pastoral Counseling Across Cultures. *Journal of Pastoral Care, 46*(2), 162–173.

Johanson, G. J. (1996). The birth and death of meaning: Selective implications of linguistics for psychotherapy. *Hakomi Forum*, (12), 45–55.

Johanson, G. J. (1999a). Far beyond psychoanalysis: Freud's repetition compulsion. *Hakomi Forum*, (13), 27–41.

Johanson, G. J. (1999b). *Making grace specific: The renewed chapter of spirituality in the history of white, mainline Protestant pastoral care in America.* (Unpublished doctoral dissertation). Drew Graduate School, Madison, New Jersey.

Johanson, G. J. (2006). A survey of the use of mindfulness in psychotherapy. *Annals of the American Psychotherapy Association, 9*(2), 15–24.

Johanson, G. J. (2008). Artistic inspirations: False colors. *Annals of the American Psychotherapy Association, 11*(3), 28.

Johanson, G. J. (2009a). Non-linear science, mindfulness, and the body in humanistic psychotherapy. *Humanistic Psychologist, 37*, 159–177.

Johanson, G. J. (2009b). Psychotherapy, science and spirit: Nonlinear systems, Hakomi therapy, and the Tao. *Journal of Spirituality in Mental Health, 11*(3), 172–212.

Johanson, G. J. (2009c). Selected bibliography on mindfulness and therapy. Retrieved from http://www.hakomi.org/resources.

Johanson, G. J. (2010a). Response to: "Existential theory and our search for spirituality" by Eliason, Samide, Williams and Lepore. *Journal of Spirituality in Mental Health, 12*, 112–117.

Johanson, G. J. (2010b). Walking into the future with hope. *Annals of the American Psychotherapy Association, 13*(2), 72–73.

Johanson, G. J. (2011a). Editorial: Ripples from a life lived. *Hakomi Forum*, (23–24), 1–2.

Johanson, G. J. (2011b). In memoriam: Ronald S. Kurtz—1934–2011. *Journal of Body, Movement and Dance in Psychotherapy, 6*(2), 175–180.

Johanson, G. J. (2011c). Mindfulness, emotions, and the organization of experience. *USA Body Psychotherapy Journal, 10*(1), 38–57.

Johanson, G. J. (2011d). Ronald S. Kurtz (1934–2011): A Remembrance. *Hakomi Forum*, 71–74.

Johanson, G. J. (2015). The organization of experience: A systems perspective on the relation of body-psychotherapies to the wider field of psychotherapy. In G. Marlock & H. Weiss, with C. Young & M. Soth, *Handbook of body psychotherapy and somatic psychology.* Berkeley: North Atlantic Books.

Johanson, G., & Kurtz, R. (1991). *Grace unfolding: Psychotherapy in the spirit of the Tao-te ching.* New York: Bell Tower.

Johanson, G., & Kurtz, R. (1993). *Sanfte Stärke—Heilung im Geiste des Tao te king.* Munich: Kösel.

Johanson, G. J., & Taylor, C. R. (1988). Hakomi therapy with seriously emotionally disturbed adolescents. In C. E. Schaefer (Ed.), *Innovative interventions in child and adolescent therapy* (pp. 232–265). New York: John Wiley.

Johnson, S. M. (1985). *Characterological transformation: The hard work miracle.* New York: Norton.

Johnson, S. M. (2009). Extravagant emotion: Understanding and transforming love relationships in emotionally focused therapy. In D. Fosha, D. J. Siegel, & M. F. Solomon (Eds.), *The healing power of emotion: Affective neuroscience, development, clinical practice* (pp. 257–279). New York: Norton.

Jones, E. E. (2000). *Therapeutic action: A guide to psychoanalytic therapy.* Northvale, NJ: Jason Aronson.

Jones, E. E., & Pulos, S. M. (1993). Comparing the process in psychodynamic and cognitive behavioral therapies. *Journal of Consulting and Clinical Psychology, 61*, 306–316.

Jordan, J. V., Kaplan, A. G., Miller, J. B., Stiver, I. P., & Surrey, J. L. (1991). *Women's growth in connection: Writings from the Stone Center.* New York: Guilford.

Juarrero, A. (1999). *Dynamics in action: Intentional behavior as a complex system.* Cambridge, MA: MIT Press.

Jung, C. G. (1958). *Complete works of C. G. Jung: Vol. 17. The development of the personality* (G. Adler & R. Hull, Eds.). London: Routledge and Kegan Paul. (Original work published 1947)

Kabat-Zinn, J. (1990). *Full catastrophe living.* New York: Dell.

Kabat-Zinn, J. (2005). *Coming to our senses: Healing ourselves and the world through mindfulness.* New York: Hyperion.

Kabat-Zinn, J., Lipworth, L., & Burney, R. (1985). The clinical use of mindfulness meditation for the self-regulation of chronic pain. *Journal of Behavioral Medicine, 8,* 163–190.

Kagen, J. (1998). How we become who we are. *Family Therapy Networker, 22*(5), 52–63.

Kahnemann, D. (2011). *Thinking, fast and slow.* London: Penguin.

Kandel, E. (2007). *In search of memory: The emergence of a new science of mind.* New York: Norton.

Kaplan, A. H. (2005). *Listening to the body: Pragmatic case studies in body-centered psychotherapy.* (Unpublished doctoral dissertation). Rutgers University, Piscataway, New Jersey.

Kaplan, A. H., & Schwartz, L. F. (2005). Listening to the body: Pragmatic case studies of body-centered psychotherapy. *USA Body Psychotherapy Journal, 4*(2), 33–67.

Kaplan-Williams, S. (1988). *Transforming childhood.* Berkeley, CA: Journey.

Karen, R. (1998). *Becoming attached: First relationships and how they shape our capacity to love.* New York: Oxford University Press.

Kauffman, S. (1995). *At home in the universe: The search for the laws of self-organization and complexity.* New York: Oxford University Press.

Kazdin, A. E. (2007). Mediators and mechanisms of change in psychotherapy research. *Annual Review of Clinical Psychology, 3,* 1–27.

Kazdin, A. E. (2008). Evidence-based treatment and practice: New opportunities to bridge clinical research and practice, enhance the knowledge base, and improve patient care. *American Psychologist, 63,* 146–159.

Kegan, R. (1982). *The evolving self: Problem and process in human development.* Cambridge, MA: Harvard University Press.

Keita, G., & Hurrell, J. (Eds.) (1994). *Job stress in a changing workforce: Investigating gender, diversity, and family issues.* Washington, DC: American Psychological Association.

Keleman, S. (1986). *Emotional anatomy: The structure of experience.* Berkeley, CA: Center Press.

Keller, C. (1986). *From a broken web: Separation, sexism, and self.* Boston: Beacon.

Keller, R. (2005). Hakomi simplified 2004: A new view of Ron Kurtz's mindfulness-based psychotherapy. *Hakomi Forum,* (14–15), 5–18.

Keltner, D., & Haidt, J. (1999). Social functions of emotions at four levels of analysis. *Cognition and Emotion, 13,* 505–521.

Keown, D. (Ed.) (2006). *Buddhist studies from India to America.* New York: Routledge.

Kepner, J. I. (1993). *Body process: Working with the body in psychotherapy.* San Francisco: Jossey-Bass.

Kernberg, O. F. (1996). Ein psychoanalytisches Modell der Klassifizierung von Persönlichkeitsstörungen (A psychoanalytic model for the classification of personality disorders). *Psychotherapeut, 41.*

Kershaw, C. J., & Wade, J. W. (2011). *Brain change therapy: Clinical interventions for self-transformation.* New York: Norton.

Kirsch, I. (2010). *The emperor's new drugs: Exploding the antidepressant myth*. New York: Basic Books.

Klein, J. (1987). *Our need for others: And its roots in infancy*. London: Tavistock.

Knight, R. T., & Grabowecky, M. (1995). Escape from linear time: Prefrontal cortex and conscious experience. In M. S. Gazzaniga, R. B. Ivry, & G. R. Mangun (Eds.), *Cognitive neuroscience: The biology of the mind* (pp. 1357–1371). Cambridge, MA: MIT Press.

Knowlan, A., & Patterson, D. (1993). *Group Leadership Training* lecture.

Koemeda-Lutz, M., Kaschke, M., Revenstorf, D., Scherrmann, T., Weiss, H., & Soeder, U. (2006). Evaluation der Wirksamkeit von ambulanten Körperpsychotherapien: EWAK, Eine Multizenter-studie in Deutchland und der Schweiz. (Evaluation of the effectiveness of body psychotherapy in outpatient settings: A multi-centre study in Germany and Switzerland). In *Psychotherapie, Psychosomatik, Medizinische Psychologie, 56*, 1–8.

Koestler, A. (1967). *The ghost in the machine*. London: Arkana.

Kohut, H. (1966). Forms and transformations of narcissism. *Journal of the American Academy of Psychoanalysis, 14*, 243–257.

Kohut, H. (1977). *The restoration of the self*. New York: International University Press.

Kohut, H. (1984). *How does analysis cure?* Chicago: University of Chicago Press.

Kornfield, J. (1993). *A path with heart*. New York: Bantam.

Kornfield, J. (1998). Even the best meditators have old wounds to heal. *Psychotherapy in Australia, 4*(3).

Korten, D. C. (2009). *Agenda for a new economy: From phantom wealth to real wealth*. San Francisco: Berrett-Koehler.

Krippner, S. (1994). Humanistic psychology and chaos theory. *Journal of Humanistic Psychology, 34*(3), 48–61.

Kris, A. O. (1982). *Free association: Methods and process*. New Haven, CT: Yale University Press.

Kurtz, R. (1978). Unlocking the map room. *Pilgrimage, 6*(1), 1–8.

Kurtz, R. (1983). *Hakomi basic level training*. Boulder, CO: Hakomi Institute.

Kurtz, R. (1985). The organization of experience. *Hakomi Forum*, (3), 3–9.

Kurtz, R. (1990a). *Body-centered psychotherapy: The Hakomi method*. Mendocino, CA: Life-Rhythm.

Kurtz, R. (1990b). *Hakomi: Eine körperorientierte Psychotherapie*. Munich: Kösel.

Kurtz, R. (2000). *Notes on Experiential Method*. Unpublished manuscript.

Kurtz, R. (2002a). *Level 2 handbook*. Ashland, OR: Ron Kurtz Trainings.

Kurtz, R. (2002b). *Psychobiological research and the practice of experiential psychotherapy*. Unpublished manuscript.

Kurtz, R. (2003). *Papers and notes on the Hakomi method of body psychotherapy*. Ashland, OR: Ron Kurtz Trainings.

Kurtz, R. (2004). *Hakomi method of mindfulness based body psychotherapy: Readings*. Ashland, OR: Ron Kurtz Trainings.

Kurtz, R. (2006). Five recent essays. *Hakomi Forum*, (16–17), 1–8.

Kurtz, R. (2008). A little history. *Hakomi Forum*, (19–21), 7–18.

Kurtz, R., & Minton, K. (1997). Essentials of Hakomi body-centered therapy. In C. Caldwell (Ed.), *Getting in touch: The guide to new body-centered therapies* (pp. 45–60). Wheaton, IL: Quest.

Kurtz, R., & Prestera, H. (1976). *The body reveals*. New York: Harper and Row.

Kvale, S. (1995). The social construction of validity. *Qualitative Inquiry, 1*, 19–20.

Laithwaite, H., Gumley, A., O'Hanlon, M., Collins, P., Doyle, P., Abraham, L., et al. (2009). Recovery after psychosis (RAP): A compassion focused programme for individuals residing in high security settings. *Behavioural and Cognitive Psychotherapy, 37,* 511–526.

Lake, F. (1966). *Clinical theology: A theological and psychiatric basis to clinical pastoral care.* London: Darton, Longman and Todd.

Lakoff, G., & Johnson, M. (1999). *Philosophy in the flesh: The embodied mind and its challenge to Western thought.* New York: Basic Books.

Lamagna, J., & Gleiser, K. (2007). Building a secure internal attachment: An intra-relational approach to ego strengthening emotional processing with chronically traumatized clients. *Journal of Trauma and Dissociation, 8,* 22–54.

Lambert, K., & Kinsley, C. (2005). *Clinical neuroscience.* New York: Worth.

Lambert, M. J., & Ogles, B. M. (2013). The efficacy and effectiveness of psychotherapy. In M. J. Lambert (Ed.), *Bergin and Garfield's handbook of psychotherapy and behavior change* (6th ed., pp. 169–218). New York: Wiley.

Langer, E. J. (1989). *Mindfulness.* Reading, MA: Addison-Wesley.

Langer, S. (1962). *Philosophy in a new key* (2nd ed.). New York: Mentor.

LaPierre, A., & Heller, L. (2012). Working with the capacity for connection in healing developmental trauma. *Hakomi Forum, (25),* 7–22.

Laszlo, E. (1987). *Evolution: The grand synthesis.* Boston: New Science Library.

Laszlo, E. (2004). *Science and the akashic field: An integral theory of everything.* Rochester, VT: Inner Traditions.

Leary, M. R., Adams, C. E., & Tate, E. B. (2006). Hypo-egoic self-regulation: Exercising self-control by diminishing the influence of the self. *Journal of Personality, 74,* 1803–1831.

Leder, D. (1984). Medicine and paradigms of embodiment. *Journal of Medicine and Philosophy, 9,* 29–43.

Leder, D. (1990). *The absent body.* Chicago: University of Chicago Press.

LeDoux, J. (1996). *The emotional brain: The mysterious underpinnings of emotional life.* New York: Simon and Schuster.

Leichsenring, F. (2005). Are psychodynamic and psychoanalytic therapies effective? *International Journal of Psychoanalysis, 86,* 841–868.

Leichsenring, F., & Leibing, E. (2003). The effectiveness of psychodynamic therapy and cognitive behavior therapy in the treatment of personality disorders: A meta-analysis. *American Journal of Psychiatry, 160,* 1223–1232.

Leichsenring, F., & Rabung, S. (2008). Effectiveness of long-term psychodynamic psychotherapy: A meta-analysis. *Journal of the American Medical Association, 300,* 1551–1565.

Leichsenring, F., Rabung, S., & Leibing, E. (2004). The efficacy of short-term psychodynamic psychotherapy in specific psychiatric disorders: A meta-analysis. *Archives of General Psychiatry, 61,* 1208–1216.

LeShan, L. (1990). *The dilemma of psychology: A psychologist looks at his troubled profession.* New York: Dutton.

LeShan, L. (1994). *Cancer as a turning point: A handbook for people with cancer, their families, and health professionals* (rev. ed.). New York: Plume.

LeShan, L., & Margenau, H. (1982). *Einstein's space and Van Gogh's sky: Physical reality and beyond.* New York: Collier.

Levine, P. A., with Frederick, A. (1997). *Waking the tiger: Healing trauma.* Berkeley, CA: North Atlantic.

Lewis, T., Amini, F., & Lannon, R. (2000). *A general theory of love.* New York: Vintage.

Lilienfeld, S. O. (2007). Psychological treatments that cause harm. *Perspectives on Psychological Science, 2,* 53–70.

Linehan, M. (1993). *Cognitive-behavioral treatment of borderline personality disorder.* New York: Guilford.

Linford, L., & Arden, J. B. (2009). Brain-based therapy and the "Pax Medica." *Psychotherapy in Australia, 15*(3), 16–23.

Linn, S., Emerson, W., Linn, D., & Linn, M. (1999). *Remembering our home: Healing hurts and receiving gifts from conception to birth.* Mahwah, NJ: Paulist.

Lipsey, M. W., & Wilson, D. B. (1993). The efficacy of psychological, educational, and behavioral treatment: Confirmation from meta-analysis. *American Psychologist, 48,* 1181–1209.

Lipton, B. (2005). *The biology of belief: Unleashing the power of consciousness, matter and miracles.* Santa Rosa, CA: Elite.

Loevinger, J. (1976). *Ego development: Conceptions and theories.* San Francisco: Jossey-Bass.

Llinás, R. (2009). *I of the vortex: From neurons to self.* Cambridge, MA: MIT Press.

Lossky, V. (1974). *In the image and likeness of God.* New York: St. Vladimir's Seminary.

Lowen, A. (1958). *The language of the body.* New York: Collier.

Lowen, A. (1967). *The betrayal of the body.* New York: Macmillan.

Lowen, A. (1975). *Bioenergetics.* New York: Coward, McCann and Geoghagan.

Luborsky, L., Singer, B., & Luborsky, L. (1975). Comparative studies of psychotherapies. *Archives of General Psychiatry, 32,* 995–1008.

Luvaas, T. (1992). *Notes from my inner child.* Mill Valley, CA: Nataraj.

Maaz, H.-J. (2006). Körperpsychotherapeutsiche Behandlung von Frühstörung. In G. Marlock & H. Weiss (Eds.), *Handbuch der Körperpsychotherapie.* Stuttgart: Schattauer.

Mace, C. (2008). *Mindfulness and mental health: Therapy, theory and science.* New York: Routledge.

Macy, J. (1983). *Despair and personal power in the nuclear age.* Philadelphia: New Society.

Macy, J. (1991). *World as lover, world as self.* Berkeley, CA: Parallax.

Mahoney, M. J. (1991). *Human change process: The scientific foundations of psychotherapy.* New York: Basic Books.

Mahoney, M. J. (2003). *Constructive psychotherapy: A practical guide.* New York: Guilford.

Mancia, M. (2006). Implicit memory and early unrepressed unconscious: Their role in the therapeutic process. *International Journal of Psychoanalysis, 87,* 83–103.

Manning, J. T., Trivers, R. L., Thornhill, R., Singh, D., Denman, J., Eklo, M. H., & Anderton, R. H. (1997). Ear asymmetry and left-side cradling. *Evolution and Behavior, 18,* 327–340.

Marcel, A. J. (2003). Introspective report: Trust, self-knowledge and science. *Journal of Consciousness Studies, 10,* 167–186.

Marks-Tarlow, T. (2011). Merging and emerging: A nonlinear portrait of intersubjectivity during psychotherapy. *Psychoanalytic Dialogues, 21,* 110–127.

Marks-Tarlow, T. (2012). *Clinical intuition in psychotherapy: The neurobiology of embodied response.* New York: Norton.

Marlock, G. (1993). Notizen über Regression (Notes on regression). In G. Marlock (Ed.), *Weder Körper noch Geist (Neither body nor Mind)* (pp. 147–166). Oldenburg: Transform Verlag.

Marlock, G., & Weiss, H. (2001). In search of the embodied self. In M. Heller (Ed.), *The flesh of the soul* (pp. 133–152). Bern: Peter Lang Verlang.

Marlock, G., & Weiss, H. (Eds.) (2006). *Handbuch der Körperpsychotherapie* (Handbook of body psychotherapy). Stuttgart: Schattauer.

Marlock, G., & Weiss, H., with Young, C., & Soth, M. (2015). *Handbook of body psychotherapy and somatic psychology.* Berkeley: North Atlantic Books.

Marsella, A. J. (1998). Toward a global psychology: Meeting the needs of a changing world. *American Psychologist, 53,* 1282–1291.

Marsella, A. J. (2009). Diversity in a global era: The context and consequences of differences. *Counselling Psychology Quarterly, 22,* 119–135.

Marsella, A. J., Bornemann, T., Ekblad, S., & Orley, J. (Eds.) (1994). *Amidst peril and pain: The mental health and well-being of the world's refugees.* Washington, DC: American Psychological Association.

Marsella, A. J., Johnson, J., Watson, P., & Gryczyski, J. (Eds.) (2008). *Ethnocultural perspectives on disaster and trauma.* New York: Springer SBM.

Martin, D. (n.d). Introduction to the practice of loving presence. Retrieved from http://www.hakomi.ca/practice.htm.

Martin, J. R. (1997). Mindfulness: A proposed common factor. *Journal of Psychotherapy Integration, 7,* 291–312.

Maslow, A. H. (1943). A theory of human motivation. *Psychological Review, 50*(4), 370–396.

Mate, G. (2003). *When the body says no: The costs of hidden stress.* Victoria, Australia: Scribe.

Matthew, M. (1998). The body as instrument. *Journal of the British Association of Psychotherapists, 35,* 17–36.

Maturana, H., & Varela, F. (1992). *The tree of knowledge: The biological roots of human understanding.* Boston: Shambala.

May, G. (1982). *Will and spirit: A contemplative psychology.* San Francisco: Harper Collins.

May, J. (2005). The outcome of body psychotherapy research. *USA Body Psychotherapy Journal, 4*(2), 93–115.

Mayo, K. R. (2009). *Creativity, spirituality, and mental health.* Burlington, VT: Ashgate.

McCrone, J. (2003, May 3). Not-so total recall. *New Scientist,* 26–29.

McGilchrist, I. (2009). *The master and his emissary: The divided brain and the making of the Western world.* New Haven, CT: Yale University Press.

McGoldrick, M., Giordano, J., & Pearce, J. K. (1996). *Ethnicity and family therapy* (2nd ed.). New York: Guilford.

McLoughlin, W. G. (1978). *Revivals, awakenings, and reform.* Chicago: University of Chicago Press.

McNeely, D. A. (1987). *Touching: Body therapy and depth psychology.* Toronto: Inner City.

Meares, R. (2005). *The metaphor of play: Origin and breakdown of personal being* (3rd ed.). New York: Routledge.

Melton, J. G., & Moore, R. L. (1982). *The cult experience: Responding to the new religious pluralism.* New York: Pilgrim.

Meyer, G. J., Finn, S. E., Eyde, L. D., Kay, G. G., Moreland, K. L, Dies, R. R., . . . Reed, G. M. (2001). Psychological testing and psychological assessment: A review of evidence and issues. *American Psychologist, 56,* 128–165.

Michell, J. (2003). The quantitative imperative: Positivism, naive realism and the place of qualitative methods in psychology. *Theory and Psychology, 13,* 5–31.

Miller, A. (1986). *Pictures of a childhood: Sixty-six watercolours and an essay.* New York: Farrar Straus.

Miller, A. (1988). *The untouched key: Tracing childhood trauma in creativity and destructiveness.* New York: Doubleday.

Miller, G. (2003). *Incorporating spirituality in counseling and psychotherapy: Theory and technique.* Hoboken, NJ: John Wiley.

Milrod, B., Leon, A. C., Busch, F., Rudden, M., Schwalberg, M., Clarkin, J., . . . Shear, M. K. (2007). A randomized control trial of psychoanalytic psychotherapy for panic disorder. *American Journal of Psychiatry, 164,* 265–272.

Missildine, W. H. (1963). *Your inner child of the past.* New York: Simon and Schuster.

Monda, L. (2000). *The practice of wholeness: Spiritual transformation in everyday life.* Placitas, NM: Golden Flower.

Mones, A. G., & Schwartz, R. C. (2007). A functional hypothesis: A family systems contribution toward an understanding of the healing process of the common factors. *Journal of Psychotherapy Integration, 17,* 314–329.

Montagu, A. (1978). *Touching: The human significance of the skin* (2nd ed.). New York: Harper and Row.

Morgan, M. (2004a). *Born to love: Hakomi psychotherapy and attachment theory.* Unpublished paper.

Morgan, M. (2004b). *The character book* (3rd ed.). Napier, New Zealand: Eastern Institute of Technology.

Morgan, M. (2006). Neuroscience and psychotherapy. *Hakomi Forum,* (16–17), 9–20.

Morgan, M. (2013). Attachment and Hakomi. *Hakomi Forum,* (26), 49–59.

Morowitz, H. J., & Singer, J. L. (1995). *The mind, the brain, and complex adaptive systems.* New York: Addison Wesley.

Moustakas, C. (1990). *Heuristic research: Design, methodology, and application.* London: Sage.

Mruk, C. J. (2010). Integrated description: A qualitative method for an evidence-based world. *Humanistic Psychologist, 38,* 305–316.

Murphy, N. C., & Brown, W. S. (2007). *Did my neurons make me do it? Philosophical and neurobiological perspectives on moral responsibility.* Oxford: Oxford University Press.

Myllerup, I. M. (2000). *From mind body fragmentation to bodymind wholeness: A call to embodied intelligence.* (Unpublished doctoral dissertation). Institute of Psychology, University of Aarhus, Denmark.

Myllerup, I. M. (2004, November). Core material as state specific learning. Lecture conducted from Hakomi Training, Atlanta, GA.

Nadel, L. (1994). Multiple memory systems: What and why. In D. T. Schacter & E. Tulving (Eds.), *Memory systems* (pp. 39–63). Cambridge, MA: MIT Press.

Nader, K. (2003). Memory traces unbound. *Trends in Neurosciences, 26*(2), 65–72.

Nader, K., Dubrow, N., & Stamm, B. (Eds.) (1999). *Honoring differences: Cultural issues in the treatment of trauma and loss.* Philadelphia: Brunner/Mazel.

Napier, A. Y. (1988). *The fragile bond: In search of an equal, intimate and enduring marriage.* New York: Harper and Row.

Nathan, P. E., & Gorman, J. M. (Eds.) (2002). *A guide to treatments that work* (2nd ed.). New York: Oxford University Press.

Natterson, J. (1991). *Beyond countertransference: The therapist's subjectivity in the therapeutic process.* Northvale, NJ: Jason Aronson.

Nauriyal, D. K., Drummond, M. S., & Lal, Y. B. (Eds.) (2006). *Buddhist thought and applied psychological research: Transcending boundaries.* Routledge: London.

Naylor, R. H., Willimon, W. H., & Oesterberg, R. (1996). *The search for meaning in the workplace.* Nashville, TN: Abingdon.

Neukrug, E. (2007). *The world of the counselor* (3rd ed.). Belmont, CA: Thomson, Brooks/Cole.

Nichols, M. P., & Schwartz, R. C. (1998). *Family therapy: Concepts and methods* (4th ed.). Boston: Allyn and Bacon.

Nisker, W. (1998). *Buddha's nature: Evolution as a practical guide to enlightenment.* New York: Bantam.

Norcross, J. C. (Ed.) (2002). *Psychotherapy relationships that work: Therapist contributions and responsiveness to patient needs.* New York: Oxford University Press.

Norcross, J. C. (2005). The psychotherapist's own psychotherapy: Educating and developing psychologists. *American Psychologist, 60,* 840–850.

Norcross, J. C., Beutler, L. E., & Levant, R. F. (Eds.) (2005). *Evidence based practices in mental health: Debate and dialogue on the fundamental questions.* Washington, DC: American Psychological Association.

Nowak, A., & Vallacher, R. R. (1998). *Dynamical social psychology.* New York: Guilford.

Nyanaponika, T. (1972). *The power of mindfulness.* San Francisco: Unity.

Nyanaponika, T. (1976). *The heart of Buddhist meditation (Satipatthana): A handbook of mental training based on the Buddha's way of mindfulness.* New York: Weiser.

Nyman, S., Nafzier, M., & Smith, T. (2010). Client outcome across counselor training levels within a multitiered supervision model. *Journal of Counseling and Development, 88,* 204–209.

Ogden, P. (1997). Hakomi integrative somatics: Hands-on psychotherapy. In C. Caldwell (Ed.), *Getting in touch: The guide to new body-centered psychotherapies* (pp. 153–178). Wheaton, IL: Quest.

Ogden, P., & Minton, K. (2000). One method for processing traumatic memory. *Traumatology, 6*(3).

Ogden, P., Minton, K., & Pain, C. (2006). *Trauma and the body.* New York: Norton.

Olendzki, A. (2005). The roots of mindfulness. In C. K. Germer, R. D. Siegel, & P. R. Fulton (Eds.), *Mindfulness and psychotherapy* (pp. 241–261). New York: Guilford.

OPD Task Force. (2006). *Operationalized psychodynamic diagnostics (OPD): Foundations and manual.* Seattle: Hogrefe.

Orlinsky, D., & Howard, K. (1986). Process and outcome in psychotherapy. In S. Garfield & A. Bergin (Eds.), *Handbook of psychotherapy and behavior change* (2nd ed., pp. 311–381). New York: Wiley.

Orlinsky, D., & Ronnestad, M. (2005). *How psychotherapists develop: A study of therapeutic work and professional growth.* Washington, DC: American Psychological Association.

Orlinsky, D. E., Ronnestad, M. H., & Willutzki, U. (2004). Fifty years of psychotherapy process-outcome research: Continuity and change. In M. J. Lambert (Ed.), *Bergin and Garfield's handbook of psychotherapy and behavior change* (5th ed., pp. 307–389). New York: Wiley.

Orsillo, S. M., Roemer, L., Block Learner, J., & Tull, M. (2004). Acceptance, mindfulness and cognitive-behavioral therapy. In S. C. Hayes, V. M. Follette, & M. M. Linehan (Eds.), *Mindfulness and acceptance: Expanding the cognitive-behavioral tradition* (pp. 66–95). New York: Guilford.

Packer, M. J., & Addison, R. B. (1989). *Entering the circle.* Albany: State University of New York Press.

Paivio, S., & Laurent, C. (2001). Empathy and emotional regulation. *Journal of Clinical Psychology, 57,* 213–226.

Paniagua, F., & Yamada, A. (Eds.) (2013). *Handbook of multicultural mental health* (2nd ed.). San Diego, CA: Academic Press.

Panksepp, J. (1998). *Affective neuroscience.* New York: Oxford University Press.

Panksepp, J. (2001). The long-term psychobiological consequences of infant emotions: Prescriptions for the 21st century. *Infant Mental Health Journal, 22,* 132–173.

Panksepp, J., & Northoff, G. (2008). The trans-species core self: The emergence of active cultural and neuro-ecological agents through self related processing within subcortical-cortical midline networks. *Conscious and Cognition, 12*(7), 259–264.

Parks, P. (1994). *The counsellor's guide to Parks inner child therapy.* London: Human Horizons.

Pattison, S. (1990). Laughter and pastoral care. *Hakomi Forum,* (8), 45–50.

Peck, M. S. (1978). *The road less traveled: A new psychology of love, traditional values and spiritual growth.* New York: Simon and Schuster.

Peloquin, S. M. (1990). Helping through touch: The embodiment of caring. *Hakomi Forum,* (8), 15–30.

Perls, F. (1973). *The Gestalt approach and eye witness to therapy.* Palo Alto, CA: Science and Behavior Books.

Perry, B., Pollard, R., Blakely, T., Baker, W., & Vigilante, D. (1995). Childhood trauma, the neurobiology of adaptation, and "use dependent" development of the brain: How "states" become "traits." *Infant Mental Health Journal, 16,* 271–291.

Pert, C. B. (1999). *Molecules of emotion.* New York: Touchstone.

Pesso, A. (1973). *Experience in action: Psychomotor psychology.* New York: New York University Press.

Pesso, A. (1990). The effects of pre- and perinatal trauma. *Hakomi Forum,* (8), 35–44.

Petzold, H. (1977). *Die neuen Körpertherapien* (The New Body Therapies). Paderborn: Junfermann.

Petzold, H. G., Wolff, H.-U., Landgrebe, B., & Josic, Z. (2002). *Das Trauma überwinden: Integrative Modelle der Traumatherapie* (Overcoming Trauma: Integrative Models of Trauma Therapy). Paderborn: Junfermann.

Phillips, J. (2003). *Using somatic tracking skills in assessment for touch in psychotherapy.* (Unpublished master's thesis). Naropa University, Boulder, CO.

Phillips, A. (2006). A mind is a terrible thing to measure. *New York Times,* February 26.

Piaget, J. (1926). *The language and thought of the child.* New York: Harcourt Brace.

Piaget, J., & Inhelder, B. (1969). *The psychology of the child.* New York: Basic Books.

Pierrakos, J. C. (1990). *Core energetics: Developing the capacity to love and heal.* Mendocino, CA: LifeRhythm.

Piers, C., Muller, J., & Brent, J. (Eds.) (2007). *Self-organizing complexity in psychological systems.* Lanham, MD: Rowman and Littlefield.

Pinderhughes, E. (1989). *Understanding race, ethnicity, and power.* New York: Free Press.

Pinker, S. (2002). *The blank slate: The modern denial of human nature.* New York: Penguin Books.

Polkinghorne, D. E. (1983). *Methodology for the human sciences: Systems of inquiry.* Albany: State University of New York Press.

Ponterotto, J. G., Casas, J. M., Suzuki, L. A., & Alexander, C. M. (2010). *Handbook of multicultural counseling* (3rd ed.). Thousand Oaks, CA: Sage.

Popper, K. R., & Eccles, J. C. (1981). *The self and its brain.* London: Springer International.

Porges, S. (2001). The polyvagal theory: Phylogenetic substrates of a social nervous system. *International Journal of Psychophysiology, 42*(2), 123–146.

Porges, S. (2003). Social engagement and attachment: A phylogenetic perspective. *Annals of the New York Academy of Sciences, 1008,* 31–47.

Porges, S. (2006). "Don't talk to me now, I'm scanning for danger." How your nervous system sabotages your ability to relate. An interview with Stephen Porges about his polyvagal theory. *Nexus,* (March/April), 30–35.

Porges, S. (2009). Reciprocal influences between body and brain in the perception and expression of affect: A polyvagal perspective. In D. Fosha, D. Siegel, & M. Solomon (Eds.), *The healing power of emotion: Affective neuroscience, development, and clinical practice* (pp. 27–54). New York: Norton.

Porges, S. (2011). *The polyvagal theory: Neurophysiological foundations of emotions, attachment, communication, and self-regulation.* New York: Norton.

Prenn, N. (2009). I second that emotion! On self-disclosure and its metaprocessing. In A. Bloomgarden & R. B. Menutti (Eds.), *The therapist revealed: Therapists speak about self-disclosure in psychotherapy* (pp. 85–99). New York: Routledge.

Prigogine, I., & Stengers, I. (1984). *Order out of chaos: Man's new dialogue with nature.* New York: Bantam.

Proust, M. (1981). *Remembrance of things past.* New York: Random House. (Original work published 1913–1927)

Rank, O. (1936). *Truth and reality: A life history of the human will.* New York: Knopf.

Raskin, N. (1948). The development of nondirective therapy. *Journal of Consulting Psychology, 12,* 92–110.

Reddemann, L. (2001). *Imagination als heilsame Kraft.* Stuttgart: Klett-Cotta.

Reich, C. A. (1970). *The greening of America.* New York: Random House.

Reich, W. (1949). *Character analysis.* New York: Farrar, Straus and Giroux.

Rizzolatti, G., & Craighero, L. (2004). The mirror-neuron system. *Annual Review of Neuroscience, 27,* 169–192.

Robbins, B. (2008). What is the good life? Positive psychology and the renaissance of humanistic psychology. *Humanistic Psychologist, 36,* 96–112.

Roberts, T. (2009). *The mindfulness workbook: A beginner's guide to overcoming fear and embracing compassion.* Oakland, CA: New Harbinger.

Robertson, R., & Combs, A. (Eds.) (1995). *Chaos theory in psychology and the life sciences.* Hillsdale, NJ: Erlbaum.

Robins, C. J., Schmidt, H., III, & Linehan, M. M. (2004). Dialectical behavior therapy: Synthesizing radical acceptance with skillful means. In S. C. Hayes, V. M. Follette, & M. M. Linehan (Eds.), *Mindfulness and acceptance: Expanding the cognitive-behavioral tradition* (pp. 30–44). New York: Guilford.

Rogers, C. R. (1942). *Counseling and psychotherapy.* Boston: Houghton Mifflin.

Rogers, C. R. (1946). Significant aspects of client-centered therapy. *American Psychologist, 1,* 415–422.

Rogers, C. R. (1951). *Client centered therapy: Its current practice, implications, and theory.* Boston: Houghton Mifflin.

Rogers, C. R. (1961). *On becoming a person.* Boston: Houghton Mifflin.

Rogers, C. R. (1980). *A way of being.* Boston: Houghton Mifflin.

Romanyshyn, R. D. (1992). The human body as historical matter and cultural symptom. In M. Sheets-Johnstone (Ed.), *Giving the body its due* (pp. 159–179). Albany: State University of New York Press.

Romanyshyn, R. D. (2007). *The wounded researcher: Research with soul in mind.* New Orleans, LA: Spring Journal.

Romanyshyn, R. D. (2010). The wounded researcher: Making a place for unconscious dynamics in the research process. *Humanistic Psychologist, 38,* 275–304.

Romme, M., & Escher, S. (2000). *Making sense of voices: A guide for mental health professionals working with voice-hearers.* London: MIND.

Rosen, E. G. (1983). *Contemporary theory and methodology in three body-centered, experiential psychotherapies.* (Unpublished master's thesis). West Georgia College, Carrolton, GA.

Rosenau, P. M. (1992). *Post-modernism and the social sciences: Insight, inroads, and intrusions.* Princeton, NJ: Princeton University Press.

Rossi, E. (1986). *The psychobiology of mind-body healing: New concepts of therapeutic hypnosis.* New York: Norton.

Rossi, E. (1996). *The symptom path to enlightenment: The new dynamics of self-organization in hypnotherapy: An advanced manual for beginners.* Phoenix, AZ: Zeig & Tucker.

Roth, G. (2003). *Fühlen, Denken, Handeln* (Feeling, thinking, acting). Frankfurt am Main: Suhrkamp.

Rothschild, B. (2000). *The body remembers: The psychophysiology of trauma and trauma treatment.* New York: Norton.

Rothschild, B. (2003). *The body remembers casebook: Unifying methods and models in the treatment of trauma and PTSD.* New York: Norton.

Rowan, J., & Cooper, M. (1999). *The plural self: Multiplicity in everyday life.* London: Sage.

Roy, D. M. (2007). Body-centered counseling and psychotherapy. In D. Capuzzi & D. R. Gross (Eds.), *Counseling and psychotherapy: Theories and interventions* (4th ed., pp. 260–289). Upper Saddle River, NJ: Pearson, Merrill/Prentice Hall.

Rubenfeld, I. (2000). *The listening hand: Self-healing through the Rubenfeld synergy method of talk and touch.* New York: Bantam.

Rubin, J. (1996). *Psychotherapy and Buddhism: Toward an integration.* New York: Plenum.

Rudolf, G. (1996). *Psychotherapeutische Medizin* (Psychotherapeutic Medicine). Stuttgart: Ferdinand Enke Verlag.

Russell, E., & Fosha, D. (2008). Transformational affects and core state in AEDP: The emergence and consolidation of joy, hope, gratitude and confidence in the (solid goodness of the) self. *Journal of Psychotherapy Integration, 18,* 167–190.

Ryan, R. M., & Brown, K. W. (2003). Why we don't need self-esteem: Basic needs, mindfulness, and the authentic self. *Psychological Inquiry, 14,* 71–76.

Sachse, R. (2002). *Histrionische und Narzisstische Persönlichkeitsstörungen* (Histrionic and Narcissistic Personality Disorders). Göttingen: Hogrefe.

Safran, J. (2003). *Psychoanalysis and Buddhism: An unfolding dialogue.* Boston: Wisdom.

Safran, J. D., & Muran, J. C. (2000). *Negotiating the therapeutic alliance: A relational treatment guide.* New York: Guilford.

Scaer, R. (2001). *The body bears the burden: Trauma, dissociation and disease.* Binghamton, NY: Haworth Medical Press.

Schacter, D. L. (1992). Understanding implicit memory: A cognitive neuroscience approach. *American Psychologist, 47,* 559–569.

Schacter, D. L. (1996). *Searching for memory: The brain, the mind, and the past.* New York: Basic Books.

Schacter, D. L., & Scarry, E. (2000). *Memory, brain and belief.* Cambridge, MA: Harvard University Press.

Schanzer, L. (1990). *Does meditation-relaxation potentiate psychotherapy?* (Unpublished doctoral dissertation). Massachusetts School of Professional Psychology, Boston.

Schellenbaum, P. (1988). *The wound of the unloved: Releasing the life energy.* Dorset, U.K.: Element.

Schmidt, W. (1994). *The development of the notion of self: Understanding the complexity of human interiority.* Lewiston, NY: Edwin Mellen.

Schore, A. (1994). *Affect regulation and the origin of the self: The neurobiology of emotional development.* Hillsdale, NJ: Erlbaum.

Schore, A. N. (2001). The effects of relational trauma on right brain development, affect regulation, and infant mental health. *Infant Mental Health Journal, 22,* 201–269.

Schore, A. N. (2003). *Affect regulation and the repair of self.* New York: Norton.

Schore, A. (2005). Back to basics: Attachment, affect regulation, and the developing right brain: Linking developmental neuroscience to pediatrics. *Pediatrics in Review, 26*(6), 204–217.

Schulmeister, M. (1988). The Hakomi method in therapy groups. *Hakomi Forum,* (6), 47–62.

Schulmeister, M. (2005). Hakomi Institute of Europe's answers to the EAP's 15 questions about scientific validation of body-psychotherapy. Retrieved from http://www.hakomi.de/.

Schulte, D., Kunzel, R., Pepping, G., & Schulte-Bahrenbert, T. (1992). Tailor-made versus standardized therapy of phobic patients. *Advanced Behavior Research and Therapy, 14,* 67–92.

Schutz, W. C. (1969). *Joy: Expanding human awareness.* New York: Grove Press.

Schwartz, J. M., & Begley, S. (2002). *The mind and the brain: Neuroplasticity and the power of mental force.* New York: Harper.

Schwartz, R. C. (1995). *Internal family systems.* New York: Guilford.

Schwartz, R. C. (2001). *Introduction to the internal family systems model.* Oak Park, IL: Trailheads.

Segal, V. S., Williams, J. M. G., & Teasdale, J. D. (2002). *Mindfulness-based cognitive therapy for depression.* New York: Guilford.

Segal, Z. V., Teasdale, J. D., & Williams, M. J. (2004). Mindfulness based cognitive therapy: Theoretical rational and empirical status. In S. C. Hayes, V. M. Follette, & M. M. Linehan (Eds.), *Mindfulness and acceptance: Expanding the cognitive-behavioral tradition* (pp. 45–65). New York: Guilford.

Seligman, M. (1998). Why therapy works. *APA Monitor On-line, 29,* 12.

Seligman, M. E. P. (1995). The effectiveness of psychotherapy. *American Psychologist, 50,* 965–974.

Seligman, M. E. P., & Csikszentmihalyi, M. (2000). Positive psychology: An introduction. *American Psychologist, 55*(1), 5–14.

Sexton, T. L., & Whiston, S. C. (1991). A review of the empirical basis for counseling: Implications for practice and training. *Counselor Education and Supervision, 30,* 330–354.

Seybold, K. S. (2007). *Explorations in neuroscience, psychology and religion.* Burlington, VT: Ashgate.

Shapiro, D. (1965). *Neurotic styles.* New York: Basic Books.

Shapiro, S. L., Brown, K. W., & Biegel, G. (2007). Teaching self-care to caregivers: The effects of mindfulness-based stress reduction on the mental health of therapists in training. *Training and Education in Professional Psychology, 1,* 105–115.

Shapiro, S. L., Carlson, C. E., Astin, J. A., & Freedman, B. (2006). Mechanisms of mindfulness. *Journal of Clinical Psychology, 62,* 373–386.

Shapiro, S. L., Schwartz, G. E., & Bonner, G. (1998). Effects of mindfulness-based stress reduction on medical and premedical students. *Journal of Behavioral Medicine, 21,* 581–599.

Shaver, P. R., Lavy, S., Saron, C. D., & Mikulincer, M. (2007). Social foundations of the capacity for mindfulness: An attachment perspective. *Psychological Inquiry: An International Journal for the Advancement of Psychological Theory, 18*(4), 264–271.

Shaw, R. (2003). *The embodied psychotherapist: The therapist's body story.* New York: Brunner-Routledge.

Shaw, R. (2004). The embodied psychotherapist: An exploration of the therapists' somatic phenomena within the therapeutic encounter. *Psychotherapy Research, 14*(3), 271–288.

Shedler, J. (2010). The efficacy of psychodynamic psychotherapy. *American Psychologist, 65*(2), 98–109.

Shedler, J., & Westen, D. (2007). Shedler-Westen Assessment Procedure (SWAP): Making personality diagnosis clinically meaningful. *Journal of Personality Assessment, 8*, 41–55.

Shiota, M., Keltner, D., Campos, B., & Hertenstein, M. (2004). Positive emotion and regulation of interpersonal relationships. In P. Phillipot & R. Feldman (Eds.), *Emotion regulation* (pp. 127–156). Mahwah, NJ: Erlbaum.

Shlain, L. (2003). *Sex, time, and power: How women's sexuality shaped human evolution.* New York: Penguin Books.

Shusterman, R. (2008). *Body consciousness: A philosophy of mindfulness and somaesthetics.* Cambridge: Cambridge University Press.

Siegel, D. J. (1999). *The developing mind: Toward a neurobiology of interpersonal experience.* New York: Guilford.

Siegel, D. J. (2003). An interpersonal neurobiology of psychotherapy: The developing mind and the resolution of trauma. In M. Solomon & D. J. Siegel (Eds.), *Healing trauma: Attachment, mind, body and brain* (pp. 1–56). New York: Norton.

Siegel, D. J. (2006). An interpersonal neurobiology approach to psychotherapy: Awareness, mirror neurons, and well-being. *Psychiatric Annals, 36*(4), 248–256.

Siegel, D. J. (2007). *The mindful brain: Reflection and attunement in the cultivation of well-being.* New York: Norton.

Siegel, D. J. (2009). Emotion as integration: A possible answer to the question, what is emotion? In D. Fosha, D. J. Siegel, & M. Solomon (Eds.), *The healing power of emotion: Affective neuroscience, development, and clinical practice* (pp. 145–171). New York: Norton.

Siegel, D. J. (2010). *The mindful therapist: A clinician's guide to mindsight and neural integration.* New York: Norton.

Siegel, D. J. (2012). *The developing mind: How relationships and the brain interact to shape who we are* (2nd ed.). New York: Guilford.

Siegel, D. J., & Hartzell, M. (2003). *Parenting from the inside out: How a deeper self-understanding can help you raise children who thrive.* New York: Tarcher/Penguin.

Siegel, D. J., & Solomon, M. (Eds.) (2013). *Healing moments in psychotherapy.* New York: Norton.

Siegel, R. D. (2010). *The mindfulness solution: Everyday practices for everyday problems.* New York: Guilford.

Simpkins, C. A., & Simpkins, A. M. (2010). *The Dao of neuroscience: Combining Eastern and Western principles for therapeutic change.* New York: Norton.

Skynner, A. C. R. (1976). *Systems of family and marital psychotherapy.* New York: Brunner/Mazel.

Smith, E. W. L., Clance, P. R., & Imes, S. (1998). *Touch in psychotherapy: Theory, research, and practice.* New York: Guilford.

Smith, K. (2005). Foreword. In C. Trungpa (Ed.), *The sanity we are born with: A Buddhist approach to psychology* (pp. ix–xvi). Boston: Shambhala.

Smith, M. L., & Glass, G. V. (1977). Meta-analysis of psychotherapy outcome studies. *American Psychologist, 32*, 752–776.

Smith, M. L., Glass, G. V., & Miller, T. I. (1980). *The benefits of psychotherapy.* Baltimore: Johns Hopkins University Press.

Smith, W. R. (1996). *The Hakomi psychotherapy system: Facilitating human change.* (Unpublished B.I.S. thesis). University of Waterloo, Canada.

Solomon, R. L., & Wynne, L. C. (1953). Traumatic avoidance learning: Acquisition in normal dogs. *Psychological Monographs: General and Applied, 67*(4), 1–19.

Sonnenmoser, M. (2005). Mindfulness-basierte Therapie: Richtungsweisende Impulse (Mindfulness-based therapy: Impulses pointing the way). In *Deutsches Ärzteblatt, 9,* 415–417.

Sorajjakool, S. (2001). *Wu wei, negativity, and depression: The principle of non-trying in the practice of pastoral care.* Binghamton, NY: Haworth.

Sorajjakool, S. (2009). *Do nothing.* West Conshohocken, PA: Templeton Foundation.

Spackman, M. P., & Williams, R. N. (2001). The affiliation of methodology with ontology in scientific psychology. *Journal of Mind and Behavior, 22,* 389–406.

Sperry, L. (2010). Psychotherapy sensitive to spiritual issues: A postmaterialist psychology perspective and developmental approach. *Psychology of Religion and Spirituality, 2,* 46–56.

Stam, H. J. (Ed.) (1998). *The body and psychology.* London: Sage.

Stark, M. (1994). *Working with resistance.* Northvale, NJ: Jason Aronson.

Stark, M. (1999). *Modes of therapeutic action: Enhancement of knowledge, provision of experience, and engagement in relationship.* Northvale, NJ: Jason Aronson.

Sterling, P. (2004). Principles of allostasis: Optimal design, predictive regulation, pathophysiology and rational therapeutics. In J. Schulkin (Ed.), *Allostasis, homeostasis, and the costs of adaptation* (pp. 17–64). Cambridge: Cambridge University Press.

Stern, D. N. (1985). *The interpersonal world of the infant: A view from psychoanalysis and developmental psychology.* New York: Basic Books.

Stern, D. N. (2002). *The first relationship—infant and mother.* Cambridge, MA: Harvard University Press.

Stern, D. N. (2004). *The present moment in psychotherapy and everyday life.* New York: Norton.

Stevens, S. E., Hynan, M. T., & Allen, M. (2000). A meta-analysis of common factors and specific treatment effects across outcome domains of the phase model of psychotherapy. *Clinical Psychology: Science and Practice, 7,* 273–290.

Stiles, W. B., Shapiro, D. A., & Elliot, R. (1986). Are all psychotherapies equivalent? *American Psychologist, 41,* 165–180.

Stolorow, R. D., Brandchaft, B., & Atwood, G. E. (1987). *Psychoanalytic treatment: An intersubjective approach.* Hillsdale, NJ: Analytic Press.

Stone, H., & Stone, S. (1989). *Embracing ourselves.* Novato, CA: New World Library.

Stone, H., & Winkleman, S. (1990). The vulnerable inner child. In J. Abrams (Ed.), *Reclaiming the inner child* (pp. 176–184). Los Angeles: Tarcher.

Stosny, S. (2014). Blue-collar therapy. *Psychotherapy Networker, 37*(6), 22–29, 54.

Stream, H. (Ed.) (1994). *The use of humor in psychotherapy.* Northvale, NJ: Jason Aronson.

Sue, D. W., & Sue, D. (1990). *Counseling the culturally different: Theory and practice.* New York: John Wiley.

Sulz, S. K. D. (2015). Cognitive-behavioral therapists discover the body. In G. Marlock & H. Weiss, with C. Young & M. Soth, *Handbook of body psychotherapy and somatic psychology.* Berkeley: North Atlantic Books.

Sundararajan, L. (2008). The plot thickens—or not: Protonarratives of emotions and the principle of savoring. *Journal of Humanistic Psychology, 48,* 243–263.

Sundararajan, L., Misra, G., & Marsella, A. (2013). Indigenous approaches to assessment, diagnosis, and treatment of mental disorders. In F. Paniagua & A. Yamada (Eds.), *Handbook of multicultural mental health* (2nd ed., pp. 69–88). Boston: Academic Press.

Szecsoedy, I. (2008). A single-case study on the process and outcome of psychoanalysis. *Scandinavian Psychoanalytic Review, 31*, 105–113.

Taft, J. (1933). *The dynamics of therapy in a controlled relationship.* New York: Macmillan.

Tart, C. T. (1987). *Waking up: Overcoming the obstacles to human potential.* Boston: Shambhala.

Taylor, K. (1995). *The ethics of caring.* Santa Cruz, CA: Hanford Mead.

Teasdale, J. D., Segal, Z. V., & Williams, J. M. G. (1995). How does cognitive therapy prevent depressive relapse and why should attentional control (mindfulness) training help? *Behavior Research and Therapy, 33*, 25–39.

Teicher, M. H. (2002). Scars that won't heal: The neurobiology of child abuse. *Scientific American, 286*(3), 54–61.

Teo, T. (2009). Editorial. *Journal of Theoretical and Philosophical Psychology, 29*, 61–62.

Thelen, E., & Smith, L. B. (2002). *A dynamic systems approach to the development of cognition and action.* Cambridge, MA: MIT Press.

Thielen, M. (2002). Narzissmus-Körperpsychotherapie zwischen Beziehungs- und Energiearbeit (Narcissism: Between relationship and energy work). In M. Thielen (Ed.), *Narzissmus: Körper-Psychotherapie zwischen Energie und Beziehung* (Narcissim: Between energy and relationship). Berlin: Leutner Verlag.

Thielen, M. (2015). Body psychotherapy with narcissistic personality disorders. In G. Marlock & H. Weiss, with C. Young & M. Soth, *Handbook of body psychotherapy and somatic psychology.* Berkeley: North Atlantic Books.

Thomas, A. J., & Schwarzbaum, S. (2006). *Culture and identity.* Thousand Oaks, CA: Sage.

Thomas, Z. (1994). *Healing touch: The church's forgotten language.* Louisville, KY: Westminster/John Knox.

Thurow, L. C. (1998). Economic community and social investment. In F. Hesselbein et al. (Eds.), *The community of the future* (pp. 19–26). San Francisco: Jossey-Bass.

Tillich, P. (1948). *Shaking the foundations.* New York: Charles Scribner's Sons.

Tipton, S. M. (1982). *Getting saved from the sixties.* Berkeley: University of California Press.

Tombs, S. K. (2001). The role of empathy in clinical practice. *Journal of Consciousness Studies, 8*, 247–258.

Torrance, R. M. (1994). *The spiritual quest: Transcendence in myth, religion, and science.* Berkeley: University of California Press.

Trevarthen, C. (2001). Intrinsic motives for companionship in understanding: Their origin, development and significance for infant mental health. *Infant Mental Health Journal, 22*(1–2), 95–131.

Tronick, E. (1989). Emotions and emotional communication in infants. *American Psychologist, 44*, 112–119.

Tronick, E. (1998). Dyadically expanded states of consciousness and the process of therapeutic change. *Infant Mental Health Journal, 19*, 290–299.

Tronick, E. (2007). *The neurobehavioral and social-emotional development of infants and children.* New York: Norton.

Tronick, E. (2009). Multilevel meaning making and dyadic expansion of consciousness theory: The emotional and polymorphic polysemic flow of meaning. In D. Fosha, D. Siegel, & M. Solomon (Eds.), *The healing power of emotion: Affective neuroscience, development, and clinical practice* (pp. 86–111). New York: Norton.

Trungpa, C. (1983). Becoming a full human being. In J. Welwood (Ed.), *Awakening the heart* (pp. 126–131). Boston: Shambhala.

Tugade, M., & Frederickson, B. L. (2004). Resilient individuals use positive emotions to bounce back from negative emotional experiences. *Journal of Personality and Social Psychology, 86,* 320–333.

Turner, E. H., Matthews, A. M., Linardatos, B. S., Tell, R. A., & Rosenthal, R. (2008). Selective publication of antidepressant trials and its influence on apparent efficacy. *New England Journal of Medicine, 358,* 252–260.

Turner, L. (2008). *Theology, psychology, and the plural self.* Burlington, VT: Ashgate.

Unno, M. (Ed.) (2006). *Buddhism and psychotherapy across cultures: Essays on theories and practices.* Boston: Wisdom.

Vallacher, R. R., & Nowak, A. (1994a). The chaos in social psychology. In R. R. Vallacher & A. Nowak (Eds.), *Dynamical systems in social psychology* (pp. 1–16). San Diego: Academic Press.

Vallacher, R. R., & Nowak, A. (1994b). *Dynamical systems in social psychology.* San Diego: Academic Press.

VandenBos, G. R., & Pino, C. D. (1980). Research in the outcome of psychotherapy. In G. R. VandenBos (Ed.), *Psychotherapy: Practice, research, policy* (pp. 23–69). Beverly Hills, CA: Sage.

Van der Hart, O., Nijenhuis, E. R. S., & Steele, K. (2006). *The haunted self: Structural dissociation and treatment of chronic traumatization.* New York: Norton.

van der Kolk, B. A. (1987). *Psychological trauma.* Washington, DC: American Psychiatric Association.

van der Kolk, B. A. (1989). The compulsion to repeat the trauma: Re-enactment, revictimization, and masochism. *Psychiatric Clinics of North America, 12*(2), 389–411.

van der Kolk, B. A. (1994). The body keeps the score: Memory and the evolving psychobiology of posttraumatic stress. *Harvard Review of Psychiatry, 1,* 253–265.

van der Kolk, B. A. (2002). *Beyond the talking cure.* Washington, DC: American Psychological Association.

van der Kolk, B. A. (2003). Posttraumatic stress disorder and the nature of trauma. In M. F. Solomon & D. J. Siegel (Eds.), *Healing trauma: Attachment, mind, body, and brain* (pp. 168–195). New York: Norton.

van der Kolk, B. A. (2005). Developmental trauma disorder: A new, rational diagnosis for children with complex trauma histories. *Psychiatric Annals, 35,* 401–408.

van der Kolk, B. A. (2014). *The body keeps the score: Brain, mind, and body in the healing of trauma.* New York: Viking.

van der Kolk, B. A., McFarlane, A. C., & Weisaeth, L. (1996). *Traumatic stress: The effects of overwhelming experience on mind, body, and society.* New York: Guilford.

Van Mistri, E. (2008). Hakomi therapy with families. *Hakomi Forum,* (19–21), 137–146.

Varela, F. J., Thompson, E., & Rosch, E. (1991). *The embodied mind: Cognitive science and human experience.* Cambridge, MA: MIT Press.

Vasquez, M. (2012). Psychology and social justice: Why we do what we do. *American Psychologist, 67*(5), 337–346.

Vocisano, C., Klein, D. F., Arnow, B., Rivera C., Blalack, J., Rothbaum, B., et al. (2004). Therapist variables that predict symptom change in psychotherapy with chronically depressed outpatients. *Psychotherapy: Theory, Research, Practice, Training, 41,* 255–265.

Vygotsky, L. S. (1962). *Thought and language.* Cambridge, MA: MIT Press.

Vygotsky, L. S. (1978). *Mind in society.* Cambridge, MA: Harvard University Press.

Wakefield, J., & Horwitz, A. (2007). *The loss of sadness: How psychiatry transformed normal sorrow into depressive disorder.* New York: Oxford University Press.

Waldrop, W. W. (1992). *Complexity: The emerging science at the edge of order and chaos.* New York: Simon and Schuster.

Wallace, B. A. (2007). *Contemplative science: Where Buddhism and neuroscience converge.* New York: Columbia University Press.

Wallerstein, I. (1979). *The capitalist world-economy.* Cambridge: Cambridge University Press.

Wallin, D. J. (2007). *Attachment in psychotherapy.* New York: Guilford.

Walsh, R. (2011). Lifestyle and mental health. *American Psychologist, 66,* 579–592.

Wampold, B. E. (2001). *The great psychotherapy debate: Models, methods, and findings.* Hillsdale, NJ: Erlbaum.

Wampold, B. E., Minami, T., Baskin, T. W., & Callen-Tirney, S. (2002). A meta-(re)analysis of the effects of cognitive therapy versus "other therapies" for depression. *Journal of Affective Disorders, 68,* 159–165.

Wampold, B. E., Mondin, G. W., Moody, M., Stich, F., Benson, K., & Ahn, H. (1997). A meta-analysis of outcome studies comparing bona fide psychotherapies: Empirically, all must have prizes. *Psychological Bulletin, 122,* 203–215.

Watkins, J. G., & Watkins, H. H. (1997). *Ego states theory and therapy.* New York: Norton.

Watt, D. (2005). Social bonds and the nature of empathy. *Journal of Consciousness Studies, 12*(8–10), 185–209.

Watzlawick, P., Beavin, J., & Jackson, D. D. (1967). *Pragmatics of human communication: A study of interactional patterns, pathologies, and paradoxes.* New York: Norton.

Watzlawick, P., Weakland, J., & Fish, R. (1974). *Change: Principles of problem formation and problem resolution.* New York: Norton.

Wehowsky, A. (2015). Affective motor schemata. In G. Marlock & H. Weiss, with C. Young & M. Soth, *Handbook of body psychotherapy and somatic psychology.* Berkeley: North Atlantic Books.

Weinhold, B. (1988). *Playing grown-up is serious business: Breaking free of addictive family patterns.* Walpole, NH: Stillpoint.

Weiss, H. (1987). Storytelling for Hakomi therapists. *Hakomi Forum,* (5), 31–37.

Weiss, H. (2008). The use of mindfulness in psychodynamic and body oriented psychotherapy. *International Journal for Body, Movement and Dance in Psychotherapy, 4*(1), 5–16.

Weiss, H., & Benz, D. (1989). *To the core of your experience.* Charlottesville, VA: Luminas.

Weiss, J. (1995). Clinical applications of control-master theory. *Current Opinion in Psychiatry, 8,* 154–156.

Welwood, J. (2002). *Toward a psychology of awakening.* Boston: Shambhala.

Wendt, D. C., Jr., & Slife, B. D. (2007). Is evidence-based practice diverse enough? Philosophy of science considerations. *American Psychologist, 62,* 613–614.

Wertz, F. J. (2005). Phenomenological research methods for counseling psychology. *Journal of Counseling Psychology, 52,* 167–177.

Wessells, M. (1999). Culture, power and community: Intercultural approaches to psychosocial assistance and healing. In K. Nader, N. Dubrow, & B. Stamm (Eds.), *Honoring differences: Cultural issues in the treatment of trauma and loss* (pp. 267–282). Philadelphia: Brunner/Mazel.

Westen, D. (1998). The scientific legacy of Sigmund Freud: Toward a psychodynamically informed psychological science. *Psychological Bulletin, 124,* 333–371.

Westen, D., Novotny, C. M., & Thompson-Brenner, H. (2004). The empirical status of empirically supported psychotherapies: Assumptions, findings, and reporting in controlled clinical trials. *Psychological Bulletin, 130,* 631–663.

Westen, D., Novotny, C. M., & Thompson-Brenner, H. (2005). EBP not equal to EST: Reply to Crits-Christoph et al. *Psychological Bulletin, 131,* 427–433.

Whiston, S. C., & Coker, J. K. (2000). Reconstructing clinical training: Implications from research. *Counselor Education and Supervision, 39,* 228–253.

Whitehead, T. (1992). Hakomi in jail: A programmatic application of the technique of "taking over" with groups of psychotic, disruptive jail inmates. *Hakomi Forum,* (9), 7–13.

Whitehead, T. (1994). Boundaries and psychotherapy: Part I. Boundary distortion and its consequences. *Hakomi Forum,* (10), 7–16.

Whitehead, T. (1995). Boundaries and psychotherapy: Part II. Healing damaged boundaries. *Hakomi Forum,* (11), 27–36.

Whitfield, C. L. (1987). *Healing the child within.* Deerfield Beach, FL: Health Communications.

Wiggins, B. J. (2009). William James and methodological pluralism: Bridging the qualitative and quantitative divide. *Journal of Mind and Behavior, 30,* 165–183.

Wiggins, B. J. (2011). Confronting the dilemma of mixed methods. *Journal of Theoretical and Philosophical Psychology, 31*(1), 44–60.

Wilber, K. (1977). *The spectrum of consciousness.* Wheaton, IL: Quest.

Wilber, K. (1979). *No boundary: Eastern and Western approaches to personal growth.* Los Angeles: Center.

Wilber, K. (1995). *Sex, ecology, spirituality: The spirit of evolution.* Boston: Shambhala.

Wilber, K. (2000). *Integral psychology: Consciousness, spirit, psychology, therapy.* Boulder, CO: Shambhala.

Wilber, K. (2006). *Integral spirituality.* Boston: Integral Books.

Williams, G. P. (1997). *Chaos theory tamed.* Washington, DC: Joseph Henry.

Williams, P. (2012). *Rethinking madness: Towards a paradigm shift in our understanding and treatment of psychosis.* San Francisco: Sky's Edge.

Wilson, T. D. (2002). *Strangers to ourselves: Discovering the adaptive unconscious.* Cambridge, MA: Harvard University Press.

Winnicott, D. W. (1965). *The maturational process and the facilitating environment: Studies in the theory of emotional development.* London: Hogarth/Institutes of Psychoanalysis.

Winnicott, D. W. (1971). *Playing and reality.* London: Tavistock.

Wisechild, L. (1988). *The obsidian mirror: An adult healing from incest.* Seattle: Seal.

Wolinsky, S. (1991). *Trances people live: Healing approaches in quantum psychology.* Falls Village, CT: Bramble.

Wolinsky, S. (2003). *The dark side of the inner child: The next step.* Norfolk, CT: Bramble.

Wulff, D. M. (1991). *Psychology of religion: Classic and contemporary views.* New York: John Wiley.

Wuthnow, R. (1998). *After heaven: Spirituality in America since the 1950s.* Berkeley: University of California Press.

Wuthnow, R. (2006). *American mythos: Why our best efforts to be a better nation fall short.* Princeton, NJ: Princeton University Press.

Wylie, M. S. (2004). Beyond talk: Using our bodies to get to the heart of the matter. *Psychotherapy Networker, 28*(4), 24–28, 31–33.

Wyss, D. (1973). *Psychoanalytic schools from the beginning to the present.* New York: Jason Aronson.

Yehuda, R., & McFarlane, A. C. (1997). *Psychobiology of traumatic stress.* New York: New Academy of Science.

Young, C. (2010). The history of science in body psychotherapy: Part 2. *United States Body Psychotherapy Journal, 8*(2), 5–15.

Zanocco, G. (2006). Sensory empathy and enactment. *International Journal of Psychoanalysis, 87,* 145–158.

Zinker, J. (1994). *In search of good form.* San Francisco: Jossey-Bass.

Zur, O. (2007). Touch in therapy and the standard of care in psychotherapy and counseling: Bringing clarity to illusive relationships. *USA Body Psychotherapy Journal, 6*(2), 61–94.

Contributors

Karen Baikie, BSc(Hons), BA, MClinPsych, PhD, MAPS, CHT, is a certified Hakomi therapist and consultant clinical psychologist with 14 years experience in private practice in Sydney, Australia. Karen is a certified Hakomi teacher with the Hakomi Institute Pacifica Team and cofacilitator with Halko Weiss in the Hakomi Embodied and Aware Relationships Training (H.E.A.R.T.). She runs workshops on aspects of Hakomi and H.E.A.R.T. throughout Australia and provides clinical supervision. Karen is coeditor of *Hakomi News*, the Hakomi Association Australia newsletter, and is a member of the Australian Psychological Society College of Clinical Psychologists. Her PhD dissertation was on expressive writing as a therapeutic tool for survivors of trauma. Karen assists individuals, couples, and therapists in using mindfulness to support deepening awareness and connection with themselves and others.

Cedar Barstow, MEd, CHT, has been a Hakomi therapist and trainer since 1989. She is also the managing editor of *Hakomi Forum* and the chair of the Hakomi International Ethics Committee. In addition to her work with the Hakomi Institute, she is the founder and director of the Right Use of Power Institute (www.rightuseofpower.org). She has authored five books, including, most recently, *Right Use of Power: The Heart of Ethics* and *Living in the Power Zone: How Right Use of Power Can Transform Your Relationships*. She teaches Hakomi therapy and ethics internationally. She and her husband, Reynold Feldman, live in Boulder, Colorado.

David Cole, LMP, CC, is a Hakomi therapist, teacher, and trainer for the Hakomi Educational Network and a founding member of the Seattle Hakomi Education Network. He is coauthor of *Mindfulness Centered Therapies: An Integrative Approach*, and produces training videos, including *Tom* with Ron Kurtz. As a certified counselor and licensed massage therapist, he synthesizes Hakomi with internal family systems and focusing in his practice and leads workshops and training in Hakomi with the Seattle Hakomi Education Network. He has been a presenter of mindfulness training for PESI, LLC. He is a member of the Hakomi Institute, the American Anthropological Association, and the Society for the Anthropology of Consciousness.

Maci Daye, EdM, EdS, is a licensed professional counselor, certified Hakomi trainer, and certified master career counselor with graduate degrees in education and counseling from Harvard and Georgia State universities. She has extensive experience as a psychotherapist, career counselor, trainer, outplacement coordinator, and consultant within government, higher education, corporate, and private practice settings. Maci has served as the editor of the Hakomi Therapy Association newsletter for nearly a decade, and on the Hakomi Institute board of directors. She is the creator of a course for couples on mindful sexuality called Passion & Presence and leads couples retreats in the United States and internationally. Her article "Have We Forgotten About Sex?" was published in *Somatic Therapy Today* and she has been interviewed on *Somatic Perspectives on Psychotherapy*.

PHIL DEL PRINCE, MA, holds professional licenses in clinical psychotherapy (LPCC) and marriage and family therapy (LMFT). He is a founding member and senior trainer of the Hakomi Institute. His first professional love is the practice of individual psychotherapy, utilizing an eclectic synthesis from certifications in Hakomi, Gestalt, hypnotherapy, psychodrama, EMDR, and the existential sense of his nature. Complementing his private practice, he has been active in training students and therapists in mindful and neuroscience-based psychology paradigms with the Hakomi Institute and other national and international programs since 1972. He is grateful to continue living and playing with his beloved partner of many years, Janna, and his deep friend and son, Julian, at the foot of the Rocky Mountains in Boulder, Colorado.

JON EISMAN, CHT, is a founding member of the Hakomi Institute, director of the Hakomi Institute of Oregon, codirector of the Hakomi Institutes of California and Canada, and a senior Hakomi trainer. For over three decades, he has taught throughout North America, Europe, New Zealand, Australia, and Japan, contributing to the Hakomi method and its teachability. Jon is also the originator of mindful experiential therapy approaches (M.E.T.A.), a comprehensive model of client woundedness and treatment, as well as the developer of Re-creation of the Self, an innovative tool for working with psychological resource, fragmentation, and Selfhood. In addition to numerous articles, he is the author of *Hakomi Institute Training Manual* and *The Re-creation of the Self as an Approach to Psychotherapy*.

ANNE FISCHER, Dipl Psych accredited professional psychotherapist, and supervisor in private practice, was a long-term Hakomi trainer until 2012. She is a member of the advisory board for the German *Journal of Sexuality Research* (*Zeitschrift für Sexualforschung*). Anne completed postgraduate training in somatic psychotherapy, psychodynamic therapy, and trauma therapy. Her special interest lies in the combination of psychodynamic concepts with mindfulness and body-psychotherapeutic approaches, as well as the potency of the therapeutic relationship. The main focus of her current work is with ethnic minorities and couples therapy. She lives and works in Hamburg, Germany.

ROB FISHER, MFT, is a certified Hakomi trainer and the author of *Experiential Psychotherapy With Couples: A Guide for the Creative Pragmatist* and of a number of articles published internationally on couples therapy and the psychodynamic use of mindfulness in journals such as *Psychotherapy Networker*, *The Therapist*, *Journal of Couples Therapy*,

USA Body Psychotherapy Journal, Psychotherapy in Australia, and others. He is an adjunct professor at JFK University, and the codeveloper and lead instructor of the Mindfulness and Compassion in Psychotherapy Certificate Program at the California Institute of Integral Studies. Rob is a speaker at conferences and workshops around the United States such as CAMFT, USABP, *Psychotherapy Networker,* and the Relationship Council, where he presents as a peer, master, or keynote speaker.

MAYA SHAW GALE, MA, BCC, is a certified Hakomi practitioner and trainer, a nationally board-certified life coach, and a certified trainer for the Circle of Life Coaching Institute. In her practice in Santa Barbara, California, her approach integrates mindfulness, eco-psychology, indigenous wisdom, and body-mind practices to midwife individuals, couples, and small organizations through crisis and transition to creative breakthrough. Since 1975, Maya has led workshops, retreats, and training sessions across the United States, Mexico, Australia, and New Zealand. For eight years, as adjunct faculty for Cambridge College Graduate School of Education, she trained educators in curriculum applications of somatic awareness, mindfulness, and emotional intelligence. A published poet and play-wright, she is currently authoring a book on the healing power of ritual, ceremony, and immersion in nature.

UTA GÜNTHER, Dipl Psych, accredited psychotherapist, and lecturer for the Bavarian Chamber of Professional Psychotherapists, is a trainer for the Hakomi Institute of Europe. She has completed postgraduate education as a psychodynamic therapist and several other psychotherapies and body-psychotherapies such as Rogerian, trauma treatment, psycho-drama, NLP, structural body therapy (Rolfing), systemic family constellations, and ego state therapy. Since 1985 she has worked in private practice with individual, couples, and group therapy, and coaching, supervision, and professional training. Uta began her career as the director of a psychological counseling center in Nuremberg, Germany. Her specific interest lies with the use of mindfulness and body-psychotherapeutic interventions for the treatment of narcissistic disorders and trauma.

JACI HULL, MA, LMFT, is a certified Hakomi trainer leading workshops and training internationally. She is alumni faculty of the Somatic Psychology Department at Naropa University and the Sensorimotor Psychotherapy Institute, and was a codeveloper with Rob Fisher of experiential couples psychotherapy. Jaci received her master's in contemplative psychotherapy from Naropa University. Her postgraduate training includes a certification in family therapy, EMDR, somatic trauma resolution, brainspotting, group genius, and certification as a relational life therapist. Jaci maintains a private psychotherapy practice in Boulder, Colorado.

GREG JOHANSON, MDiv, PhD, LPC, NCC, a founding trainer of the Hakomi Institute, has a background in therapy as well as theology. He is a member of the American Psychological Association as well as the American Association of Pastoral Counselors. He has been active in writing, publishing over 175 items in the fields of psychotherapy and pastoral theology including (with Ron Kurtz) *Grace Unfolding: Psychotherapy in the Spirit of the Tao-te ching*. Greg has served on the editorial board of six professional journals and as editor of *Hakomi Forum* and has taught as an adjunct in a number of graduate schools. He has a special interest in integral psychology, which relates spirituality to individual consciousness and behavior in the context of social and cultural issues.

RON KURTZ was the originator of Hakomi therapy and the founder of the Hakomi Institute. He was the first to pioneer integrating the use of mindfulness in psychotherapy. Ron was the author or coauthor of three books that have been influential in the world of experiential psychotherapy: *The Body Reveals* with Hector Prestera, *Body-Centered Psychotherapy: The Hakomi Method*, and *Grace Unfolding: Psychotherapy in the Spirit of the Tao-te ching* with Greg Johanson. After resigning as executive director of the Hakomi Institute, he also founded Ron Kurtz Trainings and the Hakomi Educational Network, based on his later work with Hakomi Refined. He received a lifetime achievement award from the United States Body Psychology Association and an honorary doctorate from the Santa Barbara Graduate Institute.

CAROL LADAS-GASKIN, MA, is a certified therapist, teacher, and trainer of the Hakomi Educational Network and a clinical member of the U.S. Association of Body Psychotherapy. She is licensed in the state of Washington as a certified counselor and a massage practitioner who has had an ongoing counseling practice in the Seattle area for many years. She teaches Hakomi workshops and courses in the Seattle area as part of the Seattle Hakomi Educational Network (www.seattlehakomi.com). She has been a certified consultant and workshop instructor in Progoff Intensive Journal, a mindfulness-based journal practice. She is the author of *Instant Stress Relief*, coauthor with J. David Cole of *Mindfulness Centered Therapies: An Integrative Approach*, and published *Unfurling*, a book of poetry (www.mindfulnessbooks.com).

SHAI LAVIE, MA, MFT, is a certified Hakomi therapist in private practice in San Rafael, California. He is also certified in the somatic experiencing method of working with trauma. Shai serves as adjunct professor at Sofia University and John F. Kennedy University and teaches in the Mindfulness and Compassion Certificate Program at the California Institute of Integral Studies. He also serves as a Hakomi teacher on the faculty of the Hakomi Institute of California. Shai enjoys leading transformational groups with adults that integrate Hakomi, somatic experiencing, group process, and dream work. His articles have appeared in *Psychotherapy Networker* and *The Therapist*.

DONNA MARTIN, MA, has been the senior Hakomi Education Network trainer in North America, England, Ireland, Japan, Mexico, Hawaii, Israel, Russia, and Buenos Aires. She has a background in stress management and addictions, and during the 1990s she was the clinical program director of outpatient services at the Phoenix Center for Alcohol and Drug Addiction in Kamloops, Canada. Donna coauthored with Ron Kurtz the *Practice of Loving Presence* series, now available as e-books (www.ronkurtz.com and www.reflective

presence.com). Other books include *Seeing Your Life Through New Eyes* (with Paul Brenner), *Simply Being* (with Marlena Field), and *Remembering Wholeness*, plus the chapter on Hakomi in *Inner Dialogue in Daily Life*, edited by Chuck Eigen (see www.hakomi .ca, www.donnamartin.net).

MANUELA MISCHKE REEDS, MFT, is a licensed psychotherapist, international Hakomi trainer, and author. Manuela specializes in integrating somatic and mindfulness-based psychotherapy with a specialization in trauma and stress. Her areas of expertise are in the fields of somatic trauma therapy, attachment psychotherapy, infant mental health, and continuum movement therapy. Her integrative teaching style is influenced by her longtime studies of Buddhist psychology and meditation practice. Manuela has developed a dharmic trauma training and teaches in Germany, Australia, Israel, and San Francisco. She is the codirector of the Hakomi Institute of California and maintains a private psychotherapy practice in the San Francisco area. Manuela is the author of *The 8 Keys to Practicing Mindfulness* in the Norton 8 Keys series.

LORENA MONDA, MS, DOM, LPCC, is a practicing psychotherapist and a doctor of oriental medicine. Lorena is a trainer for the Hakomi Institute and adjunct faculty at the AOMA Graduate School of Integrative Medicine in Austin, Texas, where she teaches courses in clinical communication integrating Hakomi skills. She is the author of *The Practice of Wholeness: Spiritual Transformation in Everyday Life*; a coauthor of *The Clinical Guide to Commonly Used Chinese Herbal Formulas* and *The Clinical Handbook of Chinese Veterinary Herbal Medicine*; and a coeditor of *I Have Arrived, I Am Home: Celebrating 20 Years of Plum Village Life*. Lorena lives in New Mexico with her husband John Scott and teaches Hakomi in the United States and internationally. She is currently working on a book called *Mindfulness, Qi, and Transformation*.

MARILYN MORGAN, MHSc (Hons), SRN, MNZAP, PhD, was a psychotherapist for 25 years. Before her untimely death, she was a certified Hakomi therapist and trainer who was program coordinator for the diploma in integrative psychology (Hakomi) at the Eastern Institute of Technology in Hawkes Bay, New Zealand. She was a beloved teacher in the Hakomi Institute who brought a special interest and talent from her medical background in nursing to relating Hakomi to the latest trends in neurophysiology and interpersonal neurobiology. She published articles in *Hakomi Forum* and her PhD dissertation was worked into a book, *The Alchemy of Love: Personal Growth Journeys in Psychotherapy Training*.

JULIE MURPHY, MA, LMFT, certified addictions treatment counselor and certified Hakomi trainer and therapist, has decades of experience consulting, teaching, and working in the healing arts. Julie trains mental health professionals in the United States, Canada, Australia, New Zealand, and Israel. She is adjunct faculty at John F. Kennedy University and was an instructor in the California Institute of Integral Studies Certificate Program in Mindfulness and Compassion in Psychotherapy. She specializes in experiential somatic psychotherapy, mindful recovery, creative process, attachment theory, and developing well-being. She is a marriage and family therapist who practices with individuals, couples, adolescents, and families in Santa Cruz.

JOHN PERRIN, CHT, has nearly 20 years experience in the practice of mindfulness-centered psychotherapy. He is a certified Hakomi therapist and trainer who holds a diploma in psychotherapy and relationship counseling from the Jansen Newman Institute in Sydney, Australia. He is a member of the Hakomi Institute South Pacific Team, is faculty for the Hakomi professional training in Sydney, Perth, and New Zealand, and leads Hakomi workshops throughout the region. He maintains a private practice in Sydney. John studied for many years in the Zen Buddhist tradition and has a particular interest in the role of embodiment in psychotherapy.

T. FLINT SPARKS, PhD, has nearly 40 years of experience in the practice and teaching of psychotherapy. Flint is a Zen teacher who leads retreats and teaches throughout the United States and Europe. His academic training includes graduate degrees in both biology and psychology, and he has extensive postdoctoral training in mindfulness-based psychotherapies and group therapy. His Zen teaching weaves together the skillful methods of both the Hakomi and internal family systems models into what he calls the practice of liberating intimacy. His traditional Zen training began at the San Francisco Zen Center and continued at the Austin Zen Center, which he founded and nourished in its early years. Currently he is a resident teacher at Appamada, a center for Zen in Austin, Texas.

HALKO WEISS, PhD, is a clinical psychologist and a lecturer for the Bavarian Licensing Board for Psychotherapists, the University of Marburg, and several other professional schools. He is a cofounder of the Hakomi Institute both in the United States and in Germany, working closely with Ron Kurtz for many years, and continues to provide new directions for Hakomi through developing programs such as a course in interpersonal skills called H.E.A.R.T. (Hakomi Embodied and Aware Relationships Training). Halko is the author and editor of six books, both in German and in English: *To the Core of your Experience* (with Dyrian Benz); *Auf den Körper hören* (with D. Benz); *Handbuch der Körperpsychotherapie* (editor, with G. Marlock); *Das Achtsamkeitsbuch. Grundlagen, Anwendungen, Übungen* (with M. Harrer and T. Dietz); *Das Achtsamkeitsübungsbuch. Für Beruf und Alltag* (with M. Harrer and T. Dietz); and *Handbook of Body Psychotherapy and Somatic Psychology* (editor, with G. Marlock, C. Young, and M. Soth). Aside from his work as a teacher of body psychotherapy and as a couples therapist, he is a frequent trainer and coach for corporate executives.

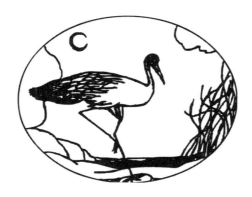

Positioning & Awareness

People always ask how to follow Tao. It is as easy and natural as the heron standing in the water. The bird moves when it must; it does not move when stillness is appropriate. The secret of its serenity is a type of vigilance, a contemplative state. The heron is not in mere dumbness or sleep. It knows a lucid stillness. It stands unmoving in the flow of the water. It gazes unperturbed and is aware. When Tao brings it something that it needs, it seizes the opportunity without hesitation or deliberation. Then it goes back to its quiescence without disturbing itself or its surroundings. Unless it found the right position in the water's flow and remained patient, it would not have succeeded.

Actions in life can be reduced to two factors: positioning and timing. If we are not in the right place at the right time, we cannot possibly take advantage of what life has to offer us. Almost anything is appropriate if an action is in accord with the time and the place. But we must be vigilant and prepared. Even if the time and the place are right, we can still miss our chance if we do not notice the moment, if we act inadequately, or if we hamper ourselves with doubts and second thoughts. When life presents an opportunity, we must be ready to seize it without hesitation or inhibition. Position is useless without awareness. If we have both, we make no mistakes.

—DENG MING-DAO

When you're not getting what you want,
there can be two reasons:
either the environment isn't offering it to you (position),
or you aren't taking in what's available (awareness).
Hakomi Therapy works with both reasons.
First we help people look at and discover
how they are organized to refuse what's available.
And, of course, since you are a part of your environment,
you can influence your environment
and help change it so that all,
including yourself, may benefit.

—RON KURTZ

Index